A Special Issue of
Memory

Neuroimaging and Memory

Edited by

Jonathan K. Foster
University of Manchester, UK

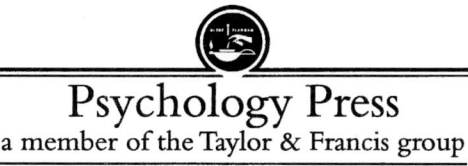

Psychology Press
a member of the Taylor & Francis group

Psychology Press Ltd, Publishers
27 Church Road
Hove
East Sussex, BN3 2FA
UK

British Library Cataloguing in Publication Data

A catalogue record for this book is available from the British Library

    ISBN 0-86377-656-6 (hbk)
    ISSN: 0965-8211

Typeset by DP Photosetting, Aylesbury, Bucks
Printed and bound in the United Kingdom by Henry Ling Ltd, Dorchester

Contents

---

*This book is also a special issue of the journal *Memory* which forms Issue 5/6 of Volume 7 (1999). The page numbers used here are taken from the journal and so begin with p. 513.

MEMORY, 1999, 7 (5/6), 513–514

Preface

The idea for this special edition emanated from a symposium that I organised at the Second International Conference on Memory, on the topic of "Neuroimaging and Memory", which was held in Padua in July 1996. Given the success of this symposium, and the enthusiasm that was generated among the contributors, we decided it would be worthwhile to follow up the symposium through another medium, which would permit a broader and more detailed discussion of some of the relevant issues.

All the contributors to the Padua symposium were invited to make a contribution to the special edition, and I am pleased to say that the vast majority were able to do so. However, in order that we did not restrict debate or the range of material that could be presented, we also invited submissions to this special edition from other contributors. In planning the special edition, a number of selection criteria were applied. The focus of the special issue would be the insights and constraints that neuroimaging data provide with respect to the functional organisation of memory. Papers reporting neuroimaging studies using the techniques of MRI, PET, SPECT, CT, EEG, or MEG and investigating all aspects of memory processing would be considered for publication. Contributions should seek to place data derived from imaging investigations within a theoretical framework of memory.

I am pleased to say that these criteria were adhered to by the 10 contributors to the special edition. This has led to contributions as diverse as studies of autobiographical memory and working memory, an investigation into "medial temporal lobe" versus "diencephalic" amnesia (combined with an evaluation of different forms of image analysis), neuroimaging and "psychogenic amnesia", an empirical review paper, a study of incidental retrieval in the context of encoding, a critique of contemporary neuroimaging research (with specific reference to the anatomical lesion literature), a neuroimaging study of memory using event-related functional neuroimaging, a paper concerned with the interpretation and meaning of psychological data obtained from contemporary neuroimaging methodologies, and a submission that questions the view that anatomically "bigger" structures necessarily subserve memory "better".

The common theme of all of these papers, submitted by 10 leading international research groups in this field, is what neuroimaging can tell us about the relationship between different types of memory and the neural substrates mediating these different mnemonic capacities. The state of our current knowledge concerning several of the most important issues in the field of imaging and memory is illustrated in this special edition. However, we are clearly in the early stages of addressing many of the most important research questions (constrained as we are both by currently available neuroimaging technologies and appropriate psychological methodologies), so that—at the current rate of progress—in 12 or 18 months' time, significant further advances will, I am sure, have been made. Even in those areas that are tackled directly by the papers reported here, as anyone working in this relatively new field would readily acknowledge, we are really still just playing in the empirical shallows and staring tentatively into the research depths beyond. It is my hope that this special edition will make a significant contribution to this ongoing exploration.

Finally, I would like to take this opportunity to thank all the contributors for the range and quality of their submissions, and Sue Gathercole and Martin Conway for facilitating the publication of this special edition.

JONATHAN K. FOSTER
University of Manchester, UK

MEMORY, 1999, 7 (5/6), 515–522

Images, Memories, and Models: Introduction to the Special Issue

Jonathan K. Foster

University of Manchester, UK

INTRODUCTION

When I first became interested in the use of neuroimaging techniques to address neuropsychological questions in the late 1980s, the volume of research in this area represented a mere blip on the experimental horizon (see Raichle, 1986). At that time, very few neuropsychological studies had been conducted using imaging techniques other than computerised tomography (CT), and few of those studies which had been conducted using the more advanced techniques that had become available focused on the neural mediation of memory. This situation changed with the publication of Press, Amaral, and Squire's (1989) paper, in *Nature*, in which—using structural Magnetic Resonance Imaging (MRI)—it was demonstrated that the size of the hippocampus could be meaningfully related to the degree of amnesics' memory dysfunction *in vivo*. The development of functional Magnetic Resonance Imaging (fMRI) in the early 1990s (see Belliveau et al., 1992) subsequently appeared to motivate researchers not only into thinking about the use of this new technique in the investigation of higher cognitive capacities, but also into using the more established technique of Positron Emission Tomography (PET) more rigorously and systematically to address questions pertaining to the neural basis of memory.

The early findings were somewhat surprising: 30 or more years of previous experimental work had nourished the view that, for an indeterminate period of time after the encoding of novel target information, the medial temporal lobe (specifically, structures within the "hippocampal system") represented the repository (or possibly the indexing system) for long-term memories, at least those of an episodic/declarative nature. However, early PET findings appeared to contradict this body of evidence: the brain regions that appeared to become most activated during memory studies using PET were located more anteriorly. In particular, evidence was put forward by the research groups based in London

---

Requests for reprints should be sent to Jonathan K. Foster, Department of Psychology, University of Manchester, Oxford Road, Manchester M13 9PL, UK.

and Toronto that the structures of the left prefrontal region were involved in encoding information into long-term memory, while regions of the right prefrontal cortex appeared to be involved in retrieving this information. Indeed, to the present day, an overwhelming majority of reported encoding and retrieval studies of memory using recently learned information produce frontal activations, while using imaging techniques to show activation in brain regions such as the medial temporal lobe and diencephalon has proved more challenging, regions that had been the focus of previous neuropsychological studies of memory and amnesia. In addition, previously mnemonically "silent" regions of the brain such as the precuneus have been cited in several neuroimaging investigations as an important component of specific memory networks.

As further research into neuroimaging and memory has been conducted through the 1990s, this picture has been extended and refined. In particular, this special edition presents the current state-of-the-art in contemporary memory neuroimaging research from the perspective of a selection of leading scientists in this field. A common feature of these papers is the use of neuroimaging technologies to investigate the relationship between phenomenological aspects of memory and their realisation in the hardware of the brain. Moreover, from the contributions presented here, it is apparent that neuroimaging data are important not only for our understanding of what can be referred to as the implementation level of cognitive neuroscience (Churchland & Sejnowski, 1988; Marr, 1982), but also for the further development of cognitive and computational models of human memory.

OVERVIEW OF CONTRIBUTIONS

In the first paper, McIntosh's theoretically insightful paper presents two evolving analytic methods for the evaluation of brain activity data—i.e. structural equation modelling and partial least squares methodologies—in the context of two specific empirical examples. McIntosh argues that recent advances in human cognitive neuroscience are at least partially due to the recent explosion in the use of functional neuroimaging techniques to investigate the neural basis of cognition. However, the author cautions that models of cognition that have been successfully developed to explain behaviour were developed without direct reference to the biology of the nervous system. He highlights the degree of redundancy known to be present in the brain, such that brain regions close to each other show overlapping functions. As McIntosh states, another no less important capacity of the nervous system is connectivity between brain regions, with a great deal of parallel and reciprocal connectivity existing within the brain. In the living brain, this means that an apparently local primary change in activity can have distinctly non-local consequences, with linear changes in input being fed back and forward to create distinctly wide-ranging and nonlinear effects. In making these observations, McIntosh re-ignites an ancient debate (see Farah, 1994; Foster, 1997): can cognitive processes can be localised to discrete regions of the brain (as some strong modularity theorists would have us believe); does the brain represent cognition in a wholly distributed fashion (as Lashley argued in the first half of this century); or are both positions true, to some degree? In this paper, McIntosh explores this fundamental question in cognitive neuroscience, within the domain of memory. More specifically, he considers the proposition that learning and memory are the direct result of interactions among large-scale neurobiological networks, with the diversity of learning and memory phenomena that are produced arising as emergent properties of the interactions between constituent brain regions. Another important concept explored in McIntosh's piece is that of ''neural context''. This refers to the notion that common levels of activity change within a specific brain region may be observed in several different situations, but because the activity of inter-related brain regions may be quite different, the emergent cognitive operations will be distinct. In other words, it is the overall pattern of activation across multiple, orchestrated brain regions that determines the cognitive operation that is ultimately subserved.

The paper written by Van der Linden et al. presents a report into the investigation of working memory using *in vivo* neuroimaging. Working memory refers to a postulated limited-capacity system, responsible for the processing and temporary storage of verbal and spatial information. In particular, according to Baddeley's (1986) influential model, working memory comprises a modality-free controlling central executive which is aided by a number of peripheral ''slave systems'' to ensure temporary maintenance of information. The two most explored of these slave systems are the phonological loop (thought to provide temporary storage for speech-based material) and the visuospatial sketchpad (thought to be involved in temporarily storing non-verbal material). The focus of Van der Linden et al.'s paper is the central executive component of the working memory system. The central executive is thought to be an attentional control system responsible for strategy selection, planning, decision making, and control and coordination of the various processes involved in short-term storage and more general processing tasks. Previous neuroimaging studies have indicated that the dorsolateral prefrontal cortex (especially areas 46 and 9) are most closely involved in central executive functioning. However, a major difficulty when exploring the neural basis of the central executive is in identifying a task in which its role can be clearly distinguished from that of the slave (i.e. storage) systems. The study reported by Van der Linden et al. makes use of the updating memory paradigm to explore this issue. This task requires participants first to watch strings of consonants of unknown length, and then to recall serially a specific number of recent items. The task is thought to require both the phonological loop and the central executive for efficient performance: the updating process requires central executive resources but not the phonological loop, while the serial recall (i.e. storage) component of the task requires the operation of the phonological loop but not the central executive. In particular, in this study, recall rather than recognition was used in order to encourage participants to use a phonological strategy in performing the task, and a sub-span four-item list was used in order to focus on the role of the phonological loop in storage of the target information.

Markowitsch notes that memory disorders occur as a consequence of a wide range of disease states, ranging from trauma, infarcts and degenerative disorders to psychogenic and psychiatric phenomena. However, Markowitsch argues that the traditional lesion-based methodology of amnesia research has been challenged by the use of functional neuroimaging techniques which, he argues, provide a more Gestalt-like, integrative view of the neuronal correlates of memory (although compare the position of Mayes & Montaldi, also in this issue). In particular, Markowitsch argues that the use of functional neuroimaging techniques has led to an acknowledgement of the role of the prefrontal cortex in episodic memory, refinement in our thinking about the role of the left and right hemispheres in long-term information processing, and the further identification of specific brain correlates of altered memory functions (especially with respect to the retrieval of autobiographical memories). Markowitsch's paper then proceeds to consider several cases of functional amnesia, the degree to which these cases are informed by a consideration of neuroimaging data, stress-related changes in the brain, and the "mnestic block syndrome".

In his paper, Nyberg presents functional neuroimaging data that are of relevance to cognitive theories and phenomena of episodic memory. The primary focus is on data obtained by Nyberg and his colleagues using positron emission tomography (PET), a technique that measures brain activity by monitoring radioactive markers of blood flow changes in the brain which take place while participants are involved in a cognitive task. By comparing the activation patterns associated with different cognitive tasks, it is assumed possible to identify brain regions that are differentially involved across different types of cognitive challenge. These differential brain responses may be due to differences in relative changes in brain activity between experimental conditions, in the way in which specific brain regions interact within each condition, or both. Types of differential response are considered in Nyberg's paper in the context of the following concepts and phenomena: retrieval mode, ecphory, encoding specificity, inhibition of task-irrelevant processing, item and source memory, conscious recollection, retrieval and the reinstatement of encoding operations, and the picture superiority effect.

The paper authored by Reed et al. presents one of a series of studies they have conducted using neuroimaging to examine patients with organic amnesia resulting from hypoxia. Reed et al. point out the complementarity of different imaging techniques: for example, it is not uncommon in patient populations to observe abnormalities using one form of neuroimaging procedure (for example, a structural technique such as CT or MRI which is designed to identify a brain "lesion") but not with another methodology (for example, using a functional imaging technique such as fMRI or PET). Moreover, the authors warn that the technical assumptions underlying different neuroimaging protocols, and problems in analysis and interpretation of neuroimaging data, are commonly underestimated in neuropsychology, with a paucity of studies comparing the findings from different forms of image analysis within a specific empirical study. Furthermore, echoing the theme of Markowitsch's paper, Reed et al. contend that patients with clear cognitive deficits sometimes fail spectacularly to manifest obvious abnormalities on MRI or PET scanning. The study reported by Reed et al. focuses on the question of the specific involvement of limbic-diencephalic brain regions in hypoxic amnesia, through an examination of both brain metabolism (using PET) and neurological pathology (using MRI). In the studies conducted by this research group, the neuroimaging analyses have been carried out in a number of different ways (and in conjunction with detailed cognitive investigations), in order to evaluate clearly the convergence of or divergence between the findings of different types of analysis.

Mayes and Montaldi point out that neuropsychological investigations of human long-term episodic and semantic memory have been conducted using two main experimental methodologies: (i) by examining the effects of selective brain lesions causing amnesia, and (ii) by functional neuroimaging in brain-damaged and in non-brain-damaged individuals. These authors proceed to argue that it is therefore possible, and indeed desirable, for researchers to adopt a convergent operations approach, in which the findings from neuroimaging studies must be reconciled with those from lesion-based experiments, before one can confidently interpret the results obtained. When there is conflict between the findings from these two literatures, it becomes essential to account for these differences in a meaningful manner before real progress can be made. One specific conflict on which Mayes and Montaldi focus concerns early neuroactivation studies of episodic encoding, in which there was a failure to obtain clear evidence for medial temporal lobe activation. Taken at face value, this finding clearly differed from what would have been predicted from the lesion literature, in which damage to the medial temporal lobes has been consistently observed to disrupt episodic memory. Although Mayes and Montaldi acknowledge that later functional imaging studies have observed medial temporal lobe activation, especially during episodic encoding, they suggest that, in future, a complete understanding of the implications of neuroimaging and lesion data requires a more thorough implementation of the converging operations methodology. In particular, they argue that in future the converging operations approach should be followed more rigorously by functional neuroimaging researchers, by using a more hypothesis-driven experimental approach. Mayes and Montaldi argue that if this approach were to be followed more faithfully, it would mean that future neuroimaging data would provide an even more powerful adjunct to the findings of other forms of neurocognitive investigation.

In the study reported by McDermott et al., the authors investigate episodic memory using event-related fMRI. As the authors point out, episodic memory encompasses both the initial acquisition of information (encoding) and the subsequent remembering of previous experiences (retrieval). These processes are thought to be closely related in functional terms (Morris, Bransford & Franks, 1977; Tulving, 1983). However, despite a recent flurry of neuroimaging investigations, due to the range and complexity of encoding and retrieval processes relatively little is yet known about the inter-relationships of these capacities at the neural level. In this study, McDermott et al. use an event-related fMRI design in order to compare the neural activation that occurs during encoding and retrieval of visually presented words. The goal of their investigation is to identify the differences and similarities in functional activation that occur between intentional, deep encoding and recognition of these materials. The authors argue that event-related fMRI provides a powerful new tool for investigating the neural mechanisms of episodic memory.

Conway et al. present an investigation of memory for the experiences of one's life, or autobiographical memory. This is one of the central aspects of cognition, contributing significantly to a sense of continuous self-identity and individuality. As the authors point out, although this field has been investigated widely by experimental psychologists, the neurobiological basis of autobiographical memory remains largely unknown. In their study, Conway et al. use a cue word procedure to elicit autobiographical memories from participants, and compare brain activation with that elicited by paired associate recall. As an additional experimental manipulation, in one condition autobiographical memories during the past 12 months were elicited, whereas in another condition autobiographical memories of events that occurred at age 15 or earlier were requested. This was done in order to evaluate whether regions of the medial temporal lobe were, according to the conventional viewpoint, active in recalling only relatively new "unconsolidated" autobiographical memories (Squire, 1992) or, according to a more recent view, whether these regions were active across all time periods (Nadel & Moscovitch, 1997).

In their paper, Fletcher and Dolan point out that the activation of right prefrontal cortex has been widely observed across a number of functional neuroimaging studies employing a range of psychological paradigms and test modalities, although the functional significance of these observations has remained rather unclear. However, there is emerging functional neuroimaging evidence concerning functional heterogeneity within right prefrontal cortex with respect to episodic memory retrieval. The experiment reported by Fletcher and Dolan was designed to explore further brain systems associated with episodic retrieval. Specifically, the authors report data using a word-pair learning task, originally employed in a previous study of encoding (Dolan & Fletcher, 1997).

The current analysis was motivated by subjective reports from the previous study that participants frequently (and spontaneously) retrieved previously presented paired items, even though the experimental task did not explicitly require this. In the current comparison, Fletcher and Dolan aim to characterise the spontaneous retrieval-related changes that occur in the right prefrontal cortex as study materials become systematically more familiar.

In the final paper in this special edition, Foster and colleagues report findings obtained from testing a sample of healthy young individuals on measures of verbal recall and then comparing individual memory performance with medial temporal brain volume, focusing on the hippocampus. As the authors point out, there has been longstanding neuropsychological interest in the relationship between a structure's volume and its functional efficiency, going back to the time of the phrenologists. However, with the advent of modern neuroimaging techniques, it is now possible to root this interest in scientific data. Studies of memory disorders have indicated that there may be a systematic relationship between the structural integrity of medial temporal lobe structures and memory performance (Press et al., 1989; Squire, 1992). The findings of recent functional brain imaging research have also implicated these brain regions in mediating aspects of long-term memory. Furthermore, there have been some recent suggestions that hippocampal circuit lesions particularly disrupt recall (Aggleton & Brown, in press; Aggleton & Shaw, 1996), although this is contentious (Reed & Squire, 1997; Rempel-Clower at al., 1996). The central objective in the study conducted by Foster et al. was therefore to determine whether the volume of the hippocampus correlated with delayed story recall in healthy normal individuals who had been preselected to show a range of memory performance, and specifically whether findings previously observed in the elderly would be replicated in healthy young individuals.

CONCLUSION

Since the late 1980s, neuroimaging techniques have enabled researchers to investigate the spatial and temporal characteristics of memory in considerable detail. All the contributors to this special edition acknowledge the intrinsically highly dynamic nature of this field. However, taken together, these papers provide an overview of where neuroimaging data currently place us with respect to the issue of the neural mediation of memory, and concerning our theorising about the cognitive architecture of memory processes. Such a review is important and timely: this research perspective, unavailable until just few years go, has already made a considerable contribution to our level of understanding, and, if harnessed appropriately, has considerably more to offer in the future.

REFERENCES

Aggleton, J.P., & Brown, M.W. (1999). Episodic memory, amnesia and the hippocampal-anterior thalamic axis. *Behavioral and Brain Sciences*, *22*, 425–489.

Aggleton, J.P., & Shaw, C. (1996). Amnesia and recognition memory: A re-analysis of psychometric data. *Neuropsychologia*, *34*, 51–62.

Baddeley, A.D. (1986). *Working memory*. Oxford: Oxford University Press.

Belliveau, J.W., Kennedy, D.N., McKinstry, R.C., Buchbinder, B.R., Weisskoff, R.M., Cohen, M.S., Vevea, J.M., Brady, T.J., & Rosen, B.R. (1992). Functional mapping of the human visual cortex by magnetic resonance imaging. *Science*, *254*, 716–719.

Churchland, P.S., & Sejnowski, T.J. (1988). Perspectives on cognitive neuroscience. *Science*, *242*, 741–745.

Dolan, R.J., & Fletcher, P.C. (1997). Dissociating prefrontal and hippocampal function in episodic memory encoding. *Nature*, *388*, 582.

Farah, M. (1994). Neuropsychological inference with an interactive brain: A critique of the "locality" assumption. *Behavioral and Brain Sciences*, *17*, 43–61.

Foster, J.K. (1997). Commentary upon M.J. Farah: 'The "locality assumption"': lessons from history and neuroscience?' *Behavioral and Brain Sciences*, *20*, 518–519.

Marr, D. (1982). *Vision*. San Francisco: WH Freeman.

Morris, C.D., Bransford, J.D., & Franks, J.J. (1977). Levels of processing versus transfer appropriate processing. *Journal of Verbal Learning and Verbal Behavior*, *16*, 519–533.

Nadel, L., & Moscovitch, M. (1997). Memory consolidation, amnesia, and the hippocampal complex. *Current Opinion in Neurobiology*, *7*, 217–227.

Press, G.A., Amaral, D.G., & Squire, L.R. (1989). Hippocampal abnormalities in amnesic patients revealed by high resolution magnetic resonance imaging. *Nature*, *341*, 54–57.

Raichle, M.E. (1986). Neuroimaging. *Trends in Neuroscience*, *9*, 525–529.

Reed, J.M., & Squire, L.R. (1997). Impaired recognition memory in patients with lesions limited to the hippocampal formation. *Behavioral Neuroscience*, *111*, 667–675.

Rempel-Clower, N.L., Zola-Morgan, S., Squire, L.R., & Amaral, D.G. (1996). Three cases of enduring memory impairment after bilateral damage limited to the hippocampal formation. *Journal of Neuroscience*, *16*, 5233–5255.

Squire, L.R. (1992). Memory and the hippocampus: A synthesis from findings with rats, monkeys and humans. *Psychological Review*, *99*, 195–231.

Tulving, E. (1983). *Elements of episodic memory*. New York: Oxford University Press.

MEMORY, 1999, 7 (5/6), 523–548

Mapping Cognition to the Brain Through Neural Interactions

Anthony Randal McIntosh

University of Toronto, Canada

Brain imaging methods, such as positron emission tomography (PET) and functional magnetic resonance imaging (fMRI), provide a unique opportunity to study the neurobiology of human memory. As these methods can measure most of the brain, it is possible to examine the operations of large-scale neural systems and their relation to cognition. Two neuroimaging studies, one concerning working memory and the other episodic memory retrieval, serve as examples of application of two analytic methods that are optimised for the quantification of neural systems, structural equation modelling, and partial least squares. Structural equation modelling was used to explore shifting prefrontal and limbic interactions from the right to the left hemisphere in a delayed match-to-sample task for faces. A feature of the functional network for short delays was strong right hemisphere interactions between hippocampus, inferior prefrontal, and anterior cingulate cortices. At longer delays, these same three areas were strongly linked, but in the left hemisphere, which was interpreted as reflecting change in task strategy from perceptual to elaborate encoding with increasing delay. The primary manipulation in the memory retrieval study was different levels of retrieval success. The partial least squares method was used to determine whether the image-wide pattern of covariances of Brodmann areas 10 and 45/47 in right prefrontal cortex (RPFC) and the left hippocampus (LGH) could be mapped on to retrieval levels. Area 10 and LGH showed an opposite pattern of functional connectivity with a large expanse of bilateral limbic cortices that was equivalent for all levels of retrieval as well as the baseline task. However, only during high retrieval was area 45/47 included in this pattern. The results suggest that activity in portions of the RPFC can reflect either memory retrieval mode or retrieval success depending on other brain regions to which it is functionally linked, and imply that regional activity must be evaluated within the neural context in which it occurs. The general hypothesis that learning and memory are emergent properties of large-scale neural network interactions is

Requests for reprints should be sent to A.R. McIntosh, PhD, Rotman Research Institute of Baycrest Centre, 3560 Bathurst Street, Toronto, Ontario M6A 2E1, Canada. Email: rmcintosh@rotman-baycrest.on.ca

The contributions of several of my colleagues to the development of the ideas expressed here are gratefully acknowledged: Drs B. Horwitz, C.L. Grady, E. Tulving, L. Nyberg, R. Cabeza, and N.J. Lobaugh. A.R. McIntosh is supported by the Natural Sciences and Engineering Council of Canada (grant OGP017034) and the Medical Research Council of Canada (grant MT-13623).

discussed, emphasising that a region can play a different role across many functions and that role is governed by its interactions with anatomically related regions.

INTRODUCTION

The past decade has seen tremendous advances in human cognitive neuroscience. Undoubtedly, part of the reason for this has been the explosion in the use of functional neuroimaging to examine the neural basis of cognition. Methods that image metabolic processes, such as positron emission tomography (PET) and most recently functional magnetic resonance imaging (fMRI), have provided wide access to the neural substrates of cognitive operations. The preferred method for determining how the brain represents cognition has been to use psychological theories of cognition to design studies for mapping the brain mechanisms. As the psychological models are by and large quite successful at explaining behaviour and guiding research, it seems reasonable that the brain areas supporting cognition should look something like these models. With the advent of the computer age, the prevailing metaphor is to view cognitive processes as a series of hierarchically organised computational modules (e.g. Baddeley, 1992; Fodor, 1983). The processes investigated are usually conceived as separable, and cognition is usually thought of as the additive result of these processes (although there are some notable exceptions, e.g. McClelland, 1979; Miller, Galanter, & Pribram, 1960).

When using these models to study the brain, it is important to keep in mind that they were developed without regard to the biology of the nervous system. Modularity in the nervous system is observed mainly in the sensory and motor systems, and even there, after a few synapses beyond the receptor organs, modularity becomes fuzzier as the cross-talk between systems increases. Within sensory and motor systems there is a great deal of redundancy, such that brain regions close to one another show overlapping functional characteristics. The partial redundancy in the nervous system allows for a great deal of flexibility in the responses of relatively small collections of cells to the internal and external world.

Another important characteristic of the nervous system is the connectivity between cells. Whereas most other systems in the body show some capacity for cell to cell communication, the nervous system is specialised for rapid transfer of chemoelectric signals. Although it is not true that every part of the brain is connected to every other part of the brain, there is a great deal of parallel and reciprocal connectivity. Physiologically, this means a single perturbation to the system is conveyed to several parts of the brain simultaneously and some of this will feed back onto the initial perturbation site. Such feedback can modify the response of the system to subsequent influence and lead to nonlinear responses despite linear changes in input.

When the question of mapping cognition to the brain is viewed in this way, the complexity of the problem seems obvious. Is it the case that cognitive processes, such as attention and memory, are localised to discrete portions of the brain, or does the brain represent cognition through the action of the whole? Is there some reasonable compromise between these views?

The purpose of this paper is to suggest that cognitive and behavioural phenomena, here learning and memory, are the direct result of the interactions among anatomically connected brain areas: neural interactions. The notion that cognition results from the operations of neural networks has a long history (Finger, 1994; Lashley, 1929), and has been put forth in recent theoretical work (e.g. Mesulam, 1998). Central to the idea of large-scale networks for learning and memory is that learning and memory are seen as a ubiquitous property of nervous tissue (Gonzalez-Lima, 1989), while the phenomenological diversity of learning and memory are emergent features of the interactions among brain regions (e.g. Edelman, 1978). A development out of the network approach is the idea of a ''neural context''. Neural context simply means that the same activity change in an isolated region may be observed across several behavioural and cognitive operations, but the activity and interactivity of related regions may be quite different. It is the relation of the activated region to other areas that determines the cognitive operation. The empirical demonstrations presented here come from studies concerning neural interactions as revealed from metabolic imaging methods, but the theoretical implications extend across all temporal and spatial scales of investigation.

MEASURING NEURAL INTERACTIONS

Neural interactions refers, in a general sense, to influences that different elements in the nervous system have on each other via synaptic communication (the term ''elements'' refers to any constituent of the nervous system, either a single neuron or collections thereof). The typical approach to the understanding of neural interactions has been to see if the activity varies systematically with some manipulated parameter. However, activity changes in one neural element usually result from a change in the influence of other connected elements, so focusing on activity in one area will miss the change in afferent influence. Furthermore, it is logically possible for the influences on an element to change without an appreciable change in measured activity. The simplest example would be where an afferent influence switches from one source to another, without a change in the strength of the influence. Monitoring regional activity alone would miss this critical shift (for experimental evidence see: Lindsey, Morris, Shannon, & Gerstein, 1997; McIntosh et al., 1994).

The alternative approach to quantifying neural interactions is to measure the relation of activity between elements. One way to do this is by measuring the covariance of activity. The foundation for covariance analysis in neuroimaging was laid by Horwitz in a number of papers that looked at regional interrelations in a pairwise manner (Horwitz, 1989; Horwitz, Duara, & Rapoport, 1984, 1986; Horwitz et al., 1991; Horwitz, Soncrant, & Haxby, 1992b). Since then, covariance analyses have been extended to the exploration of interacting neural systems (McIntosh & Gonzalez-Lima, 1994), and to the identification of spatial and temporal clustering with various multivariate techniques (Friston, 1994; McIntosh, Bookstein, Haxby, & Grady, 1996a; McLaughlin et al., 1992).

The measurement of neural interactions in neuroimaging has proceeded under two general approaches. The first emphasises pairwise interactions, often in terms of correlations or covariances. The second incorporates additional information, such as anatomical connections, and considers interactions of several neural elements simultaneously to explicitly quantify the effect one element has on another. These two approaches are known as *functional* and *effective connectivity* respectively. Both terms were introduced in the context of electrophysiological recordings from multiple cells (Aertsen, Gerstein, Habib, & Palm, 1989; Gerstein, Perkel, & Subramanian, 1978). More recently, they have been used in reference to neuroimaging data (Friston, 1994). Two methods that will be discussed here typify the use of covariance tools in the analysis of neuroimaging data: structural equation modelling, which provides a measure of effective connectivity, and partial least squares (PLS), which can be used to assessed functional connectivity (for technical details see McIntosh et al., 1996a; McIntosh & Gonzalez-Lima, 1992, 1994; McIntosh et al., 1994). Both methods have been used in other scientific disciplines and are discussed here as they pertain to neuroimaging. The present focus is on how to use the methods to ask specific questions about the functional organisation of the nervous system. An example using structural equation modelling is described first.

CHANGING NETWORKS IN WORKING MEMORY

The neural basis of working memory has been researched extensively in functional neuroimaging and in monkey electrophysiological and lesion studies (e.g. Goldman-Rakic, 1990; Jonides et al., 1993; Kirkby, Van Horn, Ostrem, Weinberger, & Berman, 1996; McCarthy et al., 1994; Petrides, 1994). (For the present experiment, working memory is defined as the process of maintaining an active representation of visual information for ongoing information processing [Baddeley & Hitch, 1974].) Consistent across most of these neurophysiological studies is a strong involvement of prefrontal cortex. A feature that has been difficult to appreciate is how the areas connected with prefrontal cortex influence working memory operations. From the perspective of interacting neural systems, working memory as a neurobiological process should engage several regions depending on task requirements. Although it may be the case that for the operation of working memory to occur, prefrontal cortex must be involved, the actual process is the interactions of prefrontal cortex with other brain regions. So rather than the function of prefrontal cortex, working memory may be best appreciated as one of the emergent properties of the interactions of prefrontal cortex with other brain areas. This possibility was examined using structural equation modelling in the study presented next (McIntosh et al., 1996b).

Structural Equation Modelling

Structural equation modelling, or path analysis, is a multivariate analytic tool that is used to test hypotheses about the causal influences among measured or latent variables. One of the main purposes is to determine whether a hypothesised set of causal relationships is consistent with the observed data. The covariances among the variables are used to provide weights to proposed causal relationships in a manner similar to a multiple linear regression, which then indexes how well the proposed causal structure represents the observed covariance. It is used extensively in psychology and other social sciences (Bollen, 1989). For example, structural equation modelling has been used to distinguish between inherited and environmentally determined influences on certain personality traits (Loehlin, 1987) and whether performance on several memory tasks is best accounted for by the influence of a unitary or bidimensional memory system (Nyberg, 1994). As applied to neuroimaging data, structural equation modelling combines interregional covariances and neuroanatomy. This is an important feature of the application of structural equation modelling to neuroimaging. The causal structure is determined from the anatomy, rather than hypothesised, and the major goal is to evaluate the experimentally induced changes in the effective connections between regions. The basic steps for structural equation modelling are illustrated in Fig. 1 and described next:

- *Select regions or nodes of the network:* The selection of areas for the model is driven by a combination of univariate analysis of changes in mean rCBF, multivariate analyses (e.g. PLS), and theoretical guidance. If there is a particular theoretical model under consideration, such as a putative network for visuospatial attention (Mesulam, 1981), the areas forming that model should be included.
  - *Obtain the anatomical model:* The anatomic connectivity between selected brain regions is derived from the neuroanatomy literature. This is not a trivial step and it is at this stage that the theoretical persuasion of the investigator must guide the decision as to which connections to include in a model. Any system of equations where there are unknowns to be solved benefits from constraints to possible solutions. Using the anatomy of the system helps to constrain solutions. However, if all major and minor paths were included most models would contain reciprocal loops at nearly every level with some interconnections

Steps in Structural Equation Modeling

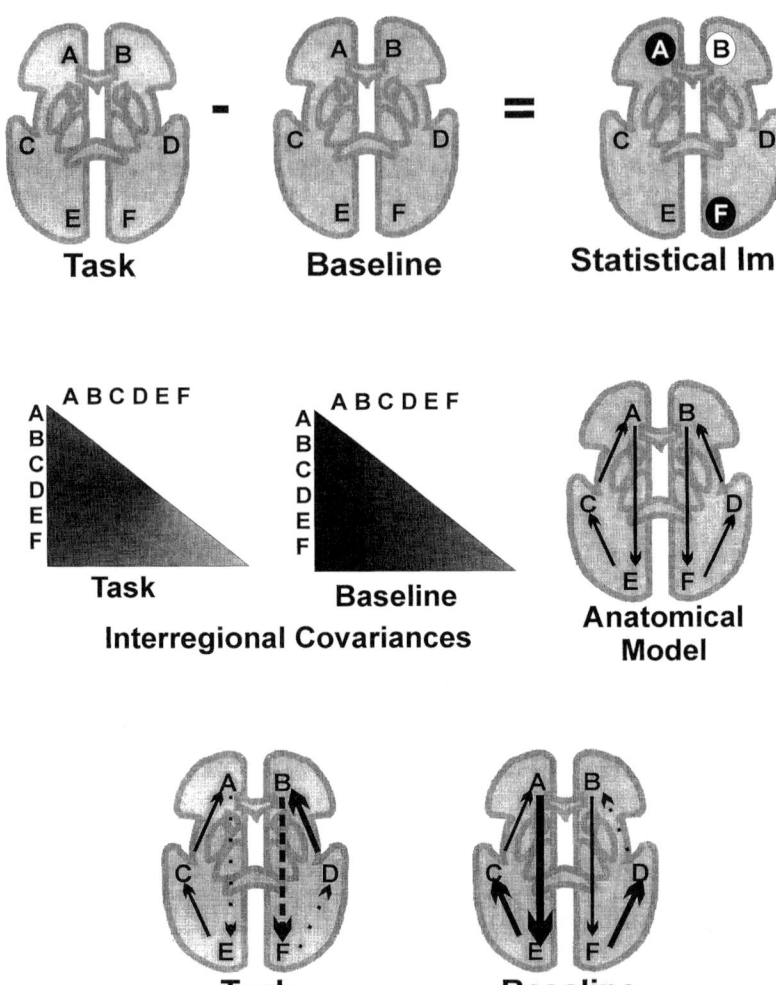

FIG. 1. Graphic representation of essential steps in structural equation modelling for imaging data. In the top row, regions for the model are selected based partly on the statistical differences between task and baseline (regions A and F showing deactivation and B showing activation) and partly on theoretical considerations, such as anatomical completeness or a theoretical model (regions C, D, and E). In the middle row, the activity correlations between areas are computed within-task and the anatomical model is constructed based on published neuroanatomical work. Finally, in the bottom row, the correlations are used to derive path coefficients for each anatomical connection within-task yielding two functional models. Positive weights are solid and negative dashed with the thickness of the line indicating the size of the weight. The ''deactivations'' identified from the subtraction image in region A correspond to a reduced involvement of region A, while the deactivation of F is because of strong negative feedback from region B. The activation in region B corresponds to its increased (suppressive) influence on F plus the stronger afferent influence from D.

between levels, both feedforward and feedback. When all possible anatomical connections are included, it is likely that an underdetermined system of equations would result, where there are either the same number of known and unknown elements or more unknown elements. In either case, unique solutions are not obtainable. In most cases, some compromise between anatomical accuracy and interpretability may be needed. There have been several published accounts where the compromises in model building have been made explicit (for further discussion see McIntosh & Gonzalez-Lima, 1992, 1994). For instance, in the example to be described next, feedforward connections were modelled first, then the path coefficients fixed at those estimates and feedback effects computed. The stability of the solution was guaranteed by ensuring the estimates were the same regardless of the order that the models were constructed. Interhemispheric effects were then estimated based on the constraints from the feedforward and feedback effects. This is obviously a compromise of what the reality of the interactions may be, and these compromises need to be made explicit for a complete understanding of the final model. Such specificity is often lacking in neurocognitive models that are loosely based on activation patterns. Any modelling effort, whether based on simulations, data fitting, or intuition, is necessarily a simplification and represents an approximation of reality. It is the degree of simplification that determines the utility of the model.

- *Calculate of interregional covariances:* For most published accounts of structural equation modelling in neuroimaging, the interregional covariances were computed within a condition and across participants. For fMRI and data from electrical or magnetic recordings (ERP or MEG), covariances can be computed for an individual subject across tasks or across trials of the same task, as many more within-subject measures can be made (for an application to fMRI see Buchel & Friston, 1997).

- *Calculate the path coefficients and comparison of functional models:* Path coefficients represent the proportion the activity in one area determined by the activity of other areas that project to it. When the coefficients are based on functional activity measured across participants, they reflect what could be thought of as an average functional influence within a given task and index the reliability and sign of the influence. The final step includes the comparison of path coefficients across tasks to determine if the interactions within the functional network differ.

The data set was obtained from a rCBF PET study of working memory using a delayed match-to-sample task for faces with a parametric manipulation of the delay interval (Haxby et al., 1995). The experiment consisted of a match-to-sample task with no delay (perceptual matching), and five scans with increasing delay (1, 6, 11, 16, and 21 s). The data from delay conditions were averaged: the 1 and 6 s delay conditions were averaged into a short delay condition, the 11 and 16 s delay into an intermediate delay condition, and the 21 s delay was the long delay condition. The grouping of conditions was based on the patterns of regional mean differences (Haxby et al., 1995).

For the working memory models, the regions chosen were those showing either a significant increase or decrease in rCBF with increasing delay as determined with the linear trend analysis and a task PLS (McIntosh et al., 1996b). The areas included ventral occipital and temporal regions (Brodmann areas [BA] 18, 37, and 21), inferior prefrontal cortices (BA 47; middle and medial prefrontal regions are part of the larger model presented in the original publication), anterior and posterior cingulate (BA 24 and 23), and the hippocampal gyrus (GH). Generally speaking, the posterior occipital and temporal areas showed decreasing rCBF with increased delay and the prefrontal and cingulate regions showed increasing activity with increasing delay. Measures of activity were obtained from both hemispheres, and interregional covariances were computed within-task and across participants.

Results

Figure 2 shows a summary of the dominant interactions for the four conditions: perceptual matching, short, intermediate, and long delay. In the perceptual matching network (top of Fig. 2), strong interactions were present bilaterally in the ventral cortical visual stream (Ungerleider & Mishkin, 1982), extending from occipital BA 18v, to occipitotemporal BA 37, to temporal BA 21 and then into ventral prefrontal BA 47. Prefrontal influences from BA 47 on GH were strong bilaterally. Cross-hemispheric effects were strongest between BA 47 and 37 with a slight asymmetry favouring the right hemisphere. The ventral stream and interhemispheric part of the network is extraordinarily similar to that of a previous path analysis from a similar perceptual matching task (McIntosh et al., 1994), which indicates that the functional networks are replicable across experiments and subjects.

The main trends of interest across the delay conditions were a change in the interactions along the ventral stream in the right hemisphere, more corticolimbic interactions in the short and intermediate delays, and more frontal involvement in the long delay. Of particular interest was the observation that several key areas, especially prefrontal cortex and anterior cingulate, showed strong interactions across all tasks, but the nature of these interactions changed as a function of delay.

The general feature of the short delay network, compared to matching, was an increase in the interactions right hemisphere involving BA 37, inferior frontal BA 47 and GH, and reduced influences in the left hemisphere (Fig. 2, bottom left). The pathway from BA 37 to BA 21 was weaker in both hemispheres and the influence of BA 37 appeared to be rerouted into the GH on the right. Within the right hemisphere, there was a strong corticolimbic trinodal loop set up with GH, BA 47, and BA 24. This loop changed at the longer delay conditions.

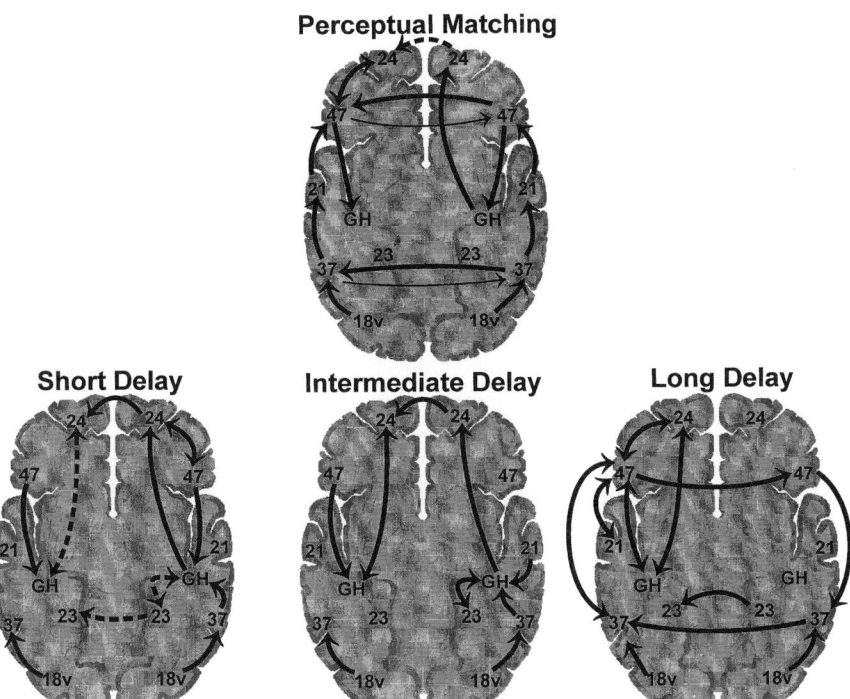

FIG. 2.   Summary diagram representing some of the dominant changes in functional interactions for the working memory tasks. Interactions are depicted on a horizontal schematic. To maintain clarity, the locations of these areas are not completely accurate and the reader is referred to the original publication for the exact location of the regions and their effects within these functional networks (McIntosh et al., 1996b). Positive path coefficients are shown as solid arrows, whereas negative ones are shown as segmented arrows. Two-headed arrows represent reciprocal and symmetric functional interactions.

The intermediate delay network (Fig. 2, bottom centre) could be characterised as showing less right inferior frontal involvement, compared to the short delay network, but still maintaining the right corticolimbic interactions with a positive loop between posterior cingulate and GH. The intermediate delay model also showed some changes in left hippocampocingulate interactions relative to the short delay model.

The long delay condition was characterised by a shift of what had been primarily right hemisphere interactions to stronger left hemisphere interactions. Right corticolimbic interactions were essentially zero, while left corticolimbic interactions increased, and a trinodal loop emerged similar to that observed in the short delay for the right hemisphere. Prefrontal effects from BA 47 seemed to play a stronger role in the long delay model compared to the other functional models (Fig. 2, bottom right). Frontal effects on occipitotemporal and temporal areas were especially strong in the long delay model. This feedback, along with the changes in interhemispheric interactions, resulted in an interesting interhemispheric circuit involving prefrontal BA 47 and posterior cortical BA 37.

Discussion

The interpretation of the change in the functional networks across delay was informed by the subject debriefing reports. The participants indicated that they could maintain a mental image of the sample face at short delays, but that it tended to degrade at the longer delays. From this, it was felt that the strategy at shorter delays was to rely on maintenance of the iconic representation of the face, whereas at longer delays an elaborative rehearsal and encoding strategy was employed. The interactions of BA 37, GH, and BA 47 during shorter delays, therefore, may partly reflect the attempt to hold the image of the face, whereas the left hemisphere interactions at the longer delay may represent elaborative rehearsal and encoding (McIntosh et al., 1996b).

The task-related network changes were not simply that certain areas interacted in one task and not in another, but in the nature of the interactions. It is important to note that the changes in neural interactions were much more striking than changes in regional mean activity. Anterior cingulate, prefrontal cortices, and GH showed strong interactions across all tasks, but the activity of these regions was not consistently higher than the control condition (Haxby et al., 1995). Even in cases where an area is not ''active'' relative to baseline, it may still show strong interactions. Activation analysis detects differences only, whereas covariance analyses reveal interesting changes in brain interactions not detectable through activation analysis.

Working memory studies have implicated three core regions: the anterior cingulate, dorsolateral prefrontal cortex, and the hippocampus (Goldman-Rakic, 1990). These regions were part of the functional networks for working memory discussed here, but they were also involved in a perceptual matching task with no obvious working memory component. An argument could be made that the interactions during perceptual matching also reflect some working memory component related to task execution, but this would require further experimental validation. Structural equation modelling results bring the suggestion that regions may play a part in more than one functional network, and that it is the interactions with other brain regions that determine what operations are being served at that time. Frontohippocampal interactions were present across all functional models. What changed between tasks was the nature of these interactions (indicated by the sign of the path coefficients). The hippocampus has been an enigma for brain imaging studies, but when examined in the context of covariance relationships, part of the reason for lack of consistent changes in activity may be that the interactions of this area are always strong and what changes with memory demand is the nature of these interactions. If this is true for the rest of the nervous system, much is to be gained by evaluating neural activity *and* interactivity related to cognition.

NEURAL CONTEXT AND RETRIEVAL MODE

One concept that arises from the network approach is that of a *neural context*. Most brain regions receive inputs from many areas and then send projections to several others. At any instance, the interactions through anatomical connections may shift from one afferent/efferent source to another, resulting in a change in cognition or behaviour. Across several different tasks, a brain area may show the same activity pattern but serve different functions because of the relation of that activity with other brain regions (for empirical examples see Chafee & Goldman-Rakic, 1998; D'Esposito, Ballard, Aguirre, & Zarahn, 1998; Zhang, Riehle, Requin, & Kornblum, 1997). The important factor is not that a particular event occurred at a particular site, but rather under what *neural context* did that event occur—in other words what was the rest of the brain doing? Neural context is closely related to the idea of "functional pluripotentialism", put forth by Filimonov (cited in Luria, 1962, pp. 24–25), which states that no formation in the central nervous system is responsible solely for a single function, and under certain conditions a given formation may be involved in other functional systems and may participate in performance of other tasks.

The notion of neural context can be illustrated by considering the activity of right prefrontal cortex (RPFC) in episodic memory retrieval (McIntosh, Nyberg, Bookstein, & Tulving, 1997). One of the most reliable results in neuroimaging of human memory is that of increased RPFC activity during episodic memory retrieval (Cabeza & Nyberg, 1997; Tulving et al., 1994). Experiments following from this observation suggest that the activation of RPFC may reflect "retrieval mode" or the act of searching memory without regard to the success of this search (Nyberg et al., 1995). In isolation, the interpretation seems reasonable. However, if cognitive states like retrieval mode are subserved by a large-scale neural network that includes RPFC, then the common pattern of RPFC activation across the retrieval tasks should reflect part of the operation of a general network for retrieval mode. Another possibility, which ties into the idea of neural context, is that RPFC activity may be similar across retrieval tasks, but result from the interactions with different brain regions depending on the act of retrieving and the success of the retrieval. Is the activation of RPFC reflecting a general retrieval mode network, or are there several networks, differentially engaged, whose interactions result in a similar pattern of RPFC activity?

One way to examine whether the same region has a consistent pattern of interactions across retrieval tasks is to explore change in the correlation of that region, or functional connectivity, with other parts of the brain. If increased

RPFC activity during retrieval represents retrieval mode, then there should be a pattern of functional connectivity for the RPFC that is similar across memory retrieval tasks. The question was addressed using PLS.

Partial Least Squares Analysis

PLS is a multivariate tool that can be used to describe the relation between a set of exogenous measures, like experimental design or behavioural measures, and a set of functional brain images (McIntosh et al., 1996a; McIntosh et al., 1998a; Schreurs et al., 1997). What results from a PLS analysis are sets of images that may be interpreted as nodes of neural systems representing some experimental effect or relating to some behaviour measure. The same analytic tool can be used to explore whether a part of the brain, represented by an image voxel, shows any task-related changes in its relation to the rest of the brain.

A highly idealised graphical description of the PLS procedure used to analyse changes in regional correlation is presented in Fig. 3. It can be regarded as an extension of the ''seed voxel'' correlation analysis proposed by Horwitz et al. (1992a). In panel A of Fig. 3, activity from a particular seed voxel (middle right of the ''image'') is correlated with the activity from the rest of the image in three tasks. This produces a correlational map for each task depicting areas that are correlated with the seed voxel.

In interpreting the correlation maps, a researcher would usually identify where the maps differ across three tasks. For example, in Fig. 3A the seed voxel shows an opposite pattern of correlations with posterior areas in tasks 2 and 3, and correlates with its contralateral homologue in task 1 only. Common correlations across the three tasks are in contralateral prefrontal regions, and, of course, of the seed voxel with itself. The extraction of commonalities and differences in the correlation maps is what the PLS analysis does. The PLS analysis of the correlation maps, or seed PLS, operates on the three correlation maps together and, through singular value decomposition (SVD), provides sets of mutually orthogonal latent variable (LV) pairs. One element of the pair contains numerical weights for each task creating a profile that depicts either a common correlation pattern or a task-related difference (i.e. a contrast)[1]. The other element of the LV pair identifies the parts of the image that show the profile across tasks and can be displayed in image space. Because it is derived from SVD, it is called a *singular image*. Within the singular image are numerical weights for each voxel, and their variation across the image shows which areas are maximally expressed on the particular LV. The weights for both the singular

---

[1] Another way to think about this is to consider an experiment with only two tasks and thus only two correlation maps. The sum of these two maps (or average) will represent areas of common correlation and a subtraction of the two maps would identify differences in correlations (McIntosh et al., 1996a). This is essentially what occurs in PLS and whether a singular image depicts common correlations or differences would be identified in the task profiles.

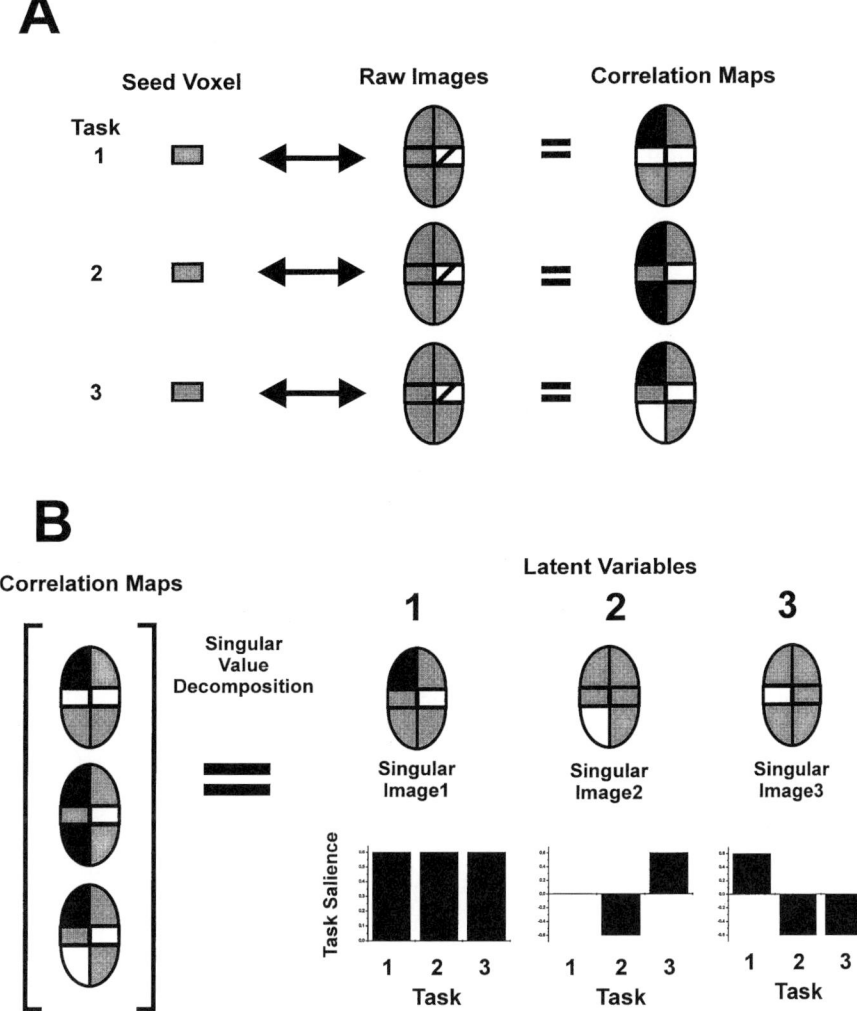

FIG. 3. Graphic representation of the steps involved in a partial least squares analysis of seed-voxel correlations. Panel A: a seed voxel is selected from the middle of the right side of the image (indicated by the black hash mark) within each of three tasks and correlated with the rest of the six-voxel image resulting in one correlation map per task. Black represents a strong negative correlation and white a strong positive. In panel B the three correlation maps are stacked into one large matrix and decomposed with singular value decomposition resulting in three latent variable (LV) pairs. Each pair consists of the singular image, which is an image representation of the weights (saliences) for voxels, and the weights or saliences across tasks or the task profile (bottom of each LV). As with the correlations, black represents a strong negative salience and white a strong positive. LV1 is a common pattern of seed voxel correlations, LV2 distinguishes the correlation maps from tasks 2 versus 3, and LV3 contrasts the map for task 1 versus tasks 2 and 3.

image and the task profile are called *saliences*. In reference to Fig. 3B, the singular image from the first LV shows positive saliences at the location of the seed voxel (middle right of the "image") and negative saliences at the contralateral prefrontal voxel. In the bar graph below the singular image, the saliences across tasks are equal, so the first LV is the common correlation of the seed voxel with itself and the contralateral frontal regions. The singular image in LV2 has a negative salience at a posterior location, and profile across the tasks contrasts tasks 2 and 3, so the LV depicts a posterior difference in seed-voxel correlation patterns. Finally, LV3 shows the salience at the contralateral homologue for the seed voxel and the task profile contrasts task 1 with 2 and 3. Although the results of the seed PLS analysis in Fig. 3 could have easily been distilled from the examination of the within-task correlation maps, it is much more difficult when images contain several thousand more voxels are analysed, as with PET or fMRI data (and real data are seldom as clean). The seed PLS analysis can also be extended to include more than one seed voxel, as in the example described next. The interpretation of the singular image and task profiles are the same as for the single seed voxel analysis, but a given singular image may show different task profiles for each seed voxel (e.g. task commonalities for one seed voxel, task differences for another).

The question of neural context and retrieval mode was examined with data from a PET rCBF study of episodic memory retrieval (Nyberg et al., 1996b; Nyberg et al., 1995). Three retrieval tasks were used with differing levels of retrieval success. Before scanning, participants were presented with two lists of words, some spoken by a male and some by a female. For one list, participants were asked to identify the gender of the speaker (shallow processing) and for the other list they were asked to decide whether the word represented a living thing (deep processing or semantic encoding). The retrieval conditions consisted of yes/no recognition (indicated by a button-press) for visually presented word lists that were either: (1) all unstudied (New); (2) from the shallow processing list (Shallow); or (3) from the deep processing list (Deep). Retrieval success would be highest in condition 3, but in all tasks participants would be in retrieval mode. A baseline task was also used, where a subject read a single word and pressed a button. Each condition was scanned twice.

Results and Discussion

For the seed voxel PLS analysis, representative voxels from three areas were selected: the two RPFC areas (BA 45/47 and BA 10, atlas [Talairach & Tournoux, 1988] XYZ coordinates: 32, 22, 0; 28, 44, 4,) and the left hippocampal gyrus (LGH: -24, -36, -8). The RPFC regions were activated to a similar degree in all retrieval tasks compared to baseline (Nyberg et al., 1995). The LGH location was activated only in the Deep condition (Nyberg et al., 1996b). The RPFC regions, assuming their activation reflects part of a retrieval mode network, should show common correlation patterns across the three retrieval conditions. The LGH, which may be more related to retrieval success, should show a pattern of correlations unique to the Deep condition. These hypotheses are presented graphically in Fig. 4 in terms of expected task profiles from a seed PLS. A profile representing retrieval mode (Fig. 4, top) would contrast the read baseline task against the three retrieval conditions, whereas a profile favouring retrieval success (Fig. 4, bottom) would contrast the New task against the Deep task with Shallow at some intermediate level.

None of the task profiles from the seed PLS was consistent with a pure retrieval mode interpretation. The singular image from the first LV is displayed in Fig. 5. Large areas of positive saliences extend across bilateral inferior temporal lobes, hippocampal and parahippocampal gyri, and retrosplenial cortex. Negative saliences are noted in left and right middle and dorsolateral prefrontal, medial occipital cortices, and midbrain. The task profiles for each seed voxel in the bar graph at the bottom of Fig. 5 indicate that the first LV was mainly a common trend in correlations for LGH and BA 10. LGH was positively correlated with areas that were positively salient in the singular image, while BA 10 was positively correlated with negatively salient areas. There was, however, an interesting addition in the Deep condition. Along with LGH and BA 10, the Deep condition showed a strong positive salience for the seed voxel at BA 45/47.

One may interpret this LV to suggest that there is a common pattern of covariances between BA 10, LGH, and the other limbic and frontal areas identified on the singular image. In the Deep condition, involving high memory retrieval following semantic encoding, another right prefrontal region, BA 45/47, shows strong covariances with limbic areas. That is to say, these three seed voxels are bound by a common pattern of functional interrelations with themselves and other brain areas only when there is successful episodic retrieval.

This interpretation of the LV may seem incongruent with the results from the activation findings, which deal with mean differences, not covariances of voxels. Recall that RPFC areas used here were relatively activated in all retrieval tasks, while the LGH activity was highest in the Deep condition. Patterns of covariation across other LVs (not presented graphically) suggested that the common task-related activation of RPFC may have arisen from different functional interrelations, as none of the LVs distinguished the retrieval tasks from baseline (e.g. Fig. 4, top). For example, LV 2 was salient for the right prefrontal regions for the Shallow and Deep conditions. The third LV was salient for BA 45/47 in the reading baseline only. In the fourth LV, the salience for BA 45/47 was strong in the New and Shallow tasks.

The results from the PLS analysis suggest that similar patterns of activation in RPFC came about through different patterns of interregional interactions. In LV 1, prefrontal BA 10 and the LGH showed common correlations across all conditions, but only when there was high memory retrieval following semantic encoding was BA 45/47 incorporated into the pattern. In light of the activation

Retrieval Mode

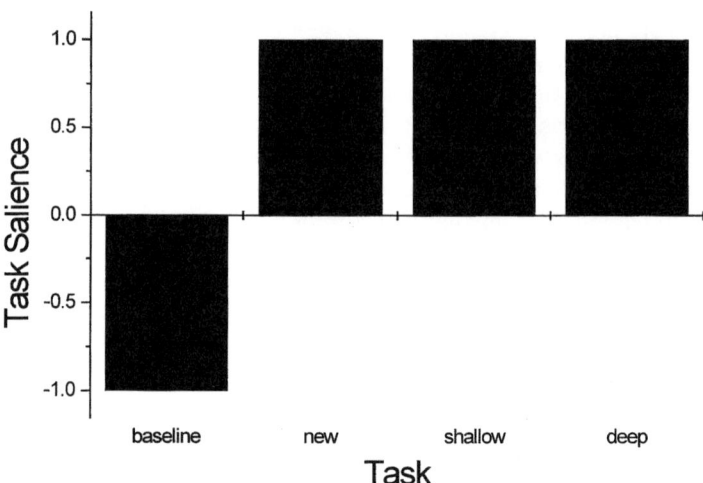

Retrieval Success

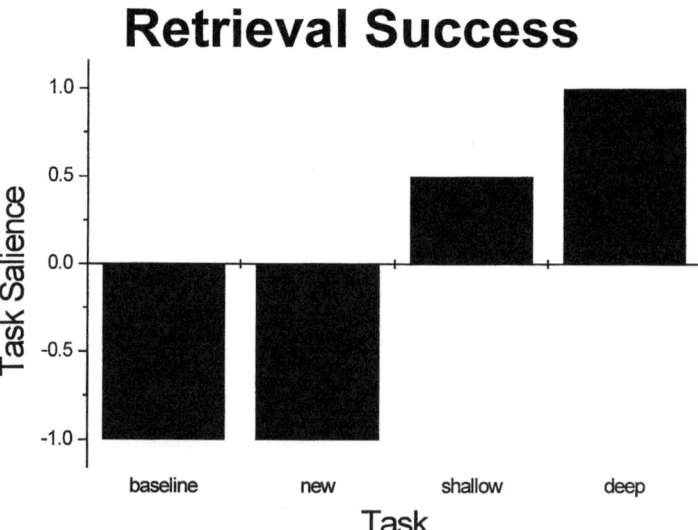

FIG. 4. Possible task profiles from a seed-voxel PLS that reflect two competing hypotheses for memory retrieval. In the top of the figure, the task profile contrasts the three retrieval tasks with the reading baseline task. This profile would be consistent with a pattern of functional connectivity for retrieval mode, or the act of retrieving independent of retrieval success. The bottom figure shows a task profile that contrasts the baseline and new task, where retrieval success is lowest, with Deep, and to a lesser degree, Shallow, where retrieval success is greatest. This is consistent with a pattern of functional connectivity representing retrieval success.

Singular Image

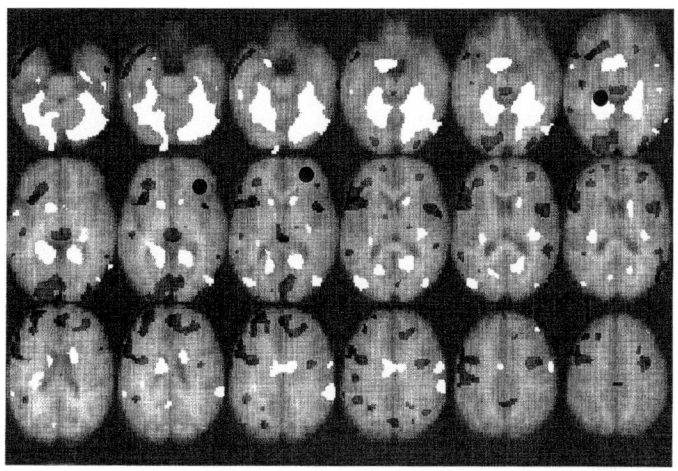

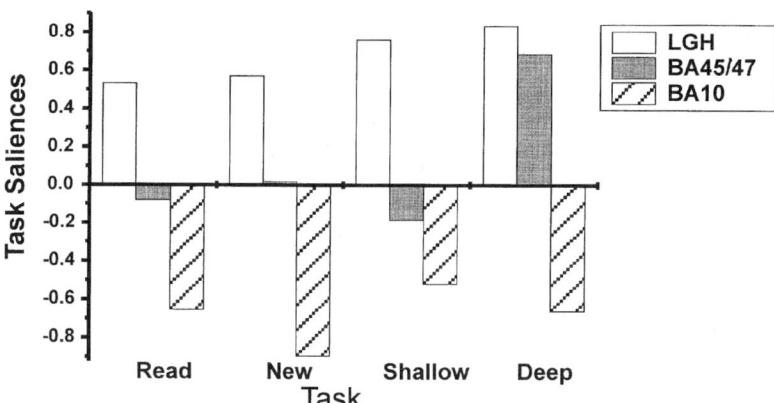

FIG. 5. First latent variable from the PLS analysis of seed voxel correlations for left hippocampus (LGH), right BA 45/47, and right BA 10. The bottom of the figure shows the task profile for each seed voxel by task, which is an index of how strongly the voxel covaries by task with the singular image at the top. This profile can be interpreted as a common pattern of correlations for LGH versus BA10 for all tasks, but Deep versus all other tasks for BA 45/47. The singular image depicts peak voxel that as a collection covaried with the task profile. Positive saliences (voxels positively correlated with LGH, i.e. greater values for higher LGH values) are drawn in white, negative saliences (voxels positively correlated with BA10 or greater values for higher BA 10 values) in black, both thresholded at a salience greater than 0.5 (absolute value). The image is displayed on horizontal sections from a structural MRI that conforms to the atlas space of Talairach and Tourneaux (1988). Slices start at −28mm from the AC–PC line at the top left slice and move in increments of 4mm to +40mm at the bottom right, and left is left and the top is anterior in the image. Black circles within the singular image mark the location of the three seed voxels and the surrounding voxels that were removed to reduce the spatial autocorrelation.

analysis, this may imply that the greater activation of the three seed voxels in the Deep condition arises through their common functional connections. For the Shallow and New tasks, however, the common activation of the two right prefrontal regions came about through other patterns of connectivity, perhaps due to increased suppressive influences on other regions (Nyberg et al., 1996a) and stronger interactions with regions identified on subordinate LVs.

The exploration of neural interactions in this study is a compelling example of the idea of neural context. Activity patterns in RPFC were common for the three retrieval conditions compared to baseline, but there was no evidence for a general retrieval mode network involving RPFC. One implication is that the equivalent activation level arose from different neural interactions across the three retrieval tasks. What distinguished the three retrieval conditions was the neural context in which the RPFC activation occurred. This result raises an interesting possibility that *neural interactions representing retrieval mode vary depending on the success of memory retrieval*. This speculation could be formally tested using methods that afford better temporal resolution, like ERP/ MEG or fMRI, with the expectation that the regions that are functionally connected with RPFC would depend on successful memory retrieval (e.g. Duzel et al., 1999).

Neural context allows regions to be part of more than one functional network. This is contrary to notions that cognitive processes like attention and memory are subserved by specific neural systems (c.f. Mesulam, 1990; Posner & Petersen, 1990). Most parts of the brain possess the rudimentary properties necessary for cognition. For instance, modification of responses related to learning and memory have been observed in several parts of the brain from single cells in isolate spinal cord preparations (Wolpaw & Lee, 1989; Wolpaw, 1997), to primary sensory and motor structures (Donoghue & Sanes, 1994; Gonzalez-Lima, 1992; Molchan et al., 1994; Recanzone, Schreiner, & Merzenich, 1992; Weinberger & Diamond, 1987). When several brain regions interact at a larger scale, these rudimentary features will combine to produce a particular cognitive function (Bressler, 1995). Whether or not a region is part of a neurocognitive system depends on the specifics of the processing demands (what is the person doing?) and the interactions with other regions (what is the rest of the brain doing?). Just as an instrument in an orchestra may switch from a lead to a support role in different pieces of music, some regions may play a more prominent role in certain cognitive functions, and then play a supporting role in others.

METHODOLOGICAL CONSIDERATIONS AND CAVEATS

The techniques presented in this paper represent two of several possible approaches to the estimation of functional and effective connectivity. Partial least squares and structural equation modelling may be employed separately or together to address specific questions about neural interactions. Indeed the combination of the two is a powerful means to go from activity changes, to functional connectivity, and then finally to the derivation of effective connectivity (e.g. McIntosh, Cabeza, & Lobaugh, 1998b). However, each approach does have its limitations. The examination of functional connectivity provides a means to address whether a region or collection of regions is interacting, but gives no information on the direction of these interactions. As such, inferences regarding the modulation of one area by another are not warranted. Estimation of effective connectivity provides some basis for inferences regarding the direction of influences, but in order to do this, assumptions on how these influences can occur are required. For example, in structural equation modelling the anatomical model constrains how regions may interact. Moreover, because it is a modelling technique certain simplifications are required as stated earlier. Both methods as presented here are restricted to exploration of linear relationships between brain areas. Although it is reasonable to assume that the scales measured in PET the predominant relationship is linear, the explicit incorporation of nonlinearities will be required for a full appreciation of neuronal components of cognition. Indeed there is some suggestion that in the time scales relevant for cognition (50–200ms) there are significant nonlinear components (Friston, 1997). Nonlinear extensions to structural equation modelling are rather straightforward (Kenny & Judd, 1984) and there has been some progress towards this in fMRI (Buchel & Friston, 1997).

There is some concern about which source of variance, across tasks or across subjects, is best for the estimation of neural interactions (see Friston, 1995; Strother, Kanno, & Rottenberg, 1995). The issue of which source of variability is "correct" is not unique to neuroscience (Mandler, 1959), and there is no necessity for a logical connection between covariances computed across tasks within-subjects and those computed across subjects within-task. However, there is also no justification for preferring one source of variability to another, particularly in cases where both can be examined as in fMRI or ERP studies. Within-subject analysis assesses the direct relation between regions, whereas across-subjects analysis provides an indication of the stability that relation. These are complementary, not contradictory, pieces of information.

For illustration, say we take 10 people of varying heights and weight, and ask them to pull on a potentiometer by flexing their arm (an arm curl). If you measured activity of the muscles in the arm for each subject, say through blood flow, and correlated them, you would probably find a strong correlation with the biceps and brachialis muscles. Although each person would differ in the amount of blood flow to the muscles, from the correlation based on this variance, you would conclude that the muscles on the ventral surface of the arm have something to do with flexion. If instead you measured muscle activity in a single subject with a progressive increase in the resistance to arm flexion, you would find a correlation between muscle activity in the ventral part of the arm. Replicating the measurement by running different subjects would lead you to the same conclusion that you had reached by using the between-subjects covariance. The point here is that computing covariances between or within subjects can lead to complementary conclusions so long as there are adequate experimental controls, and the statistical analysis ensures the answers are reliable.

CONCLUSIONS

The paper began by presenting the possibility that with neuroimaging we can investigate the operations of neural networks supporting cognition. Creating activity maps can give hints about the constituents of these distributed systems, but an appreciation for their interactions can only come from investigation of something like interregional covariances. Two covariance-based methods, structural equation modelling and partial least squares, were presented as ways to quantify neural interactions. Structural equation modelling was used to demonstrate the dependence of the functional network interactions on memory load. Partial least squares was used to show how right prefrontal cortical activity could be associated with the act of searching memory (retrieval mode) or successful retrieval depending on its relation to other brain regions, or neural context. Common in both examples is the possibility that learning and memory, very broadly defined, may emerge from neural interactions rather than being the responsibility of particular brain areas.

The idea that learning and memory are ubiquitous properties of the brain is counter to the parcellated view of nervous system functional organisation. However, physiological data have consistently shown that almost all parts of the nervous system show the capacity for learning and memory. There may, therefore, be several "types" of learning and memory depending on which regions are interacting. This is not to say that the brain contains several memory systems that are independent of perceptual operations, as has been implied by some theories in cognitive psychology (Schacter & Tulving, 1994). Instead, higher-order memory will involve interactions among different brain regions depending on the stimuli, the process, and what must be done with the information. This idea is similar to psychological theories that view memory as the dynamic combination of several processes rather than a discrete system (Jacoby, 1991). The interactions between brain regions lead to formation of memory. Memory *per se* is an emergent behaviour of the central nervous system—it is something the brain does.

At first pass, this may seem in direct opposition to data demonstrating severe and permanent deficits in learning and memory following damage to specific parts of the brain. However, it should be clear that the idea of emergent properties from neural interactions is neutral with respect to the lesion findings. Lesion findings give clues about functional organisation, but are silent as to how the function is carried out. This point is underscored by the following excerpt (John, 1961, p.480):

> The fact an animal can learn or retain the [conditioned] response after a lesion does not of itself warrant the conclusion that the structure normally played no role in the response. The engram, we suspect, is wily enough to elude the subcortical shot as easily as the cortical knife. Memory seems more likely to be set processes, which define a state, than a ''bit'' in a place. That places participate in process is apparent, but we may more legitimately expect the lesion of a region to alter the process than to abolish the state. That lesions can alter process we know, witness the effect of septal lesions on slow hippocampal waves. The problem that confronts us is to unravel how the condition response is produced by the process.

Substituting the words ''conditioned response'' with something like ''memory trace'' makes this point quite relevant to human cognitive neuroscience.

Some valuable insights could be gained from the exploration of network interactions in the damaged nervous system to see how the networks reorganise themselves in an attempt to compensate. When interpreted in light of interactions in the normal brain, such research could provide the important link between lesion data and normative experiments by explaining the lesion effect. For example, is the lesioned area a convergence site for functional interactions (Damasio, 1989)? Some strides towards this end have been made in examining ageing and Alzheimer's disease effects from a network perspective (Horwitz et al., 1995).

The idea of a neural context has important implications for how neuroimaging data are evaluated. If one is willing to accept that brain regions communicate with one another in the course of cognitive operations, then what one brain area does must be determined by what other areas connected to it are doing. When an area is more active in a cognitive task relative to a control task, that change must arise from neural interactions. Undoubtedly, there are consistencies in these activations as the realisation of the Hemispheric Encoding/Retrieval Asymmetry (HERA) model (Tulving et al., 1994), and the more recent Hippocampal Encoding/Retrieval model (HIPER, Lepage, Habib, & Tulving, 1998) attest. The next reasonable step would be to determine whether such consistent activations arise from the interactions of common neural systems.

Neuroimaging studies often present data in terms of ''activated'' regions that are considered independent of deactivated regions. However, relative deactivations are just as important as activations in setting up a neural context. An activation that occurs in one case may mean a different thing in the company of different deactivations. An illustrative example is selective attention. In PET studies of visual selective attention, rCBF in auditory and somatosensory regions decreases while visual regions are activated (Haxby et al., 1994). Consider another study where the same visual activation occurs without concomitant deactivation of auditory cortex. This pattern may signal quite a different cognitive process, perhaps that both visual and auditory domains are being attended to. If activations alone were examined, there would be no difference between studies. Deactivations are problematic for those who strictly adhere to the cognitive subtraction paradigm, but from a physiological perspective, increases and decreases in neural activity are equally important for nervous system operation. Deactivations can result from an active suppressive influence or from reduced interactions in the task of interest (as with regions F and A in Fig. 1, respectively; it is worth noting that these interpretation ambiguities are also there for activations). A recent paper from our lab demonstrates how it is possible to evaluate the source of deactivations with structural equation modelling (Nyberg et al., 1996a), leading to network models of cognitive operations that are more congruent with neurophysiology (Abeles, 1982; Douglas et al., 1995; Somers, Nelson, & Sur, 1995; Tsodyks, Skaggs, Sejnowski, & McNaughton, 1997; Turova, 1997; van Vreeswijk & Sompolinsky, 1996).

The complexity of data analysis and interpretation is great when covariance-based approaches are used. However, most questions in neuroimaging are phrased such that the answer is best provided by some sort of covariance analysis. Data interpretations are often made from the perspective of interacting networks, even if the network structure is never specified (Fink et al., 1996). To appreciate neural interactions does not require a drastic change in experimental questions, rather it requires a change in how the answers are provided. For example, top-down modulation in studies of selective attention is best explored through a covariance-based approach. Activation of higher-order areas (prefrontal) may arise from increased input or output, and without further analysis these possibilities are not distinguishable (e.g. Shulman et al., 1997). Covariance analyses like structural equation modelling can sort out these possibilities. Neuroimaging is in the peculiar position of having the answers to experimental questions constrained by the analytic methods. With the intellectual and financial investment needed from functional imaging studies, it is a shame that the fate of an entire experiment rests on a t-test. The subtraction method in PET, its carryover to fMRI, and the related statistical tools, have become the default for imaging experiments, but neuroimaging has matured beyond this. The choice of the analytic tool should be dictated by the particular experimental question. If the question is about neurocognitive networks , then the answer should come from something like a covariance-based analyses. If questions are phrased at a regional level (e.g. does an area contribute to an operation?), then activation analyses will provide an appropriate answer. Removed from the constraints of convention, the theoretical issues addressable by neuroimaging expand greatly.

REFERENCES

Abeles, M. (1982). Role of the cortical neuron: Integrator or coincidence detector? *Israel Journal of Medical Science, 18*(1), 83–92.

Aertsen, A.M.H.J., Gerstein, G. L., Habib, M.K., & Palm, G. (1989). Dynamics of neuronal firing correlation: Modulation of "effective connectivity". *Journal of Neurophysiology, 61*, 900–917.

Baddeley, A. (1992). Working memory. *Science, 255*, 556–559.

Baddeley, A.D., & Hitch, G.J. (1974). Working memory. In G. Bower (Ed.), *The psychology of learning and motivation* (pp. 47–90). San Diego, CA: Academic Press.

Bollen, K.A. (1989). *Structural equations with latent variables.* New York: Wiley.

Bressler, S.L. (1995). Large-scale cortical networks and cognition. *Brain Research Reviews, 20*, 288–904.

Buchel, C., & Friston, K. (1997). Modulation of connectivity in visual pathways by attention: Cortical interactions evaluated with structural equation modeling and fMRI. *Cerebral Cortex, 7*(8), 768–778.

Cabeza, R., & Nyberg, L. (1997). Imaging cognition: An empirical review of PET studies with normal subjects. *Journal of Cognitive Neuroscience, 9*(1), 1–26.

Chafee, M.V., & Goldman-Rakic, P.S. (1998). Matching patterns of activity in primate prefrontal area 8a and parietal area 7ip neurons during a spatial working memorytask. *Journal of Neurophysiology, 79*(6), 2919–2940.

Damasio, A.R. (1989). The brain binds entities and events by multiregional activation from convergence zones. *Neural Computation, 1*, 123–132.

D'Esposito, M., Ballard, D., Aguirre, G.K., & Zarahn, E. (1998). Human prefrontal cortex is not specific for working memory: A functional MRI study. *Neuroimage, 8*(3), 274–282.

Donoghue, J.P., & Sanes, J.N. (1994). Motor areas of cerebral cortex. *Journal of Clinical Neurophysiology, 11*(4), 382–396.

Douglas, R., Koch, C., Mahowald, M., Martin, K., & Suarez, H. (1995). Recurrent excitation in neocortical circuits. *Science, 269*, 981–985.

Duzel, E., Cabeza, R., Picton, T.W., Yonelinas, A.P., Heinze, H.-J., Scheich, H., & Tulving, E. (1999). Task-related and item related processes in episodic and semantic retrieval: A combined PET and ERP study. *Proceedings of the National Academy of Science USA, 96*, 1794–1799.

Edelman, G.M. (1978). Group selection and phasic re-entrant signalling: A theory of higher brain function. In V. Mountcastle & G.M. Edelman (Eds.), *The mindful brain* (pp. 55–100). Cambridge, MA: MIT Press.

Finger, S. (1994). *Origins of neuroscience: A history of explorations into brain function.* New York: Oxford University Press.

Fink, G., Markowitsch, H., Reinkemeier, M., Bruckbauer, T., Kessler, J., & Heiss, W. (1996). Cerebral representation of One's Own Past: Neural Networks Involved in Autobiographical Memory. Journal of neuroscience, *16*(13), 4275–4282.

Fodor, J.A. (1983). *The modularity of mind.* Cambridge, MA: MIT Press.

Friston, K. (1994). Functional and effective connectivity: A synthesis. *Human Brain Mapping, 2*(1&2), 56–78.

Friston, K.J. (1995). Statistical parametric mapping: Ontology and current issues. *Journal of Cerebral Blood Flow and Metabolism, 15*, 361–370.

Friston, K.J. (1997). Another neural code? *Neuroimage, 5*(3), 213–220.

Gerstein, G.L., Perkel, D.H., & Subramanian, K.N. (1978). Identification of functionally related neural assemblies. *Brain Research, 140*, 43–62.

Goldman-Rakic, P.S. (1990). Cellular and circuit basis of working memory in prefrontal cortex of nonhuman primates. In H.B.M. Uylings, C.G. Van Eden, J.P.C. De Bruin, M.A. Corner, & M.G.P. Feenstra (Eds.), Progress in brain research (Vol. 85, pp. 325–336). Amsterdam: Elsevier Science Publishers.

Gonzalez-Lima, F. (1989). Functional brain circuitry related to arousal and learning in rats. In M.A. Arbib & J.P. Ewert (Eds.), *Visuomotor coordination: Amphibians, comparisons, models and robots* (pp. 729–765). New York: Plenum Press.

Gonzalez-Lima, F. (1992). Brain imaging of auditory learning functions in rats: Studies with fluorodeoxyglucose autoradiography and cytochrome oxidase histochemistry. In F. Gonzalez-Lima, T. Finkenstaedt, & H. Scheich (Eds.), *Advances in metabolic mapping techniques for brain imaging of behavioral and learning functions* (Vol. 68, pp. 39–109). Dordrecht: Kluwer Academic Publishers.

Haxby, J.V., Horwitz, B., Ungerleider, L.G., Maisog, J.M., Pietrini, P., & Grady, C.L. (1994). The functional organization of human extrastriate cortex: A PET-rCBF study of selective attention to faces and locations. *Journal of Neuroscience, 14,* 6336–6353.

Haxby, J.V., Ungerleider, L.G., Horwitz, B., Rapoport, S.I., & Grady, C.L. (1995). Hemispheric differences in neural systems for face working memory: A PET–rCBF Study. *Human Brain Mapping, 3,* 68–82.

Horwitz, B. (1989). Functional neural systems analyzed by use of interregional correlations of glucose metabolism. In J.-P. Ewert & M.A. Arbib (Eds.), *Visuomotor coordination* (pp. 873–892). New York: Plenum Press.

Horwitz, B., Duara, R., & Rapoport, S.I. (1984). Intercorrelations of glucose metabolic rates between brain regions: Application to healthy males in a state of reduced sensory input. *Journal of Cerebral Blood Flow and Metabolism, 4,* 484–499.

Horwitz, B., Duara, R., & Rapoport, S.I. (1986). Age differences in intercorrelations between regional cerebral metabolic rates for glucose. *Annals of Neurology, 19,* 60–67.

Horwitz, B., Grady, C., Haxby, J., Schapiro, M., Carson, R., Herscovitch, P., Ungerleider, L., Mishkin, M., & Rapoport, S.I. (1991). Object and spatial visual processing: Intercorrelations of regional cerebral blood flow among posterior brain regions. *Journal of Cerebral Blood Flow and Metabolism, 11 (Suppl. 2),* S380.

Horwitz, B., Grady, C.L., Haxby, J.V., Ungerleider, L.G., Schapiro, M.B., Mishkin, M., & Rapoport, S.I. (1992a). Functional associations among human posterior extrastriate brain regions during object and spatial vision. *Journal of Cognitive Neuroscience, 4,* 311–322.

Horwitz, B., McIntosh, A.R., Haxby, J.V., Furey, M., Salerno, J.A., Schapiro, M.B., Rapoport, S.I., & Grady, C.L. (1995). Network analysis of PET-mapped visual pathways in Alzheimer type dementia. *Neuroreport, 6,* 2287–2292.

Horwitz, B., Soncrant, T.T., & Haxby, J.V. (1992b). Covariance analysis of functional interactions in the brain using metabolic and blood flow data. In F. Gonzalez-Lima, T. Finkenstaedt, & H. Scheich (Eds.), *Advances in metabolic mapping techniques for brain imaging of behavioral and learning functions* (pp. 189–217). Dordrecht, The Netherlands: Kluwer Academic Publishers.

Jacoby, L.L. (1991). A process dissociation framework: Separating automatic from intentional uses of memory. *Journal of Memory and Language, 30,* 513–541.

John, E. (1961). High nervous functions: Brain functions and learning. *Annual Review of Physiology, 23,* 451–484.

Jonides, J., Smith, E.E., Koeppe, R.A., Awh, E., Minoshima, S., & Mintun, M.A. (1993). Spatial working memory in humans as revealed by PET. *Nature, 363,* 623–625.

Kenny, D.A., & Judd, C.M. (1984). Estimating nonlinear and interactive effects of latent variables. *Psychological Bulletin, 96,* 201–210.

Kirkby, B., Van Horn, J., Ostrem, J., Weinberger, D., & Berman, K. (1996). Cognitive activation during PET: A case study of monozygotic twins discordant for closed head injury. *Neuropsychologia, 34*(7), 689–697.

Lashley, K.S. (1929). *Brain mechanisms and intelligence.* New York: Hafner Publishing Co., Inc.

Lepage, M., Habib, R., & Tulving, E. (1998). Hippocampal PET activations of memory encoding and retrieval: The HIPER model. *Hippocampus, 8*(4), 313–322.

Lindsey, B.G., Morris, K.F., Shannon, R., & Gerstein, G.L. (1997). Repeated patterns of distributed synchrony in neuronal assemblies. *Journal of Neurophysiology, 78*, 1714–1719.

Loehlin, J.C. (1987). Latent variable models. An introduction to factor, path, and structural analysis. Hillsdale, NJ: Lawrence Erlbaum Associates.

Luria, A.R. (1962). *Higher cortical functions in man*. New York: Basic Books.

Mandler, G. (1959). Stimulus variables and subject variables: A caution. *Psychological Review, 55*, 145–149.

McCarthy, G.M., Blamire, A.M., Puce, A., Nobre, A.C., Bloch, G., Hyder, F., Goldman-Rakic, P., & Shulman, R.G. (1994). Functional magnetic resonance imaging of human prefrontal cortex activation during a spatial working memory task. *Proceedings of the National Academy of Science USA, 91*, 8690–8694.

McClelland, J.L. (1979). On the time relations of mental processes: An examination of systems of processes in cascade. *Psychological Review, 86*, 287–330.

McIntosh, A., Nyberg, L., Bookstein, F., & Tulving, E. (1997). Differential functional connectivity of prefrontal and medial temporal cortices during episodic memory retrieval. *Human Brain Mapping, 5*(4), 323–327.

McIntosh, A.R., Bookstein, F.L., Haxby, J.V., & Grady, C.L. (1996a). Spatial pattern analysis of functional brain images using Partial Least Squares. *Neuroimage, 3*, 143–157.

McIntosh, A.R., Cabeza, R.E., & Lobaugh, N.J. (1998b). Analysis of neural interactions explains the activation of occipital cortex by an auditory stimulus. *Journal of Neurophysiology, 80*, 2790–2796.

McIntosh, A.R., Cabeza, R., Lobaugh, N.J., Bookstein, F.L., & Houle, S. (1998a). Convergence of neural systems processing stimulus associations and coordinating motor responses. *Cerebral Cortex, 8*, 648–659.

McIntosh, A.R., & Gonzalez-Lima, F. (1992). The application of structural modeling to metabolic mapping of functional neural systems. In F. Gonzalez-Lima, T. Finkenstadt, & H. Scheich (Eds.), *Advances in metabolic mapping techniques for brain imaging of behavioral and learning functions* (pp. 219–255). Dordrecht, Germany: Kluwer Academic Publishers.

McIntosh, A.R., & Gonzalez-Lima, F. (1994). Structural equation modeling and its application to network analysis in functional brain imaging. *Human Brain Mapping, 2*(1–2), 2–22.

McIntosh, A.R., Grady, C.L., Haxby, J.V., Ungerleider, L.G., & Horwitz, B. (1996b). Changes in limbic and prefrontal functional interactions in a working memory task for faces. *Cerebral Cortex, 6*, 571–584.

McIntosh, A.R., Grady, C.L., Ungerleider, L.G., Haxby, J.V., Rapoport, S.I., & Horwitz, B. (1994). Network analysis of cortical visual pathways mapped with PET. *Journal of Neuroscience, 14*, 655–666.

McLaughlin, T., Steinberg, B., Christensen, B., Law, I., Parving, A., & Friberg, L. (1992). Potential language and attentional networks revealed through factor analysis of rCBF data measured with SPECT. *Journal of Cerebral Blood Flow and Metabolism, 12*, 535–545.

Mesulam, M.M. (1981). A cortical network for directed attention and unilateral neglect. *Annals of Neurology, 10*, 309–325.

Mesulam, M.M. (1990). Large-scale neurocognitive networks and distributed processing for attention, language, and memory. *Annals of Neurology, 28*(5), 597–613.

Mesulam, M.M. (1998). From sensation to cognition. *Brain, 121*(Pt 6), 1013–52.

Miller, G.A., Galanter, E., & Pribram, K.H. (1960). *Plans and the structure of behavior*. New York: Holt, Rinehart, & Winston.

Molchan, S.E., Sunderland, T., McIntosh, A.R., Herscovitch, P., & Schreurs, B.G. (1994). A functional anatomical study of associative learning in humans. *Proceedings of the National Academy of Science USA, 91*, 8122–8126.

Nyberg, L. (1994). A structural equation modeling approach to the multiple memory systems question. *Journal of Experimental Psychology: Learning, Memory, and Cognition, 20*(2), 485–491.

Nyberg, L., McIntosh, A.R., Cabeza, R., Nilsson, L.-G., Houle, S., Habib, R., & Tulving, E. (1996a). Network analysis of positron emission tomography regional cerebral blood flow data: Ensemble inhibition during episodic memory retrieval. *Journal of Neuroscience, 16,* 3753–3759.

Nyberg, L., McIntosh, A.R., Houle, S., Nilsson, L.-G., & Tulving, E. (1996b). Activation of medial temporal structures during episodic memory retrieval. *Nature, 380,* 715–717.

Nyberg, L., Tulving, E., Habib, R., Nilsson, L.-G., Kapur, S., Houle, S., Cabeza, R., & McIntosh, A.R. (1995). Functional brain maps of retrieval mode and recovery of episodic information. *NeuroReport, 7,* 249–252.

Petrides, M. (1994). Frontal lobes and working memory: Evidence from investigations of the effects of cortical excisions in nonhuman primates. In F. Boller & J. Grafman (Eds.), *Handbook of neuropsychology* (Vol. 9, pp. 59–82). Amsterdam: Elsevier Science B.V.

Posner, M.I., & Petersen, S.E. (1990). The attention system of the human brain. *Annual Review of Neuroscience, 13,* 25–42.

Recanzone, G.H., Schreiner, C.E., & Merzenich, M.M. (1992). Plasticity in the frequency representation of primary auditory cortex following discrimination training in adult owl monkeys. *Journal of Neuroscience, 13*(1), 87–103.

Schacter, D.L., & Tulving, E. (1994). What are the memory systems of 1994? In D.L. Schacter & E. Tulving (Eds.), *Memory systems 1994* (pp. 1–38). Cambridge, MA: MIT Press.

Schreurs, B.G., McIntosh, A.R., Bahron, M., Herscovitch, P., Sunderland, T., & Molchan, S.E. (1997). Lateralization and behavioral correlation of changes in regional cerebral blood flow with classical conditioning of the human eyeblink response. *Journal of Neurophysiology, 77,* 2153–2163.

Shulman, G., Corbetta, M., Buckner, R., Raichle, M., Fiez, J., Miezin, F., & Petersen, S. (1997). Top-down modulation of early sensory cortex. *Cerebral Cortex, 7*(3), 193–206.

Somers, D., Nelson, S., & Sur, M. (1995). An emergent model of orientation selectivity in cat visual cortical simple cells. *Journal of Neuroscience, 15,* 5448–5465.

Strother, S.C., Kanno, I., & Rottenberg, D.A. (1995). Principal components analysis, variance partioning, and "functional connectivity". *Journal of Cerebral Blood Flow and Metabolism, 15,* 353–360.

Talairach, J., & Tournoux, P. (1988). Co-planar stereotaxic atlas of the human brain [Mark Rayport, Trans.]. New York: Thieme Medical Publishers, Inc.

Tsodyks, M., Skaggs, W., Sejnowski, T., & McNaughton, B. (1997). Paradoxical effects of external modulation of inhibitory interneurons. *Journal of Neuroscience, 17*(11), 4382–4388.

Tulving, E., Kapur, S., Craik, F.I.M., Moscovitch, M., & Houle, S. (1994). Hemispheric encoding/retrieval asymmetry in episodic memory: Positron emission tomography findings. *Proceedings of the National Academy of Science USA, 91*(6), 2016–2020.

Turova, T. (1997). Stochastic dynamics of a neural network with inhibitory and excitatory connections. *Biosystems, 40*(1–2), 197–202.

Ungerleider, L.G., & Mishkin, M. (1982). Two cortical visual systems. In D.J. Ingle, M.A. Goodale, & R.J.W. Mansfield (Eds.), *Analysis of visual behavior* (pp. 549–586). Cambridge, MA: MIT Press.

van Vreeswijk, C., & Sompolinsky, H. (1996). Chaos in neuronal networks with balanced excitatory and inhibitory activity. *Science, 274,* 1724–1726.

Weinberger, N.M., & Diamond, D.M. (1987). Physiological plasticity in auditory cortex: Rapid induction by learning. *Progress in Neurobiology, 29*(1), 1–55.

Wolpaw, J., & Lee, C. (1989). Memory traces in primate spinal cord produced by operant conditioning of H-reflex. *Journal of Neuroscience, 61*(3), 563–572.

Wolpaw, J.R. (1997). The complex structure of a simple memory. *Trends in Neuroscience, 20*(12), 588–594.

Zhang, J., Riehle, A., Requin, J., & Kornblum, S. (1997). Dynamics of single neuron activity in monkey primary motor cortex related to sensorimotor transformation. *Journal of Neuroscience, 17*(6), 2227–2246.

MEMORY, 1999, 7 (5/6), 549–560

The Neural Correlates of Updating Information in Verbal Working Memory

Martial Van der Linden and Fabienne Collette

Neuropsychology Unit, University of Liège, Belgium

Eric Salmon

*Cyclotron Research Centre, and Department of Neurology,
University of Liège, Belgium*

Guy Delfiore, Christian Degueldre, and A. Luxen

Cyclotron Research Centre, University of Liège, Belgium

G. Franck

Department of Neurology, University of Liège, Belgium

The aim of the present study was to re-examine cerebral areas subserving the updating function of the central executive with a running span task requiring subjects to watch strings of consonants of unknown length and then to recall serially a specific number of recent items. In order to dissociate more precisely the updating process from the storage function, a four-item instead of a six-item memory load was used, contrary to our previous study (Salmon et al., 1996). In addition, a serial recall procedure was preferred to a recognition procedure in order to suppress the use of visuospatial strategies. The most significant increase of rCBF occurred in the left frontopolar cortex (Brodmann's area 10), spreading to the left middle frontal (Brodmann's area 46). Results suggest that frontopolar activation underlies an updating process in working memory.

INTRODUCTION

Working memory refers to a limited capacity system which is responsible for the processing and temporary storage of information. Baddeley's model represents a current and influential attempt to define the structure and functioning of working

Requests for reprints should be sent to M. Van der Linden, Neuropsychology Unit, University of Liège, B33 Sart Tilman, B-4000 Liège, Belgium. Email: mvanderlinden@ulg.ac.be

This work was supported by the Belgian National Fund for Scientific Research (FNRS), the "Fondation Médicale Reine Elisabeth", and the Interuniversity Pole of Attraction Program P4/22, Belgian State, Prime Minister's Office, Federal Office for Scientific, Technical and Cultural Affairs. F. Collette is Aspirant at the FNRS.

memory (Baddeley, 1986). This model comprises a modality-free controlling central executive which is aided by a number of peripheral slave systems ensuring temporary maintenance of information. Two such systems have been more deeply explored: the phonological loop and the visuospatial sketchpad. The visuospatial sketchpad system is assumed to be involved in setting up and maintaining visuospatial material. The phonological loop system provides temporary storage for speech-based material and is composed of two subsystems: a passive phonological input store and an active articulatory rehearsal process. The central executive is assumed to be an attentional control system responsible for strategy selection, planning, decision making, and for control and co-ordination of the various processes involved in short-term storage and more general processing tasks.

In recent years, a large number of neuroimaging studies have contributed to identifying the physiological substrate of the different components of working memory (for a review, see Smith & Jonides, 1997). Several experiments have studied a variety of central executive processes such as random number generation (Petrides, Alivastos, Evans, & Meyer, 1993a; Petrides, Alivastos, Meyer, & Evans, 1993b) or co-ordination of dual tasks (D'Esposito et al., 1995). All these studies support the involvement of the dorsolateral prefrontal cortex (especially Brodmann's areas [BA] 46 and 9) in the central executive functioning.

However, a major difficulty in the exploration of the neural basis of the central executive is finding a task in which the role of the central executive can be clearly distinguished from that of the slave (storage) systems. In that perspective, the updating memory paradigm initially used by Pollack, Johnson, and Knaff (1959) and investigated by Morris and Jones (1990) appears to meet this requirement. The task requires subjects to watch strings of consonants of unknown length, and to recall serially a specific number of recent items. It requires considerable flexibility and a progressive shift of attention, i.e. discarding some items while new ones are registered. Morris and Jones (1990) showed that the updating memory task requires two independent mechanisms: the phonological loop and the central executive. The updating process requires central executive resources but not the phonological loop. Conversely, the serial recall (storage) component of the task requires the phonological loop but not the central executive.

In a recent PET study, we investigated the neural basis of this central executive updating process (Salmon et al., 1996) by using a working-memory updating task adapted from Morris and Jones (1990). In this task, lists of eight, nine, and ten consonants were presented at a rate of one per second. Subjects were not informed of the length of each list before presentation. They were asked to remember serially only the last six items (a six-item memory load). In the phonological short-term memory (control) task, sequences of six consonants were presented and the subjects were instructed to remember them serially.

When the updating task (requiring both the central executive and the phonological loop) was compared with the phonological short-term memory task (requiring the phonological loop), activation in a set of frontal and parietal regions was observed. An increase of rCBF occurred in the right mid-dorsal prefrontal cortex (BA 9), in left middle frontal regions (BA 46 and possibly BA 10) and in the right frontal pole (BA 10). Increased rCBF was found in a broad area of the right inferior parietal and angula gyri (BA 40/39), and in the left supramarginal gyrus (BA 40). We also observed activation foci in cuneus/ precuneus and superior occipital gyri on both sides (BA 18/19), in the right thalamus, and in the cerebellum.

However, a problem with this study was that we changed the Morris and Jones (1990) original updating procedure by converting the serial recall task into a short-term memory recognition task . This was made in order to be close to the procedure used by Paulesu, Frith, and Frackowiak (1993) to explore the neural substrates of the phonological loop. More specifically, instead of asking the subjects to recall serially the last six items of a sequence, they were asked to judge whether a consonant displayed two seconds after each list was present in the six last consonants for this particular list (a similar recognition procedure was used in the phonological short-term memory task). We recently obtained preliminary data suggesting that the recognition and the recall procedures promote the preferential utilisation of visuospatial and phonological strategies, respectively. In addition, post hoc questioning of the subjects examined in our initial PET study indicated that half of them used a phonological strategy in the updating memory experiment, while the other half used a visual imagery strategy or a combination of phonological and visuospatial strategies. As it appears that the subjects have frequently adopted a visuospatial strategy in our experimental updating condition, some of the observed activation (e.g. parietal and occipital activation) might be related to generation and short-term storage of visuospatial images rather than to central executive functioning. Another problem was that the subjects were asked to remember the last six items, a memory load close to, or beyond their memory span. According to Baddeley (1986; see also Vallar & Baddeley, 1984), span performance depends on both the phonological loop system and the central executive. The phonological loop system is able to store only a limited number of items but the central executive may increase this number either by improving the working of the phonological loop (for example, by grouping items into higher-level units) or even by using long-term memory information. In that perspective, it is plausible that holding a six-item memory load is very dependent on central executive resources and consequently, in our updating experiment, the central executive system would have been involved not only in the updating process but also in the storage function.

The present PET experiment was carried out to re-examine the brain regions involved in working-memory updating by using a serial recall procedure instead of a recognition procedure and by using a sub-span (four-item) memory load which is presumably less dependent on the central executive.

MATERIALS AND METHODS

Subjects

Six male, European, right-handed volunteers (age range 20–25 years) gave written informed consent to take part in this study, which was approved by the University of Liège Ethics Committee. None had any past medical history nor used any medication.

PET Scanning

Scans of regional cerebral blood flow (rCBF) were obtained for each subject using a CTI model 951/31 R PET scanner (CTI, Knoxville, Tenn., USA) with collimating septa extended. The physical characteristics of the tomograph have been described previously (Degueldre & Quaglia, 1992). Subjects wore an individual thermoplastic face mask for head stabilisation. A transmission scan was acquired for attenuation correction using three rotating sources of 68Ge. Emission scans were reconstructed using a Hanning filter at a cut-off frequency of 0.5 cycles per pixels giving a transaxial resolution of 8.7mm full width at half maximum and an axial resolution of 5mm for each of 31 planes with a total field of view of 10.8cm in this direction.

Volunteers received a 60 seconds intravenous infusion of $H_2^{15}O$ (total activity 35mCi) through a left forearm cannula. A dynamic PET scan consisting of two frames was collected over a period of three minutes (background frame duration, one minute, second frame duration, two minutes). The infusion of ^{15}O labelled water began 45 seconds after acquisition start time (Lammersta et al., 1990). Cognitive activation started upon $H_2^{15}O$ infusion, 15 seconds before the second scan. The integrated counts per pixel recorded during the second scan were used as an index of rCBF (Fox & Mintum, 1989; Mazziota et al., 1985). All subjects underwent six consecutive rCBF measurements (three for each experimental and control condition). Fifteen minutes elapsed between the scans. The order of memory tasks was fixed so that control and experimental tasks alternated.

Memory Tasks

In the control verbal working-memory task (see Fig. 1a), randomised sequences of four consonants were displayed on a computer screen at a rate of one per second. Subjects were instructed to rehearse the stimuli silently and to remember them serially, in order to repeat the sequence aloud after presentation of each list (the end of the list being indicated by a question mark). The presentation of each sequence began after the subjects pressed a key-response.

In the updating working-memory task (adapted from Morris & Jones, 1990; see also Van der Linden, Brédart, & Beerten, 1994; see Fig. 1b), lists of 4, 6, 8, 10 consonants were presented at a rate of one per second. Subjects were not informed of the length of each list before presentation. They were asked to rehearse silently and to remember serially only the last four items. They had to repeat those four items aloud after presentation of each list (the end of the list being indicated by a question mark). The presentation of each sequence began after the subjects pressed a key-response.

Sequences sounding like words and abbreviations were avoided, and for the updating task, the various lists were presented in a randomised order, with the restriction that no more than two lists of the same length were presented successively. Subject responses were recorded on a tape microphone. Patients were trained five or six days before the PET session. Five minutes before each acquisition, instructions were rehearsed. The control task consisted of 16 sequences, the experimental task of 10 sequences, each task lasting between 210 and 240 seconds.

Data Analysis

Image analysis was performed on a SPARC workstation (Sun Microsystems Inc., Surrey, UK) using statistical parametric mapping software 95 (Friston et al., 1995). Each reconstructed rCBF scan consisting of 31 primary transverse planes was interpolated to 43 planes to render the voxels isotropic. The six

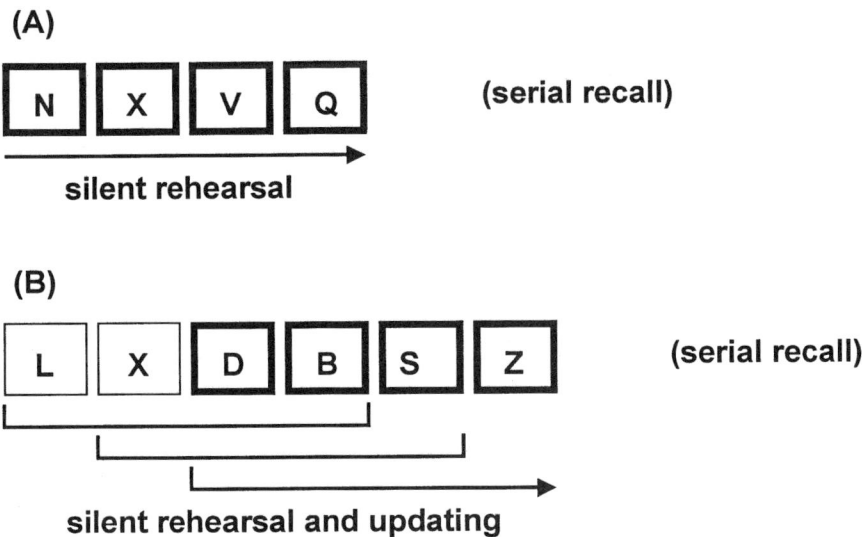

FIG. 1.   Schematic illustration of cognitive components involved in control and experimental tasks.

acquisitions from each subject were realigned using the first as reference (Woods, Cherry, & Mazziotta, 1992). The data were then transformed into a standard stereotactic space (Talairach & Tournoux, 1988). A gaussian filter (16mm full width at half maximum) was applied to smooth each image to accommodate inter-subject differences in gyral and functional anatomy and to suppress high-frequency noise in the images. Such transformation of the data enables pixel-by-pixel averaging of data across subjects and for direct cross-reference to the anatomical features in the standard stereotactic atlas.

Differences in global activity within and between subjects were removed by analysis of covariance on a pixel-by-pixel basis with global count as covariate and regional activity across subjects for each task as treatment (Friston et al., 1990). The across-task comparisons were first performed by averaging paired measurements. For each pixel in stereotactic space, the analysis of covariance (ANCOVA) generated a condition-specific adjusted mean rCBF value (normalised to 50ml/100ml/min) and an associated adjusted error variance. The ANCOVA enabled comparison of the means across conditions on a pixel-by-pixel basis using the t statistic. The resulting sets of t values constituted statistical parametric maps [SPM(t)] (Friston, Frith, Liddle, & Frackowiak, 1991). The SPM(t) were transformed to the unit normal distribution [SPM(Z)]. The design of our study was the comparison of a task implicating both the phonological loop and the central executive to a task implicating only the phonological loop. Besides this main effect, we looked for time or position effects in the repeated measurements, and for interactions between task and "time" effects. For all analyses, we used a SPM thresholded at $P < .001$, with a further correction for multiple comparisons ($P < .05$). We anticipated bilateral frontopolar activation and/or dorsolateral frontal activation in the updating task (Salmon et al., 1996). For this additional hypothesis-driven analysis, we used a statistical threshold of $P < .05$, corrected for the number of regions interrogated (n = 4) (Poline, Holmes, Worsley, & Friston, 1997).

RESULTS

Neuropsychological Performance

Subjects made only a few errors in the various tasks. There was no significant difference in the number of errors between the phonological short-term memory task (correctly recalled letters: $98.11 \pm 1.17\%$) and the updating working-memory task (correctly recalled letters: $91.33 \pm 7.80\%$; $Z = 1.75$, $P = .08$). Questioning the subjects about the way they carried out the tasks revealed that all subjects but one used verbal rehearsal, the last subject using mixed verbal and visual strategy. All subjects performed the updating task by removing successively the first letter(s) of the sequence for each presentation of a novel item after the fourth consonant was presented.

PET Data

When the updating working-memory task was compared with the phonological working-memory task, significant activation appeared in the left frontopolar cortex (BA 10), spreading to the left middle frontal cortex (BA 46). A significant activation was also observed in the right frontopolar cortex. Activation was located in the left frontopolar region when we used a SPM thresholded at $P < .001$ (see Plate 1, and Table 1). In order to assess an eventual effect of task difficulty (as the difference between the error rates in the updating and control condition approached significance), the metabolic changes between these conditions were assessed with the error score as a confounding covariate. The cerebral areas found in that analysis were similar to those found in the first analysis ($P < .01$, non-corrected for multiple comparisons).

A relative decrease of rCBF was observed in the right postcentral gyrus (40, –20, 32, $Z = 4.58$) for the updating working-memory task. There was also a trend for deactivation in the posterior cingulate cortex and the precuneus.

When looking for a temporal or position effect (Tables 2 and 3), we observed a decrease of rCBF from the initial to the last pair of tasks (first performance on both experimental and control tasks to the third performance on the tasks) in the left (fusiform) temporal inferior gyrus (BA 20). There was a rCBF increase

TABLE 1

Regions in Which There Was More Activation During Updating Condition
Than Control Condition

Area	X	Y	Z	Z score
Left frontopolar (BA 10)*	–24	50	4	4.32
Left middle frontal (BA 46)**	–50	24	24	3.15
Right frontopolar (BA 10)**	30	56	–4	3.57

Coordinates (in mm, relative to the anterior commissure) and Z scores.
* P value < .001, corrected for multiple comparisons.
** P value < .05, non-corrected for multiple comparisons.

TABLE 2

Regions in Which There Was a Decreased Activation From First Performance on Both
Experimental and Control Tasks to Last

Area	X	Y	Z	Z score
Left fusiform gyrus/inferior temporal (BA 20)	–54	–16	24	4.40

Coordinates (in mm, relative to the anterior commissure) and Z scores.
P value < .001, corrected for multiple comparisons.

TABLE 3
Regions in Which There Was an Increased Activation From First Performance on Both Experimental and Control Tasks to Last

Area	X	Y	Z	Z score
Right post central gyrus (BA 1/3)	46	−18	44	5.12
Right precentral gyrus (BA 4)	42	−18	36	4.98
Right precentral gyrus (BA 6)	46	−8	28	4.68

Coordinates (in mm, relative to the anterior commissure) and Z scores.
P value < .001, corrected for multiple comparisons.

(from the first to the third performance on the tasks) in the right postcentral (BA 1/3) and precentral (BA 4/6) gyri. The main point was that no significant interaction existed between task and time.

DISCUSSION

The aim of the present study was to re-examine the cerebral susbstrate of what appears to be an important function of the central executive component of working memory, i.e. the updating of information. In order to obtain a better dissociation between the updating process, requiring mainly central executive resources, and the storage function, requiring mainly the phonological loop, we used a serial recall procedure and a four-item memory load instead of a recognition procedure and a six-item memory load used in our previous study (Salmon et al., 1996).

The comparison of phonological short-term memory with working-memory updating confirmed that the prefrontal cortex is a key structure for central executive functioning. However, the most significant increase of rCBF occurred more specifically in the left frontopolar cortex (BA 10). Activation spread to the left middle frontal cortex (BA 46), and it was also observed in the right frontopolar cortex.

The dorsolateral prefrontal cortex (especially BA 9 and 46) is the region the most often implicated in working-memory tasks (Cohen et al., 1994; Mellers et al., 1995; Petrides et al., 1993a, b). Several functions have been attributed to this region, such as the co-ordination of dual tasks (D'Esposito et al., 1995), the temporal coding of items (Cohen et al., 1997), storage functions (Braver et al., 1997; Smith, Jonides, & Koeppe, 1996) or, in a more general way, the manipulation of information in working memory (Cohen et al., 1994 ; Owen, Evans, & Petrides, 1996 ; Petrides et al., 1993a, b; Salmon et al., 1996). However, some of the working-memory tasks used in those studies were multi-compound and did not permit researchers to isolate a specific function of the central executive or to separate precisely executive function from storage processing. In the present study, a specific function of the central executive, the updating of information, was explored and the region the most implicated in that function was the left frontopolar cortex (BA 10).

Increase of rCBF in the frontopolar cortex has been reported in several other working-memory activation studies, along with a dorsolateral prefrontal cortex activation (Owen et al., 1996; Petrides et al., 1993b; Salmon et al., 1996), but the role of those regions in working-memory tasks has not been specifically discussed. An intervention of the frontopolar cortex was also found in word recall tasks when the number of items to memorise was near to or above the span level (Becker et al., 1994; Grasby et al., 1993, 1994). In this context, it could be argued that the frontopolar cortex is related to the contribution of the central executive in storage function when the subjects are submitted to a memory load close to or beyond the memory span (see Salmon et al., 1996). However, in the present study, it seems unlikely that the frontopolar cortex was implicated in a specific storage function. Indeed, the memory load used in the present study (four items) was low and would plausibly not require an intervention of the ''storage'' function of the central executive. In addition, Braver et al. (1997) and Smith and Jonides (1997) showed a linear increase of metabolic activity, related to the memory load, in the prefrontal dorsolateral cortex bilaterally (BA 9/46), and not in the frontopolar cortex. Finally, it should be noted that no frontopolar cortex activation has been related to the phonological loop of working memory. Indeed, previous studies (e.g. Salmon et al., 1996; Paulesu et al., 1993) showed that the neural substrates of tasks involving only the phonological loop were located in the premotor cortex and adjacent Broca's area (BA 6/44), in the left temporal gyrus (BA 22/42), in the left and right insula, and in the inferior part of the left inferior parietal gyrus (BA 40).

Accordingly, the frontopolar cortex activation observed in the present study could be specifically related to the updating of working memory. The function of this updating process is to continuously modify the content of working memory according to newer external (sensory input) or internal (long-term memory retrieval) information. Interestingly, Grasby et al. (1994) showed that activation in the frontopolar cortex increased in relation to the number of times that subjects had to repeat a single word. It appears that this task also involves a continuous updating process, that is to control how many times the word was repeated and had again to be repeated, and the updating process becomes more important as the number of repetitions increases.

However, it remains to be determined whether the activation observed in the frontopolar cortex is related to a general updating process (independent of the type of updated information; i.e. semantic, visual, or phonological) or to an updating operation specifically devoted to serial verbal recall. Furthermore, it could be argued that the attribution of an updating function to the frontopolar cortex is not related to the specific involvement of the central executive component but rather to a greater difficulty in the updating task than in the serial recall task. Accordingly, recall performance tended to be lower in the updating task than in the serial recall task. However, when the error score of the subjects is taken as the covariate, similar activations were observed in the comparison of the updating and serial recall task.

In conclusion, the present study shows that, when the influence of the storage function is removed, specific cerebral regions can be isolated in tasks implicating the central executive, a structure nevertheless considered to have highly integrated functioning. In the same vein, Owen et al. (1996) demonstrated the existence of two functionally distinct subdivisions of the lateral frontal cortex, subserving different aspects of spatial working memory, with the ventrolateral frontal cortex (BA 47) related to the organisation and execution of a sequence of spatial moves and the mid-dorsolateral frontal cortex (BA 46/9) related to active monitoring and manipulation of spatial information. These findings suggest that the exploration of the central executive by means of functional imagery will be fruitful only if the experimental designs succeed in isolating specific components of this system. Moreover, given the integrative functioning of the central executive, the study of the relationships existing between several cerebral areas implicated in working-memory tasks will be particularly interesting. Indeed, it seems probable that the central executive function involves different interactions between a network of regions rather than specific regions devoted to each task. So, the frontopolar region appears to be involved in updating processes, but dorsolateral cortices are recruited when memory load increases. Moreover, the relative lateralisation of activation depends on the preferential use of verbal or visual strategies.

REFERENCES

Baddeley, A.D. (1986). *Working memory*. Oxford: Clarendon Press.

Becker, J.T., Mintum, M.A., Diehl, D.J., Dobkin, J., Martidis, A., Madoff, D.C., & DeKosky, S.T. (1994). Functional neuroanatomy of verbal free recall: A replication study. *Human Brain Mapping, 1*, 284–292.

Braver, T.S., Cohen, J.D., Nystrom, L.E., Jonides, J., Smith, E.E., & Noll, D.C. (1997). A parametric study of prefrontal cortex involvement in human working memory. *Neuroimage, 5*, 49–62.

Cohen, J.D., Forman, S.D., Braver, T.S., Casey, B.J., Servan-Schreiber, D., & Noll, D.C. (1994). Activation of the prefrontal cortex in a nonspatial working memory task with functional MRI. *Human Brain Mapping, 1*, 293–304.

Cohen, J.D., Perlstein, W.M., Braver, T.S., Nystrom, L.E., Noll, D.C., Jonides, J., & Smith, E.E. (1997). Temporal dynamics of brain activation during a working memory task. *Nature, 386*, 604–607.

Degueldre, C., & Quaglia, L. (1992). Performance evaluation of a new whole body position tomograph: the ECAT 951/31 R. Proceedings of the 14th Annual International Conference of the IEEE. *Engineering in Medicine and Biology Society, 14*, 1831–1833.

D'Esposito, M., Detre, J.A., Alsop, C.D., Shin, R.K., Atlas, S., & Grossman, M. (1995). The neural basis of the central executive of working memory. *Nature, 378*, 279–281.

Fox, P.T., & Mintum, M.A. (1989). Noninvasive functional brain mapping by change-distribution analysis of averaged PET images of $H_2^{15}O$ tissue activity. *Journal of Nuclear Medicine, 30*, 141–149.

Friston, K.J., Frith, C.D., Liddle, P.F., Dolan, R.J., Lammertsma, A.A., & Frackowiak, R.S.J. (1990). The relationship between global and local changes in PET scans. *Journal of Cerebral Blood Flow and Metabolism, 10*, 458–466.

Friston, K.J., Frith, C.D., Liddle, P.F., & Frackowiak, R.S.J. (1991). Comparing functional (PET) images: The assessment of significant changes. *Journal of Cerebral Blood Flow and Metabolism, 11*, 690–699.

Friston, K.J., Holmes, A.P., Worsley, K.J., Poline, J.-B., Frith, C.D., & Frackowiak, R.S.J. (1995). Statistical parametric maps in functional imaging: A general linear approach. *Human Brain Mapping, 2*, 189–210.

Grasby, P.M., Frith, C.D., Friston, K.J., Bench, C., Frackowiak, R.S.J., & Dolan, J.R. (1993). Functional mapping of brain areas implicated in auditory–verbal memory function. *Brain, 116*, 1–20.

Grasby, P.M., Frith, C.D., Friston, K.J., Simpson, J., Fletcher, P.C., Frackowiak, R.S.J., & Dolan, J.R. (1994). A graded task approach to the functional mapping of brain areas implicated in auditoty-verbal memory. *Brain, 117*, 1271–1282.

Lammertsma, A.A., Cunningham, V.J., Deiber, M.P., Heather, J.D., Bloomfield, P.M., & Nutt, J. (1990). Combination of dynamic and integral methods for generating reproducible functional CBF images. *Journal of Cerebral Blood Flow and Metabolism, 10*, 675–686.

Mazziotta, J.C., Huang, S.C., Phelps, M.E., Carson, R.E., MacDonald, N.S., & Mahoney, K. (1985). A noninvasive positron computed tomography technique using oxygen-15 labeled water for the evaluation of neurobehavioral task batteries. *Journal of Cerebral Blood Flow and Metabolism, 5*, 70–78.

Mellers, J.C.D., Bullmore, E., Brammer, M., Williams, S.C.R., Andrew, C., Sachs, N., Andrews, C., Cox, T.S., Simmons, A., Woodruff, P., David, A.S., & Howard, R. (1995). Neural correlates of working memory in a visual letter monitoring task: An fMRI study. *Neuroreport, 7*, 109–112.

Morris, N., & Jones, D.M. (1990). Memory updating in working memory: The role of the central executive. *British Journal of Psychology, 81*, 111–121.

Owen, A.M., Evans, A.C., & Petrides, M. (1996). Evidence for a two-stage model of spatial working memory processing within the lateral frontal cortex: A positon emission tomography study. *Cerebral Cortex, 6*, 31–38.

Paulesu, E., Frith, C.D., & Frackowiak, R.S.J. (1993). The neural correlates of the verbal component of working memory. *Nature, 362*, 342–345.

Petrides, M., Alivastos, B., Evans, A.C., & Meyer, E. (1993a). Dissociation of human mid-dorsolateral from posterior dorsolateral frontal cortex in memory processing. *Proceedings of National Academy of Sciences, USA, 90*, 873–877.

Petrides, M., Alivastos, B., Meyer, E., & Evans, A.C. (1993b). Functional activation of the human frontal cortex during the performance of verbal working memory tasks. *Proceedings of National Academy of Sciences, USA, 90*, 878–882.

Poline, J.B., Holmes, A., Worsley, K., & Friston, K.J. (1997). Making statistical inferences. In R.S.J. Frackowiak, K.J. Friston, C.D. Frith, R.J. Dolan, & J.C. Mazziotta (Eds.), *Human brain function* (pp. 85–106), San Diego: Academic Press.

Pollack, I., Johnson, L.B., & Knaff, P.R. (1959). Running memory span. *Journal of Experimental Psychology, 57*, 137–146.

Salmon, E., Van der Linden, M., Collette, F., Delfiore, G., Maquet, P., Degueldre, C., Luxen, A., & Franck, G. (1996). Regional brain activity during working memory tasks. *Brain, 119*, 1617–1625.

Smith, E.E., & Jonides, J. (1997). Working memory: A view from neuroimaging. *Cognitive Psychology, 33*, 5–42.

Smith, E.E., Jonides, J., & Koeppe, R.A. (1996). Dissociating verbal and spatial working memory using PET. *Cerebral Cortex, 6*, 11–20.

Talairach, J., & Tournoux, P. (1988). *Co-planar stereotaxic atlas of the human brain: 3-dimensional proportional system: An approach to cerebral imaging.* Stuttgart: Thieme.

Vallar, G., & Baddeley, A.D. (1984). Fractionation of working memory: Neuropsychological evidence for a phonological short-term store. *Journal of Verbal Learning and Verbal Behavior, 23*, 151–161.

Van der Linden, M., Brédart, S., & Beerten, A. (1994). Age-related differences in updating working memory. *British Journal of Psychology, 85*, 145–152.

Woods, R.P., Cherry, S.R., & Mazziotta, J.C. (1992). Rapid automated algorithm for aligning and reslicing PET images. *Journal of Computed Assisted Tomography, 16*, 620–633.

MEMORY, 1999, 7 (5/6), 561–583

Functional Neuroimaging Correlates of Functional Amnesia

Hans J. Markowitsch

University of Bielefeld, Germany

Especially in the field of memory encoding and retrieval, the results of functional neuroimaging have provided new insights in anatomico-functional interactions. In particular this holds true for the role of the prefrontal cortex in mnestic information processing, for the contribution and participation of the two hemispheres in various processes of information transmission, and for views on disturbed information processing after organically obvious and so-called psychogenic forms of memory impairments. This report particularly stresses the insights obtained by functional neuroimaging for probably environmentally triggered deficiencies in memory processing and discusses possible subtle neuroanatomical correlates of functional amnesias. It is especially emphasised that stress conditions and depressive states may modify the release of steroids (glucocorticoids) and transmitter agonists at the brain level with the consequence of selective memory disturbances which may manifest as a ''mnestic block syndrome''.

INTRODUCTION

Memory disorders occur as a consequence of a wide range of disease conditions ranging for example from traumata, over infarcts and degenerative illnesses, to psychogenic and psychiatric phenomena (Markowitsch, 1995a, 1996, in press). Not all disease processes have the same consequences—both quantitatively and qualitatively—on memory. Some may lead to only transient disturbances such as in transient global amnesia (Markowitsch, 1990a), others may affect either predominantly verbal or predominantly non-verbal forms of memory, or mainly information stored for a long time (retrograde amnesia), or information to be stored anew (anterograde amnesia).

Requests for reprints should be sent to Hans J. Markowitsch, Physiological Psychology, University of Bielefeld, P.O. Box 10 01 31, D-33501 Bielefeld, Germany. Email: *hjmarkowitsch@post.uni-bielefeld.de*

I sincerely thank all my co-workers without whom this report would not have appeared. Similarly, without the kind co-operation of the patients this paper could not have appeared. My work was supported by grants from the Deutsche Forschungsgemeinschaft (German Research Council; He 2664/1; Ir 17/5; Ma 795/24).

The subdivision of memory along content-based domains (Tulving, 1995; Tulving & Markowitsch, 1998) led to refined behavioural analyses and provided evidence for intimate relations between distinct forms of brain damage and disturbances in one memory subdivision (e.g. episodic memory), but not others (e.g. priming or procedural memory) (Calabrese et al., 1996; Markowitsch, von Cramon, & Schuri, 1993b).

Traditionally, the correlation between focal brain damage—both in humans and animals—and disorders in learning and memory has been favoured, although a number of structure–function inferences based on this model have been questioned (Chow, 1967; Isaacson, 1988; Markowitsch & Calabrese, 1996).

The advent and steep progression of functional neuroimaging techniques changed the picture and provided the basis for a more *Gestalt*-like, integrative view of neuronal correlates of complex behaviour. In particular the study of aspects of learning and memory profited by the possibilities inherent in the dynamic imaging techniques—single photon emission computed tomography (SPECT), positron-emission-tomography (PET) and functional magnetic resonance imaging (fMRI)—and enhanced our understanding of brain networks implicated in memory processing (Fuster, 1997a). Using these, a number of unexpected relations between brain and behaviour became overt, among them (a) a changed view on the role of the prefrontal cortex in memory, (b) a refined relation between hemisphere-specific roles in long-term information processing, and (c) specific metabolic brain correlates of altered mnestic functions, particularly with respect to the retrieval of autobiographic episodes. In the following I will comment briefly on the first two relations, before dealing in detail with the third one.

Role of the Prefrontal Cortex in Memory

The prefrontal cortex has expanded considerably in evolution (Markowitsch, 1988) and consequently in its anatomical parcellation and functional involvements (Fuster, 1997b). The orbitofrontal portion is largely implicated in social-emotional and personality dimensions (Cicerone & Tanenbaum, 1997; Damasio, Tranel, & Damasio, 1990; Harrington, Salloway, & Malloy, 1997), the dorsolateral aspects are dominantly related to the initiation and control of willful and effortful acts, and to the temporary sequencing and organising of information (Jetter, Poser, Freeman, & Markowitsch, 1986; Milner, Petrides, & Smith, 1985; Stuss et al., 1994). Memory impairments after prefrontal damage were consequently attributed to changes along the dimensions just named. Jetter et al. (1986), for instance, found that patients with frontal, as opposed to patients with posterior, cortical damage were strongly impaired in retrieving a learned word list after one day under free recall, but not under recognition conditions (Fig. 1). The authors (1986, p. 238) interpreted this finding as indicative of an

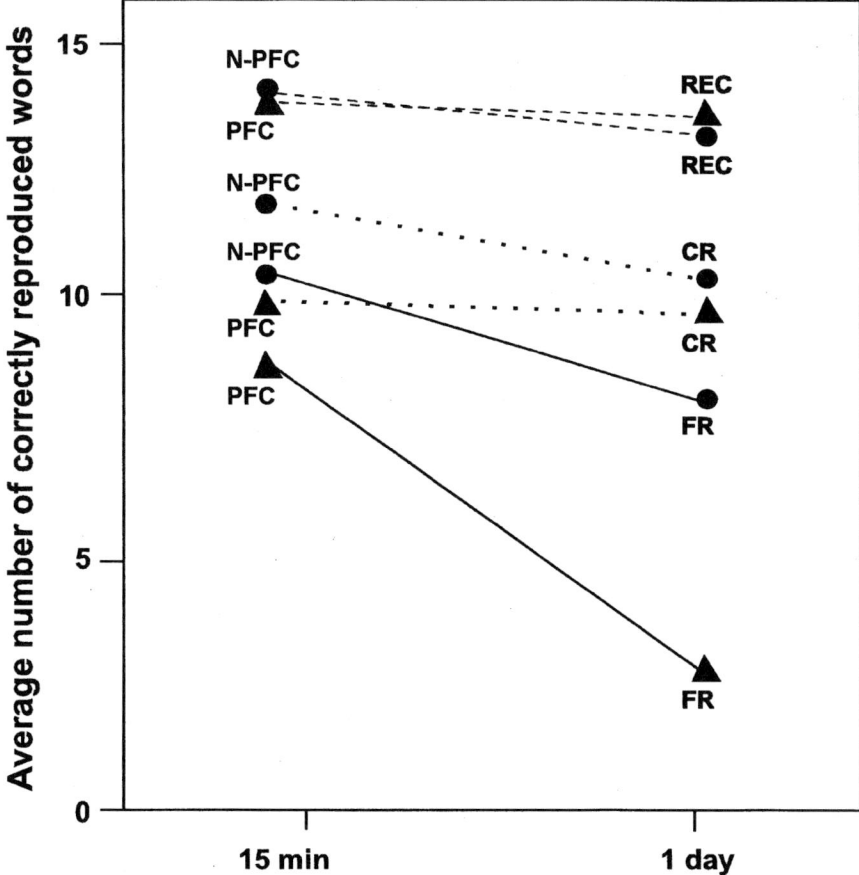

FIG. 1.   Memory performance of patient groups with prefrontal (PFC) or posterior cortical damage (N-PFC) under conditions of free recall (FR), cued recall (CR), and recognition (REC). (Data from Jetter et al., 1986.)

''impaired ability to generate adequate retrieval cues following a delay of one day.''

While functional neuroimaging studies measuring the brain's glucose metabolism in general confirmed such relations (J. Kessler et al., 1999), those measuring blood flow and using subtraction techniques (i.e. subtracting blood flow activations obtained during one condition of measurement from those obtained during a different, but related one; Raichle, 1994), found more direct involvements of prefrontal regions in memory encoding and retrieval (Fink et al., 1996; Fletcher, Frith, & Rugg, 1997; Markowitsch et al., 1997b; Shallice et al., 1994; Tulving et al., 1994a, b).

The prefrontal cortex consequently was found to be engaged both when it comes to the encoding of new information and to the retrieval of old information. Both conditions require active engagement of the brain; for encoding, the information most likely has to be transmitted further to limbic regions to then be associated, synchronised and related to the motivational and emotional state of the organism (Markowitsch, 1997a, in press). Retrieval is an active process as well, which Tulving (1983), in accordance with Semon (1904), prefers to term ecphory, in order to cover the process by which retrieval cues interact with stored information so that an image or a representation of the information in question appears.

Most interestingly, it was found that, at least for left-hemispherically dominant individuals, encoding and ecphorising information are coupled to different hemispheres, the former to the left and the latter to the right hemisphere.

Hemispheric Asymmetry in Mnestic Processing

Tulving and co-workers (1994a) first proposed what they termed the HERA-model, HERA standing for "Hemispheric Encoding Retrieval Asymmetry", and meaning that the left hemisphere is relevant for information encoding (both episodic and semantic information in the terminology of Tulving & Markowitsch, 1998), while the right one is relevant particularly for retrieving episodic information. Evidence consistent with this model was described in a number of reports summarised by Fletcher et al. (1997) and Markowitsch (1995b).

METABOLIC CORRELATES OF PSYCHIC VERSUS ORGANIC AMNESIA

We are used to viewing our present life, knowledge, and behaviour as caused by the experiences we had in the past. Furthermore, we have the firm belief that we can plan our future on the basis of the knowledge and the events we have processed and stored as memories. The time-embedding of memories is one of the most basic experiences, and it is only rarely reflected that our sense of time in particular provides and supports a reliable consciousness which allows us to travel back in time and to order, sequence, associate, and categorise experiences. This ability to travel back in time is one of the principal features of episodic memory and distinguishes this memory system from others—the knowledge system (or semantic memory), procedural memory, and the priming system (Tulving, 1995; Tulving & Markowitsch, 1998).

Patients with bilateral limbic brain damage, that is with a destruction of medial diencephalic or medial temporal lobe regions, have lost this basic ability with regard to their post-morbid life (Markowitsch, 1995a, in press). Patients with other kinds of brain damage, in particular with combined damage to temporopolar and infero-lateral prefrontal regions (Markowitsch, 1995b), may show a selective inability to retrieve information from their personal past. This inability is selective, in that those patients are still able to rely on memory subsystems different from the episodic (autobiographic) one (Markowitsch, in press). That is, they still can read, write, and calculate, and are able to maintain and even develop procedural skills. The discrepancy between preservation of some forms of memory and loss of other forms has been noted repeatedly since the turn of the century (see descriptions in Markowitsch, 1992).

Also, since the last century it has been noted that there are patients without obvious brain damage who nevertheless show widely similar amnesic disturbances, namely an inability to retrieve or ecphorise information, or an inability to acquire new episodic information long term (Markowitsch, 1990a, 1996). Such patients, in whom manifest brain damage could not be detected or suspected, have frequently been subsumed under the heading of psychogenic amnesia. However this label requires an explanation as well: What are the causes leading to psychogenic amnesia? It is assumed that a labile personality and stressful life events that cannot be adequately compensated or processed may lead to a retrieval block for personal past memories. Breuer and Freud (1895) and others (Janet, 1894; Mai, 1995) used the term "hysterical amnesia" to classify this condition. Freud (1901; Breuer & Freud, 1895) also emphasised that the forgetting may be selective (e.g. referring only to certain events or a certain time period or epoch). Furthermore, false memories may occur, that is, a subject may be of the opinion that something has happened which in fact did never occur, or that something happened in a different way than it did in reality.

All such biases in information processing can usually be traced back to certain personality dimensions or to certain environmental events. Usually, inappropriate affective or emotional processing is a prerequisite for such mnestic blocks. As an example, a subject who had most likely been sexually abused by her relatives had lost conscious access to her life period between ages 10 and 16 (Markowitsch et al., 1997c). Her therapist suggested to her that she produce drawings that would most likely correspond to or represent actual life situations of that time. She produced some drawings whose contents she could explain verbally, and others where for instance she only had strong negative emotional feelings. Measuring her regional cerebral blood flow during actual inspection of these drawings and during imagery of possible corresponding situations revealed a strong activation in the region of the right temporo-polar cortex which probably reflected her attempt to imagine the emotionally agitating mental image.

Organic Versus Psychogenic Amnesias

The phenomenon of psychogenic amnesia is usually related to a selective inability to retrieve episodic material of the personal past (Markowitsch, 1990b). Although a number of early, but also some recent reports (Mayes, Daum,

Markowitsch, & Sauter, 1997; Rempel-Clower, Zola-Morgan, Squire, & Amaral, 1996; Schmidtke & Vollmer, 1997), emphasised a strong inter-relation between anterograde and retrograde amnesia, there is more recently increasing evidence for a possible independence of the two (Kapur, 1993; Markowitsch, 1995b). Most of the cases with more selective retrograde amnesia after organic damage have a brain trauma-based etiology (Fink & Markowitsch, in press; Kapur et al., 1992; Kroll, Markowitsch, Knight, & von Cramon, 1997; Markowitsch et al., 1993a; Markowitsch & Ewald, 1997; Russell, 1971).

On the other hand, for cases with minor head concussions or other accidents not resulting in major bodily injury, associations between memory block conditions and the previous events seemed questionable (e.g. Härtl, 1916; Kohnstamm, 1917; Müller-Suur, 1949). The numerous labels used by psychiatrists to classify patients with specific biases in memory processing (e.g. "hysterical amnesia", "Wanderlust", "fugue-condition", "multiple personality", "Ganser-syndrome") were scrupulously separated from those labels attributed to cases with a known organic basis.

Patients with selective or largely selective retrograde (or anterograde) amnesia of an organic basis appear changed in their personality—primarily emotionally flattened (cf. Table 1). This makes them similar to patients with psychogenic or functional amnesia. (De Renzi, Lucchelli, Muggia, & Spinnler, 1997, introduced the term "functional amnesia" to describe amnesic conditions of unknown or unclear origin.) Consequently, the hypothesis was proposed that there is a basic similarity between amnesias based on a clear organic basis (manifest brain damage) and amnesias considered to be of principally psychic origin (Markowitsch, 1996). Furthermore, it was hypothesised that locus and extent of brain damage is not directly related to the severity of retrograde amnesia (Markowitsch, 1996, 1997b; Markowitsch et al., 1999a). Instead, biochemical or other changes might at least be co-factors of the amnesia.

Furthermore, the frequently involved prefrontal damage might modulate amnesia by provoking motivational changes, and changes in initiative, drive, and will (Jetter et al., 1986; Markowitsch, 1997a). As mentioned earlier, results from functional neuroimaging underline the importance of the prefrontal cortex for information recall (Fink et al., 1996; Fletcher et al., 1997; Shallice et al., 1994; Tulving et al., 1994a, b).

On the other hand, the often affected anterior temporal lobe region points to the importance of the emotional dimension (Damasio, 1994; Franzen & Myers, 1973). Starkstein, Fedoroff, Berthier, and Robinson (1991) found that particularly patients with damage to the orbitofrontal and temporobasal cortex of the right hemisphere were easily affected by unipolar manic disturbances. Within the temporal lobe, the amygdala has a special importance for the coupling of emotion and memory (Cahill, Babinsky, Markowitsch, & McGaugh, 1995; Markowitsch et al., 1994). Especially the amygdala and surrounding regions of the right hemisphere seem to be engaged in the processing of

TABLE 1
Case Descriptions: Emotional Flattening

Study	Remarks on the Patient's Affective Behaviour
Wechsler (1973)	"... cerebral dysfunction due to organic disease results in a comparatively selective inability to recall emotionally charged, ... material" (p.134) [varous kinds of brain damage]
Markowitsch et al. (1993b)	"The quite constant mood of the patient underlined the impression of somnambulism" (p.648) [diencephalic infarct]
Calabrese et al. (1996)	"Emotional flattening is a frequent concomitant in patients with retrograde amnesia, both of organic and psychogenic origin" (p.309) [encephalitis]
Kessler et al. (1997)	"During the interviews [with a psychiatrist], his retreat from social bonds was reflected by his keeping a certain distance, only occasionally entering into a more warm and emotional conversation" (p.609) [functional amnesia]
Markowitsch et al. (1997b)	"... he repeatedly mentioned that life events were apparently of much less importance to him than to his wife and children" (p.152) [psychogenic fugue]
Kroll et al. (1977)	"His memories seem 'flat' " (p.1380) [traumatic organic retrograde amnesia]

Examples of case descriptions of patients with organic or functional amnesia indicating emotional flattening.

autobiographical-emotional information (Davidson & Sutton, 1995; Fink et al., 1996; Shin et al., 1997).

Of special interest is to what degree stress-evoking events block the recall of old episodic information, or to what degree stress-related events have a higher chance than neutral to be blocked from recall (or ecphory) (Cacioppo, 1994). The multiple nature of stress makes a concise definition impossible. Selye (1956) pointed to the subjectivity in the treatment of stimuli within and between individuals: what is stressful for one person on one occasion may not be so on another. Similarly, what one person considers stressful, another needs not. Furthermore, the consequences of stress may differ over time: in the short term, stress may induce positive, adaptive changes; in the long-term, it may become maladaptive. There exist physical, psychic, and social stressors (stress-evoking agents). The most widely accepted definition of stress relies on a person's response and takes the activation of the pituitary-adrenal axis as measure of stress (Akil et al., 1999; Dunn, 1987).

Southwick, Morgan, Nicolaou, and Charney (1997) found distortions and omission of trauma-related events in soldiers from the Kuwait war, and Sutker, Winstead, Galina, and Allain (1991) reported cognitive deficits in prisoners of war and participants in the Korean war. Possible neural mechanisms may lie in the release of stress-related hormones (glucocorticoids) which are especially active in the anterior temporal lobe region (Lupien & McEwen, 1997; McGaugh, Cahill, & Roozendaal, 1996; Roozendaal, Portillo Marquez, & McGaugh, 1996). Furthermore, direct changes in the brain's norepinephrine level (Southwick et al., 1993) and an increased action of GABA-agonists are postulated. Our own findings demonstrate that reactive stress can block the action of multiple brain regions (Markowitsch et al., 1998).

Cases with Functional Amnesia

Table 2 lists case descriptions of others on patients with functional amnesia as defined by De Renzi et al. (1997). Although it is unjustified to generalise from a sample of 10 patients, there are nevertheless certain remarkable features among these individuals. All but one were 38 years or younger (median and mode: 20 years), eight had minor accidents which immediately induced their amnesic condition, and all showed an unexpected discrepancy between the severity of their amnesia and the failure to detect any brain injury with static neuroimaging methods. Dynamic imaging techniques (SPECT, PET) revealed changes in brain metabolism for three patients. All patients showed a clear dissociation between their largely preserved anterograde memory abilities and their profound retrograde amnesia, which nevertheless was usually restricted to the autobiographical domain. Although the possibility of malingering was addressed in all reports, the overall conclusion was that pure malingering could be excluded or was very unlikely. (A thoughtful discussion of the topic of malingering in such patients is made in Barbarotto, Laiacona, & Cocchini, 1996.)

Together, these reports underline the necessity to question the dichotomy between organic and psychogenic amnesia and indicate that even minor traumatic conditions can induce lasting amnesia.

In the following, our own cases manifesting retrograde or anterograde amnesia or a combination of both will be described. Table 3 gives a summary of the described cases. Plate 2 illustrates the overall similarity in metabolic brain changes in cases with amnesia of a probable organic and probable psychogenic basis.

Case AA (J. Kessler et al., 1997). A 29-year-old student developed within a month a complete inability to form lasting new episodic memories while his intelligence, his retrograde memory ability, and his short-term memory remained preserved. In spite of major attempts to find a brain correlate for his amnesia, this could not be established: Doppler-sonography, magnetic resonance imaging, $2(^{18}F)$-fluorodeoxyglucose (FDG) positron-emission-tomography and electrophysiological recordings (EEG, evoked potentials) all remained within

TABLE 2

Cases with Functional Amnesia Described by Others

Study	Patient Characteristics	Trauma condition	Brain Damage	Follow-up	Type of Amnesia
Barbarotto et al. (1996) (case PA)	38-year-old woman	Slipped and fell in her office	CT: normal	$^{1}/_{2}$ year	Pure RA
Dalla Barba et al. (1997) (case RM)	17-year-old girl	?	EEG, CT, MRI, FDG-PET: all normal	~ 1 year	Pure RA
De Renzi and Lucchelli (1993) (case PI)	26-year-old man	Fell from a tractor	MRI normal PET: hypometabolism of posterior temporal lobes	2 years	Pure RA, abnormally fast forgetting
De Renzi et al. (1995) (case MA)	19-year-man	Car accident without apparent brain damage	CT, MRI normal	29 months	Pure RA
De Renzi et al. (1997) (case Andrea)	59-year-old man	Car accident	CT, MRI, SPECT: all normal	4 years	Pure RA
Stracciari et al. (1994) (case ML)	20-year-old man	Road accident	EEG, MRI normal, SPECT showed hypoperfusion on the left frontal region	1 year	Autobiographical RA
(case DR)	20-year-old man	Car accident	Closed head trauma EEG, CT: normal; SPECT: modest left parietal abnormalities; PET: no definite abnormalities		Autobiographical RA
Lucchelli et al. (1998) (case CDA)	20-year-old man	Falling or fight	CT, MRI, EEG: all normal	11 months	Pure RA with recovery over time
(case GC)	38-year-old man	Fugue	CT, MRI, SPECT, EEG: all normal	?	Pure RA with recovery over time
(case AF)	15-year-old boy	Minor head bumping	CT, EEG: normal	1 month	Pure RA with recovery over time

EEG, electroencephalography; CT, computed tomography; MRI, magnetic resonance tomography; FDG-PET, 2(^{18}F)-fluorodeoxyglucose positron-emission-tomography; RA, retrograde amnesia; SPECT, single photon emission computed tomography.

569

TABLE 3
Cases with Functional Amnesia Described by Our Research Group

Study	Patient Characteristics	Trauma Condition	Brain Damage	Follow-up	Type of Amnesia
J. Kessler et al. (1997) (case AA)	29-years-old	?	EEG, MRI, FDG-PET all normal	1 year	AA
Markowitsch et al. (1997b) (case NN)	37-years-old	Personality problems since childhood	EEG, MRI normal; ^{15}O-PET shows abnormal autobiographical memory processing	1 year	Episodic RA
Markowitsch et al. (1998) (case AMN)	23-years-old	Singular childhood trauma and related trauma at present	EEG, MRI normal, FDG-PET drastically reduced in memory processing regions	1 year	Episodic AA, episodic RA for the last 6 years
Markowitsch et al. (1999a) (case FA)	46-years-old	Stressful life situations throughout his life	EEG, MRI, FDG-PET normal	~ 1 year	Episodic AA, reduced STM
Markowitsch et al. (1997a) (case BT)	30-years-old	Probably stressful life situations since childhood	CT, MRI normal, past meningitis?, SPECT: right temporo-frontal hypometabolism, ^{15}O-PET: abnormal processing of learned information	~ 1 year	Episodic RA
Markowitsch et al. (1997c) (case DO)	59-years-old	Probable multiply sexually abused as child	MRI normal, ^{15}O-PET: temporopolar activation during ephory of affective memories	~ 3 years	Selective RA for life period 10–16 years of age
Markowitsch et al. (1999b) (case TA)	30-years-old	Trauma due to whiplash injury (about $3^{1}/_{2}$ years prior to the present examination)	MRI, FDG-PET, EEG, EPs normal	~ 6 months	Severe AA for time periods beyond 1 hour; severe RA for events from about the last $3^{1}/_{2}$ years

EPs, evoked potentials; EEG, electroencephalography; CT, computed tomography; MRI, magnetic resonance tomography; FDG-PET, $2(^{18}$F)-fluorodeoxyglucose positron-emission-tomography; SPECT, single photon emission computed tomography; RA, retrograde amnesia; AA, anterograde amnesia; STM, short-term memory.

the normal range. The condition was followed up for more than a year and remained unchanged within this time period. We assumed that a complex chain of interacting variables produced the syndrome which appeared phenomenologically as anterograde amnesia. A grossly reduced drive to consolidate or ecphorise memories was probably a major determinant of his deficit.

Case NN (Markowitsch et al., 1997b). The patient came to our attention because of a persistent retrograde amnesia after a fugue condition. He rode his bicycle for several days along the river Rhine without knowing who he was or why he did it. This condition remained unchanged for more than one year. NN had had a poor childhood. His mother would have preferred a daughter and put him into female clothes for the first five years of his life. Later she frequently told him that he would ruin their restaurant and would be unable to lead a successful life. He had spontaneously "escaped" from his life situation before the present fugue (by driving e.g. 700 kilometres away from home), but had not lost his identity during those occasions. The patient was of above average intelligence and had good anterograde memory abilities. After the fugue, he changed his life habits and manifested other somatic changes (e.g. he gained 15kg of body weight within a short time, lost his allergy and asthma, changed his profession and no longer wanted to drive or ride in cars because of their speed).

NN did not reveal any brain abnormalities under (static) magnetic resonance imaging or when recording EEGs. However, a ^{15}O-positron-emission-tomographic activation study, during which his brain activity was compared during imagery of sentences containing autobiographical events and containing biographic events from somebody else, revealed that he processed both kinds of information in a similar way and different from normals (Fink et al., 1996).

Case AMN (Markowitsch et al., 1998). A 23-year-old patient had major and persistent anterograde amnesia and six years of retrograde amnesia after a shock experience. The patient saw the outbreak of a fire in his house and the next morning he was severely disturbed and amnesic. This condition remained unchanged for about eight months and manifested as severe verbal and nonverbal amnesia in both anterograde and retrograde directions. Four weeks after the shock condition, the patient could report that he had seen a man burning to death in his car when he was 4 years old. As he mentioned further, since then fire meant a life-threatening situation to him. Apparently, the new fire situation had resulted in a sudden and major release of stress hormones (glucocorticoids) leading to a block of the normal mnestic information flow. After about 8 months AMN somewhat improved cognitively, but even after 12 months he was severely disturbed especially with respect to long-term memory. His FDG-PET had returned to normal glucose scores for subjects of his age and sex; his mnestic condition, however, did not allow him to return to work (Markowitsch et al., submitted).

Case FA (Markowitsch et al., 1999a). A 46-year-old independent engineer had apparently lost his ability to acquire new episodic information long term. Furthermore, he had a drastically reduced short-term memory, disturbances in old memories, acalculia, and word-finding difficulties. Otherwise, his intellectual capacity was in the normal range (that is he was not pseudo-demented, for example). Neither neuromonitoring nor static or dynamic neuroimaging methods demonstrated any brain abnormality. The patient was diagnosed as depressive. However, various forms of drug treatment and psychotherapy—given over a period of altogether more than a year—failed to improve his condition. The patient's personal history indicated that he had had a complicated stressful life from childhood to the present.

Case BT (Markowitsch et al., 1997a). A 30-year-old male patient complained of having lost his personal memory for his total life time. The patient otherwise had normal intelligence and normal anterograde memory abilities. His retrograde semantic memory (''world knowledge'') was within the normal range as well. He did not regain access to his autobiography over several months of follow-up. BT behaved cooperatively in neuropsychological tests. Initial computer tomography and magnetic resonance imaging revealed no brain damage. Investigation of his cerebrospinal fluid showed a slightly elevated cell count which was interpreted as a possible past meningitis. Under single photon emission computed tomography (SPECT), there was a reduction in cerebral blood flow in the anterior temporal and infero-lateral prefrontal cortex of the right hemisphere, corresponding to that seen in a patient with massive and selective retrograde amnesia due to encephalitis (Calabrese et al., 1996) (see Plate 2). Measurements of regional cerebral blood flow with PET during episodic memory retrieval revealed a pattern of activated brain structures which differed in several of the regions with enhanced or decreased blood flow from that seen in normal subjects exposed to the same experimental design (Tulving et al., 1994b). It was concluded that BT represented a case of probable psychogenic amnesia.

Case TA (Markowitsch, Kessler, Kalbe, & Herholz, 1999b). TA was a 30-year-old right-handed former university student who had led an active life with multiple interests. Three and a half years prior to the present examination she was involved in a car accident, with another individual driving into her car. The accident provoked a whiplash injury and hearing disturbances, but no skull damage. Since this accident TA had severe and persisting anterograde amnesia which, however, occurred only after about $\frac{1}{2}$ to 2 hours after information acquisition. She was disoriented with respect to time and had to learn about her situation every morning anew. Multiple CT and MRI scans remained negative. EEG was normal, showing a 10Hz alpha EEG with vigilance changes, no signs of general or focal changes, and no hypersynchronous potentials. An FDG-PET performed $3^1/_2$ years after the injury was insignificant as well compared to age and sex matched normals.

TA performed neuropsychological tests slowly but with high concentration. She gained high scores for intelligence and anterograde memory. In the revised Wechsler Memory Scale she obtained the highest possible General Memory Index for a subject of her age. In spite of this, she could not recall any acquired information after periods of more than one or two hours. Her retrograde semantic and episodic memories were excellent until the time of the injury. Thereafter they were practically zero. For instance she remembered events that had happened half a year prior to her injury, but not events that had happened two or three months thereafter.

General remarks on these cases. Again, as stated for the cases in Table 2, the existence of tendencies to malinger are difficult to exclude, especially in patients of high intelligence. Nevertheless—as for the cases in Tables 2 and 3—there was usually little evidence from the outcome of the test examinations performed. Possible influences of malingering on the test results were nevertheless discussed.

Interestingly, only patients who had retrograde amnesia (or both retrograde and anterograde amnesia) manifested metabolic brain changes. It is, however, still premature to conclude from this observation that functional retrograde amnesia involved different brain mechanisms (e.g. biochemical changes) than functional anterograde amnesia. Retrograde memory processing most likely engages more compact cortical regions (Kroll et al., 1997; Markowitsch, 1995b) (which are more easily reflected by functional imaging deviations), while anterograde memory processing relies on wide-spanned limbic networks (Markowitsch, in press).

Only future research can determine why the retrograde (compared to the anterograde) memory domain seems to be affected to a higher degree in functional amnesia (cf. Tables 2 and 3), whether the underlying mechanisms are principally similar, and whether the individual manifestation of one form or the other (or of varying degrees of both forms) can be related to the patients' past experience or to their future perspective.

STRESS-RELATED CHANGES IN THE BRAIN, LEADING TO A MNESTIC BLOCK SYNDROME

Taken together, these cases indicate that there are similarities between amnesic patients with a manifest organic basis and those lacking such a basis (Markowitsch, 1996). Under both conditions (organic amnesia, psychic amnesia) emotional changes such an indifference towards one's own condition and a reduced affect in general are not uncommon (cf. Table 1). Most interestingly, our results obtained with dynamic imaging techniques indicate that affective mnestic processing is accompanied by a right hemispheric temporo-frontal activation (Fink et al., 1996; Markowitsch, 1997a; Markowitsch et al., 1997c), whereas vice versa a reduced affective state and retrograde amnesia for autobiographic events are followed by a reduced right hemispheric temporo-frontal activation (Markowitsch et al., 1997a, b). This reduced affective condition can be observed both in patients with a manifest neural basis for their amnesia (Markowitsch et al., 1993a; Markowitsch & Ewald, 1997), and in patients with a psychogenic diagnosis for their amnesia (cf. Tables 2 and 3). Interestingly, Iidaka and co-workers (1997) similarly found with dynamic imaging a reduced right-hemispheric temporo-frontal activation in patients with mood disorders. Recently, Bicik et al. (1998) demonstrated that in patients with late whiplash injury (of which Case TA, described earlier, is an example) frontopolar and lateral temporal regions may show decreased FDG uptake. However, the authors had to conclude from their data that FDG PET does not allow a reliable diagnosis of metabolic disturbances for individual patients and should not be recommended for routine examinations of late whiplash syndrome patients. Again, Case TA seems to confirm this recommendation. Alexander (1998), furthermore, pointed to possible relations between mild traumatic brain injury and mood disorders in patients after whiplash injury.

Patients with functional amnesia manifest as their principal syndrome a disproportionally heavy amnesic condition, but may show other cognitive deviations as well (Barbarotto et al., 1996; De Renzi, Luccelli, Muggia, & Spinnler, 1995; De Renzi et al., 1997; J. Kessler et al., 1997; Markowitsch, 1995b; Markowitsch et al., 1998; Mattioli et al., 1996). In some cases, psychiatric symptoms may be manifest which are a further correlate for the usually rapidly occurring cognitive defects. As an example, a patient with massive anterograde and retrograde amnesia had had a major depression since his early adulthood which had been (unsuccessfully) treated with drugs and electroconvulsive therapy. Four of his relatives, including his mother, had committed suicide due to depressive conditions (Markowitsch, 1997b). This patient had shown a symmetrical degeneration of his medial temporal lobe region, whose etiology was obscure. It can be speculated that his brain damage had a relation to his depression and amnesia. Recently, Gurvits et al. (1996) reported a significant reduction (up to 25%)—compared to control subjects—in the hippocampal volumes of combat veterans who had been subjected to life-threatening and consequently quite stressful situations. Most likely these reductions are due to a shrunken hippocampal neuropil (Magariños, McEwen, Flügge, & Fuchs, 1996; Magariños, Verdugo, & McEwen, 1997).

There are a number of studies which demonstrate that massive stress conditions increase the release of glucocorticoids to such a degree that they finally change the neuronal metabolism (Bremner, Krystal, Southwick, & Charney, 1995a; Bremner et al., 1993, 1995b, c, 1997a, b; Sapolsky, 1994, 1996a, b; Sapolsky, Uno, Rebert, & Finch, 1990). As a consequence, neural tissue degenerations, especially in regions with a high glucocorticoid receptor density—the anterior temporal lobe with amygdaloid complex and hippocampal formation—may occur (Haas & Schauenstein, 1997; Joëls & de Kloet, 1992; Lupien & McEwen, 1997; Majewska, 1992; O'Brien, 1997; Vidal, Jordan, & Zieglgänsberger, 1986).

Effects of massive stress conditions on cognitive performance and brain function have been frequently documented (aside from the work of Bremner and of Sapolsky and their co-workers the following examples may be listed: Barrett et al., 1996; Carlier, Lamberts, Fouwels, & Gersons, 1996; Elder, Shanahan, & Clipp, 1997; King, 1997; Layton & Wardi-Zonna, 1995; Skodol et al., 1996; van der Kolk, 1994). The reductions in cognitive performance were attributed to reduced capacities in information-processing and information-evaluating neuronal nets (Brewin, Dagleish, & Joseph, 1996; Layton & Wardi-Zonna, 1995; Markowitsch, 1996; Pitman, 1988).

A number of reports propose that a predisposition for the development of stress-related cognitive changes in adulthood is enforced by mechanisms present in childhood (Aldenhoff, 1997; Kuyken & Brewin, 1995; Liotti, 1992; Parks & Balon, 1995; Schacter, Koutstall, & Norman, 1996; Teicher, Glod, Surrey, & Swett, 1993). Teicher et al. (1993), for instance, showed highly significantly that early physical or sexual abuse hinders the development of the limbic system. The case history of our patient AMN who had seen the outbreak of a fire as an adult and had seen a person burning to death at age 4 is another example (Markowitsch et al., 1998).

The central importance of the hypothalamic-hypophyseal-adrenocortical axis (Herman & Cullinan, 1997; Holsboer, 1989) has been repeatedly emphasised for these mechanisms, and ineffective coping strategies (Heim, 1988) may foster the outbreak of the illness. (Stress conditions have even been proposed to be related to the manifestation of Creutzfeldt-Jakob-disease: Brandel & Delasnerie-Laupretre, 1997.)

Depressive conditions are also known to change the glucocorticoid feedback on the brain level (Young et al., 1991) with the consequence of changes in the cellular immune response (Dorian & Garfinkel, 1989; Herbert & Cohen, 1993; O'Leary 1990). The intimate relation between changes in biochemical brain processes leading to behavioural alterations, particularly depression, was emphasised by McAllister-Williams, Ferrier, and Young (1998) as well as by Aldenhoff (1997). Similarly, severe memory disturbances have been linked to the excessive and prolonged release of glucocorticoids in patients without a clear organic base for amnesia (Markowitsch et al., 1999a; Sapolsky, 1996). It is assumed that prolonged glucosteroid release (as in chronic stress conditions or depression) may alter neuronal functioning in the memory-processing bottleneck structures of the medial temporal lobe, and will eventually result in exhaustion-related neuronal degeneration (O'Brien, 1997; Vidal et al., 1986). Both the reduced hippocampal volumes in combat-veterans (Bremner et al., 1995b) and the grossly reduced metabolism in these (plus medial diencephalic) regions found in a patient suffering from massive psychic shock (Markowitsch et al., 1998), strongly favour such a model which is also supported by the results of animal experiments (de Quervain, Roozendaal, & McGaugh, 1998; Diamond & Rose, 1994; Kaufer, Friedman, Seldman, & Soreq, 1998; Xu, Anwyl, & Rowan, 1997). Kaufer et al. (1998) demonstrated the modulation of genes that regulate acetylcholine after stress and the blockade of acetylcholinesterase. They suggested that robust cholinergic stimulation may trigger the rapid induction of the gene encoding the transcription factor c-Fos. C-Fos then might mediate selective regulatory effects on the long-lasting activities of genes involved in acetylcholine metabolism.

Presently results from a considerable number of studies indicate a close association between stress and depression, and show a heightened risk for post traumatic stress disorder patients to develop depression (Breslau, Davis, Peterson, & Schultz, 1997; Fawzi et al., 1997; R.C. Kessler, 1997; Peck, Robertson & Zeffert, 1996; Silove et al., 1997). The findings from patients with minor brain injury and amnesia, given in Tables 2 and 3, and the discussion of such relations in patients with late whiplash injury (Alexander, 1998; Bicik et al., 1998) underline what might be named the development of a "somato-psychic" illness (Alexander, 1998; Radanov, Di Stefano, Schnidrig, & Sturzenegger, 1994).

The Mnestic Block Syndrome

It is commonplace to say that memory disturbances that lead to a general (or selective) inability to encode or recall (ecphorise) information are determined by a corresponding brain activity. For a number of cases, specific brain damage can be traced as cause, although both the selectivity of disturbances (e.g. confined to episodic memories) and their generality (e.g. the total autobiographical old memories across the whole past life) are astonishing and question a complete "organic" attribution (Markowitsch, 1996). For other cases, evidence for an "organicity" is obtained only indirectly or even not at all. Nevertheless, a changed brain metabolism is also assumed to be the cause for the memory block. To what degree this changed metabolism is the consequence of inner body conditions or is induced by the environment (and may then later manifest itself independent of environmental conditions) has been recognised only very rudimentarily up to now. It can, however, be assumed that there are more cases with a "mnestic block syndrome" (Markowitsch et al., 1999a, b) than described up to now. This mnestic block syndrome can be visualised as a kind of disconnection which undermines the access to the engrams or storage places. As long as there are no clearer or more straightforward possibilities to explain the multitude of suddenly occurring and globally acting amnesias without manifest brain tissue damage, the assumption of a mnestic block condition can be taken as a preliminary model to attack the multitude of manifestations of functional amnesia.

The term ''mnestic block syndrome'' is introduced here as a label that is devoid of associations coupled to subforms such as hysterical amnesia. The term ''mnestic block syndrome'' is intended to bridge the former division into ''organic'' and ''psychogenic'' memory disorders (Kisely, Goldberg, & Simon, 1997; Markowitsch, 1996; White & Moorey, 1997). It makes no implicit assumptions on underlying psychiatric illnesses, such as depression. In fact, there may be profound differences in the cognitive patterns of patients with depressive disorders and patients with mnestic block syndrome: Patient FA, described earlier, for example, with a combination of severe memory impairments accompanied by a general slowing of psychic and psychomotor functions, demonstrated above-average reasoning levels (IQ = 118) and unimpaired visuo-constructive abilities, a highly unusual configuration of deficits, which deviated considerably from that of groups of patients with depression, or Alzheimer's disease, and (of course) from normal controls (Markowitsch et al., 1999a).

REFERENCES

Akil, H., Campeau, S., Cullinan, W.E., Lechan, R.M., Toni, R., Watson, S.J., & Moore, R.Y. (1999). Neuroendocrine systems I: Overview—thyroid and adrenal axes. In M. J. Zigmond, F.E. Bloom, S.C. Landis, J.L. Roberts, & L.R. Squire (Eds.), *Fundamental neuroscience* (pp. 1127–1150). San Diego: Academic Press.

Aldenhoff, J. (1997). Überlegungen zur Psychobiologie der Depression. *Nervenarzt, 68*, 379–389.

Alexander, M.P. (1998). In the pursuit of proof of brain damage after whiplash injury. *Neurology, 51*, 336–340.

Barbarotto, R., Laiacona, M., & Cocchini, G. (1996). A case of simulated, psychogenic or focal pure retrograde amnesia: Did an entire life become unconscious? *Neuropsychologia, 34*, 575–585.

Barrett, D.H., Green, M.L., Morris, R., Giles, W.H., & Croft, J.B. (1996). Cognitive functioning and posttraumatic stress disorder. *American Journal of Psychiatry, 153*, 1492–1494.

Bicik, I., Radanov, B.P., Schäfer, N., Dvorak, J., Blum, B., Weber, B., Burger, C., von Schulthess, G.K., & Buck, A. (1998). PET with [18]fluorodeoxyglucose and hexamethylpropylene amine oxime SPECT in late whiplash syndrome. *Neurology, 51*, 345–350.

Brandel, J.-P., & Delasnerie-Laupretre, N. (1997). Creutzfeldt-Jakob disease and stress. *Journal of Neurology, Neurosurgery, and Psychiatry, 62*, 541–548.

Bremner, J.D., Innis, R.B., Ng, C.K., Staib, L.H., Salomon, R.M., Bronen, R.A., Duncan, J., Southwick, S.M., Krystal, J.H., Rich, D., Zubal, G., Dey, H., Soufer, R., & Charney, D.S. (1997a). Positron emission tomography measurement of cerebral metabolic correlates of yohimbine administration in combat-related posttraumatic stress disorder. *Archives of General Psychiatry, 54*, 246–254.

Bremner, J.D., Krystal, J.H., Southwick, S.M., & Charney, D.S. (1995a). Functional neuroanatomical correlates of the effects of stress on memory. *Journal of Traumatic Stress, 8*, 527–553.

Bremner, J.D., Randall, P., Scott, T.M., Bronen, R.A., Seibyl, J.P., Southwick, S.M., Delaney, R.C., McCarthy, G., Charney, D.S., & Innis, R.B. (1995b). MRI-based measurement of hippocampal volume in patients with combat-related posttraumatic stress disorder. *American Journal of Psychiatry, 152*, 973–981.

Bremner, J.D., Randall, P., Scott, T.M., Capelli, S., Delaney, R., McCarthy, G., & Charney, D.S. (1995c). Deficits in short-term memory in adult survivors of childhood abuse. *Psychiatry Research, 59*, 97–107.

Bremner, J.D., Randall, P., Vermetten, E., Staib, L., Bronen, R.A., Mazure, C., Capelli, S., McCarthy, G., Innis, R.B., & Charney, D.S. (1997b). Magnetic resonance imaging-based measurement of hippocampal volume in posttraumatic stress disorder related to childhood physical and sexual abuse—a preliminary report. *Biological Psychiatry, 41*, 23–2.

Bremner, J.D., Scott, T.M., Delaney, R.C., Southwick, S.M., Mason, J.W., Johnson, D.R., Innis, R.B., McCarthy, G., & Charney, D.S. (1993). Deficits in short-term memory in posttraumatic stress disorder. *American Journal of Psychiatry, 150*, 1015–1019.

Breslau, N., Davis, G.C., Peterson, E.L., & Schultz, L. (1997). Psychiatric sequelae of posttraumatic stress disorder in women. *Archives of General Psychiatry, 54*, 81–87.

Breuer, J., & Freud, S. (1895). *Studien über Hysterie.* Wien: Deuticke.

Brewin, C.R., Dalgleish, T., & Joseph, S. (1996). A dual representation theory of posttraumatic stress disorder. *Psychological Review, 103*, 670–686.

Cacioppo, J.T. (1994). Social neuroscience: Autonomic, neuroendocrine, and immune responses to stress. *Psychophysiology, 31*, 113–128.

Cahill, L., Babinsky, R., Markowitsch, H.J., & McGaugh, J.L. (1995). Involvement of the amygdaloid complex in emotional memory. *Nature, 377*, 295–296.

Calabrese, P., Markowitsch, H.J., Durwen, H.F., Widlitzek, B., Haupts, M., Holinka, B., & Gehlen, W. (1996). Right temporofrontal cortex as critical locus for the ecphory of old episodic memories. *Journal of Neurology, Neurosurgery, and Psychiatry, 61*, 304–310.

Carlier, I.V.E., Lamberts, R.D., Fouwels, A.J., & Gersons, B.P.R. (1996). PTSD in relation to dissociation in traumatized police officers. *American Journal of Psychiatry, 153*, 1325–1328.

Chow, K.L. (1967). Effects of ablation. In G.C. Quarton, T. Melnechuk, F.O. Schmitt (Eds.), *The neurosciences* (pp. 705–713). New York: Rockefeller University Press.

Cicerone, K.D., & Tanenbaum, L.N. (1997). Disturbance of social cognition after traumatic orbitofrontal brain injury. *Archives of Clinical Neuropsychology, 12*, 173–188.

Dalla Barba, G., Mantovan, M.C., Ferruzza, E., & Denes, G. (1997). Remembering and knowing the past: A case study of isolated retrograde amnesia. *Cortex, 33*, 143–154.

Damasio, A.R. (1994). *Descartes' error. Emotion, reason and the human brain.* New York: Putnam's Son.

Damasio, A.R., Tranel, D., & Damasio, H. (1990). Individuals with sociopathic behavior caused by frontal damage fail to respond autonomically to social stimuli. *Behavioural Brain Research, 41*, 81–94.

Davidson, R.J., & Sutton, S.K. (1995). Affective neuroscience: The emergence of a discipline. *Current Opinion in Neurobiology, 6,* 217–224.

de Quervain, D.J.-F., Roozendaal, B., & McGaugh, J.L. (1998). Stress and glucocorticoids impair retrieval of long-term spatial memory. *Nature, 394*, 787–790.

De Renzi, E., & Lucchelli, F. (1993). Dense retrograde amnesia, intact learning capability and abnormal forgetting rate: A consolidation deficit? *Cortex, 29*, 449–466.

De Renzi, E., Lucchelli, F., Muggia, S., & Spinnler, H. (1995). Persistent retrograde amnesia following a minor head trauma. *Cortex, 31*, 531–542.

De Renzi, E., Lucchelli, F., Muggia, S., & Spinnler, H. (1997). Is memory without anatomical damage tantamount to a psychogenic deficit? The case of pure retrograde amnesia. *Neuropsychologia, 35*, 781–794.

Diamond, D.M., & Rose, G.M. (1994). Stress impairs LTP and hippocampal-dependent memory. *Annals of the New York Academy of Sciences, 746*, 411–414.

Dorian, B., & Garfinkel, P.E. (1989). Stress, immunity and illness—a review. *Psychological Medicine, 17*, 393–407.

Dunn, A.J. (1987). Neurochemistry of stress. In G. Adelman (Ed.), *Encyclopedia of neuroscience* (pp. 1146–1148). Boston: Birkhäuser.

Elder, G.H, Shanahan, M.J., & Clipp, E.C. (1997). Linking combat and physical health: The legacy of World War II in men's lives. *American Journal of Psychiatry, 154,* 330–336.

Fawzi, M.C.S., Murphy, E., Pham, T., Lin, L., Poole, C., & Mollica, R.F. (1997). The validity of screening for post-traumatic stress disorder and major depression among Vietnamese former political prisoners. *Acta Psychiatrica Scandinavica, 95,* 87–93.

Fink, G.R., & Markowitsch, H.J. (in press). Hirntraumata. In H. Förstl (Ed.), *Klinische Neuro-Psychiatrie: Hirnerkrankungen und psychische Störungen.* Stuttgart: F. EnkeVerlag.

Fink, G.R., Markowitsch, H.J., Reinkemeier, M., Bruckbauer, T., Kessler, J., & Heiss, W.-D. (1996). Cerebral representation of one's own past: neural networks involved in autobiographical memory. *Journal of Neuroscience, 16,* 4275–4282.

Fletcher, P.C., Frith, C.D., & Rugg, M.D. (1997). The functional neuroanatomy of episodic memory. *Trends in Neurosciences, 20,* 213–218.

Franzen, E.A., & Myers, R.E. (1973). Neural control of socical behavior: Prefrontal and anterior temporal cortex. *Neuropsychologia, 11,* 141–157.

Freud, S. (1901). Zur Psychopathologie des Alltagslebens (Vergessen, Versprechen, Vergreifen) nebst Bemerkungen über eine Wurzel des Aberglaubens. *Monatsschrift für Psychiatrie und Neurologie, 10,* 95–143.

Fuster, J.M. (1997a). Network memory. *Trends in Neurosciences, 20,* 451–459.

Fuster, J.M. (1997b). *The prefrontal cortex* (3rd Edn.). Philadelphia, PA: Lippincott-Raven.

Gurvits, T.V., Shenton, M.E., Hokama, H., Ohta, H., Lasko, N.B., Gilbertson, M.W., Orr, S.P., Kikinis, R., Jolesz, F.A., McCarley, R.W., & Pitman, R.K. (1996). Magnetic resonance imanging study of hippocampal volume in chronic, combat-related posttraumatic stress disorder. *Biological Psychiatry, 40,* 1091–1099.

Haas, H.S., & Schauenstein, K. (1997). Neuroimmunomodulation via limbic structures—The neuroanatomy of psychoimmunology. *Progress in Neurobiology, 51,* 195–222.

Harrington, C., Salloway, S., & Malloy, P. (1997). Dramatic neurobehavioral disorder in two cases following bilateral anteromedial frontal lobe injury: Delayed psychosis and marked change in personality. *Neurocase, 3,* 137–149.

Härtl, J. (1916). Fehlende Erinnerung des Verletzten für einen Schädelschuss. Verkannter Mordversuch. *Deutsche Medizinische Wochenschrift, 42,* 1352–1353.

Heim, E. (1988). Coping und Adaptivität: Gibt es geeignetes oder ungeeignetes Coping? *Psychotherapie und medizinische Psycholologie; 38,* 8-18.

Herbert, T. B., & Cohen, S. (1993). Depression and immunity: A meta-analytic review. *Psychological Bulletin, 113,* 472–486.

Herman, J.P., & Cullinan, W.E. (1997). Neurocircuitry of stress: central control of the hypothalamo-pituitary-adrenocortical axis. *Trends in Neurosciences, 20,* 78–84.

Holsboer, F. (1989). Psychiatric implications of altered limbic-hypothalamic-pituitary-adrenocortical activity. *European Archives of Psychiatry and Neurological Sciences, 238,* 302–322.

Iidaka, T., Nakajima, T., Suzuki, Y., Okazaki, A., Maehara, T., & Shiraishi, H. (1997). Quantitative regional cerebral blood flow measured by Tc-99m HMPAO SPECT in mood disorder. *Psychiatry Research: Neuroimaging Section, 68,* 143–154.

Isaacson, R.L. (1988). Brain lesion studies related to memory: A critique of strategies and interpretations. In H. J. Markowitsch (Ed.), *Information processing by the brain* (pp. 87–105). Toronto: Huber.

Janet P. (1894). *Der Geisteszustand der Hysteriker (Die psychischen Stigmata).* Leipzig: Deuticke.

Jetter, J., Poser, U., Freeman, R.B. Jr., & Markowitsch, H.J. (1986). A verbal long term memory deficit in frontal lobe damaged patients. *Cortex, 22,* 229–242.

Joëls, M., & de Kloet, E.R. (1992). Control of neuronal excitability by corticosteroid hormones. *Trends in Neurosciences, 15,* 25–30.

Kapur, N. (1993). Focal retrograde amnesia in neurological disease: A critical review. *Cortex, 29*, 217–234.

Kapur, N., Ellison, D., Smith, M.P., McLellan, D.L., & Burrows, E.H. (1992). Focal retrograde amnesia following bilateral temporal lobe pathology. *Brain, 115*, 73–85.

Kaufer, D., Friedman, A., Seldman, S., & Soreq, H. (1998). Acute stress facilitates long-lasting changes in cholinergic gene expression. *Nature 393*, 373–377.

Kessler, J., Markowitsch, H.J., Ghaemi, M., Rudolf, J., Weniger, W.D., & Heiss,W.-D. (1999). Degenerative prefrontal damage in a young adult: Static and dynamic imaging and neuropsychological correlates. *Neurocase, 5*, 173–179.

Kessler, J., Markowitsch, H.J., Huber, R., Kalbe, E., Weber-Luxenburger, G., & Kolk, P. (1997). Massive and persistent anterograde amnesia in the absence of detectable brain damage—anterograde psychogenic amnesia or gross reduction in sustained effort? *Journal of Clinical and Experimental Neuropsychology, 19*, 604–614.

Kessler, R.C. (1997). The effects of stressful life events on depression. *Annual Reviews of Psychology, 48*, 191–214.

King, N.S. (1997). Post-traumatic stress disorder and head injury as a dual diagnosis: "Islands" of memory as a mechanism. *Journal of Neurology, Neurosurgery & Psychiatry, 62*, 82–84.

Kisely, S., Goldberg, D., & Simon, G. (1997). A comparison between somatic symptoms with and without clear organic cause: Results of an international study. *Psychological Medicine, 27*, 1011–1019.

Kohnstamm, O. (1917). Über das Krankheitsbild der retro-anterograden Amnesie und die Unterscheidung des spontanen und lernenden Merkens. *Monatsschrift für Psychiatrie und Neurologie, 41*, 373–382.

Kroll, N., Markowitsch, H.J., Knight, R. & von Cramon, D.Y. (1997). Retrieval of old memories—the temporo-frontal hypothesis. *Brain, 120*, 1377–1399.

Kuyken, W., & Brewin, C.R. (1995). Autobiographical memory functioning in depression and reports of early abuse. *Journal of Abnormal Psychology, 104*, 585–591.

Layton, B.S., & Wardi-Zonna, K. (1995). Posttraumatic stress disorder with neurogenic amnesia for the traumatic event. *Clinical Neuropsychologist, 9*, 2–10.

Liotti, G. (1992). Disorganized/disoriented attachment in the etiology of the dissociative disorders. *Dissociation, V*, 196–204.

Lucchelli, F., Muggia, S., & Spinnler, H. (1998). The syndrome of pure retrograde amnesia. *Cognitive Neuropsychiatry, 3*, 91–118.

Lupien, S.J., & McEwen, B.S. (1997). The acute effects of corticosteroids on cognition: Integration of animal and human model studies. *Brain Research Reviews, 24*, 1–27.

Magariños, A.M., McEwen, B.S., Flügge, G., & Fuchs, E. (1996). Chronic psychosocial stress causes apical dendritic atrophy of hippocampal CA3 pyramidal neurons in subordinate tree shrews. *Journal of Neuroscience, 16*, 3534–3540.

Magariños, A.M., Verdugo, J.M.G., & McEwen, B.S. (1997). Chronic stress alters synaptic terminal structure in hippocampus. *Proceedings of the National Academy of Sciences of the USA, 94*, 14002–14008.

Mai, F.M. (1995). "Hysteria" in clinical neurology. *Canadian Journal of Neurological Sciences, 22*, 101–110.

Majewska, M.D. (1992). Neurosteroids: Endogenous bimodal modulators of the GABAA receptor. Mechanism of action and physiological significance. *Progress in Neurobiology, 38*, 379–395.

Markowitsch, H.J. (1988). Anatomical and functional organization of the primate prefrontal cortical system. In H.D. Steklis, & J. Erwin (Eds.), *Comparative primate biology, Vol. IV: Neurosciences* (pp. 99–153). New York: Alan R. Liss.

Markowitsch, H.J. (Ed.). (1990a). *Transient global amnesia and related disorders*. Toronto: Hogrefe & Huber.

Markowitsch, H.J. (1990b). Transient psychogenic amnesic states. In H.J. Markowitsch (Ed.), *Transient global amnesia and related disorders* (pp. 181–190). Toronto: Hogrefe & Huber.

Markowitsch, H.J. (1992). *Intellectual functions and the brain. An historical perspective.* Toronto: Hogrefe & Huber.

Markowitsch, H.J. (1995a). The anatomical basis of memory disorders. In M.S. Gazzaniga (Ed.), *The cognitive neurosciences* (pp. 665–679). Cambridge, MA: MIT Press.

Markowitsch, H.J. (1995b). Which brain regions are critically involved in the retrieval of old episodic memory? *Brain Research Reviews, 21,* 117–127.

Markowitsch, H.J. (1996). Organic and psychogenic retrograde amnesia: Two sides of the same coin? *Neurocase, 2,* 357–371.

Markowitsch, H.J. (1997a). The functional neuroanatomy of episodic memory retrieval. *Trends in Neurosciences, 20,* 557–558.

Markowitsch, H.J. (1997b). Varieties of memory: Systems, structures, mechanisms of disturbance. *Neurology, Psychiatry and Brain Sciences, 5,* 37–56.

Markowitsch, H.J. (in press). Memory and amnesia. In M.-M. Mesulam (Ed.), *Principles of cognitive and behavioral neurology.* Philadelphia, PA: F.A. Davis Comp.

Markowitsch, H.J., & Calabrese, P. (1996). Commonalities and discrepancies in the relationship between behavioural outcome and the results of neuroimaging in brain-damaged patients. *Behavioural Neurology, 9,* 45–55.

Markowitsch, H.J., Calabrese, P., Fink, G.R., Durwen, H.F., Kessler, J., Härting, C., König, M., Mirzaian, E.B., Heiss, W-D., Heuser, L., & Gehlen, W. (1997a). Impaired episodic memory retrieval in a case of probable psychogenic amnesia. *Psychiatry Research: Neuroimaging Section, 74,* 119–126.

Markowitsch, H.J., Calabrese, P., Haupts, M., Durwen, H.F., Liess, J., & Gehlen, W. (1993a). Searching for the anatomical basis of retrograde amnesia. *Journal of Clinical and Experimental Neuropsychology, 15,* 947–967.

Markowitsch, H.J., Calabrese, P., Würker, M. Durwen, H.F., Kessler, J., Babinsky, R., Brechtelsbauer, D., Heuser, L., & Gehlen, W. (1994). The amygdala's contribution to memory—A PET-study on two patients with Urbach-Wiethe disease. *NeuroReport, 5,* 1349–1352.

Markowitsch, H.J., & Ewald, K. (1997). Right-hemispheric fronto-temporal injury leading to severe autobiographical retrograde and moderate anterograde episodic amnesia. *Neurology, Psychiatry and Brain Sciences, 5,* 71–78.

Markowitsch, H.J., Fink, G.R., Thöne, A.I.M., Kessler, J., & Heiss, W.-D. (1997b). Persistent psychogenic amnesia with a PET-proen organic basis. *Cognitive Neuropsychiatry, 2,* 135–158.

Markowitsch, H.J., Kessler, J., Kalbe, E., & Herholz, K. (1999b). Functional amnesia and memory consolidation: A case of severe and persistent anterograde amnesia with rapid forgetting following whiplash injury. *Neurocase, 5,* 189–200.

Markowitsch, H.J., Kessler, J., Russ, M.O., Frölich, L., Schneider, B., & Maurer, K. (1999a). Mnestic block syndrome. *Cortex, 35,* 219–230.

Markowitsch, H.J., Kessler, J., Van der Ven, C., Weber-Luxenburger, G., & Heiss, W.-D. (1998). Psychic trauma causing grossly reduced brain metabolism and cognitive deterioration. *Neuropsychologia, 36,* 77–82.

Markowitsch, H.J., Kessler, J., Van der Ven, C., Weber-Luxenburger, G., & Heiss, W.-D. (submitted). Neuroimaging and behavioral correlates of recovery from 'mnestic block syndrome'.

Markowitsch, H.J., Thiel, A., Kessler, J., & Heiss. W-D. (1997c). Ecphorizing semi-conscious episodic information via the right temporopolar cortex—a PET study. *Neurocase, 3,* 445–449.

Markowitsch, H.J., von Cramon, D.Y., & Schuri, U. (1993b). Mnestic performance profile of a bilateral diencephalic infarct patient with preserved intelligence and severe amnesic disturbances. *Journal of Clinical and Experimental Neuropsychology, 15,* 627–652.

Mattioli, F., Grassi, F., Perani, D., Cappa, S.F., Miozzo, A., & Fazio, F. (1996). Persistent post-traumatic retrograde amnesia: A neuropsychological and (18F)FDG PET study. *Cortex, 32*, 121–129.

Mayes, A.R., Daum, I., Markowitsch, H.J., & Sauter, B. (1997). The relationship between retrograde and anterograde amnesia in patients with typical global amnesia. *Cortex, 33*, 197-217.

McAllister-Williams, R.H., Ferrier, I.N., & Young, A.H. (1998). Mood and neuropsychological function in depression: The role of corticosteroids and serotonin. *Psychological Medicine, 28*, 573–584.

McGaugh, J.L., Cahill, L., & Roozendaal, B. (1996). Involvement of the amygdala in memory storage: Interaction with other brain systems. *Proceedings of the National Academy of Sciences of the USA, 93*, 13508–13514.

Milner, B., Petrides, M., & Smith, M.L. (1985). Frontal lobes and the temporal organization of memory. *Human Neurobiology, 4*, 137–142.

Müller-Suur, H. (1949). Beitrag zur Frage des Korsakow-Syndroms und zur Analyse der amnestisch-strukturellen Demenz. *Archiv für Psychiatrie und Nervenkrankheiten, 181*, 683–711.

O'Brien, J.T. (1997). The 'glucocorticoid cascade' hypothesis in man. *British Journal of Psychiatry, 170*, 199–201.

O'Leary, A. (1990). Stress, emotion, and human immune function. *Psychological Bulletin, 108*, 363–382.

Parks, E.D., & Balon, R. (1995). Autobiographical memory for childhood events: Patterns of recall in psychiatric patients with a history of alleged trauma. *Psychiatry, 58*, 199–208.

Peck, D.F., Robertson, A., & Zeffert, S. (1996). Psychological sequelae of mountain accidents: A preliminary study. *Journal of Psychosomatic Research, 41*, 55–63.

Pitman, R.K. (1988). Post-traumatic stress disorder, conditioning, and network theory. *Psychiatric Annals, 18*, 182–189.

Radanov, B.P., Di Stefano, G., Schnidrig, A., & Sturzenegger, M. (1994). Common whiplash: Psychosomatic or somatopsychic? *Journal of Neurology, Neurosurgery, and Psychiatry, 57*, 486–490.

Raichle, M.E. (1994). Visualizing the mind. *Scientific American, 270*(4), 58–64.

Rempel-Clower, N.L., Zola-Morgan, S., Squire, L.R., Amaral, D.G. (1996). Three cases of enduring memory impairment after bilateral damage limited to the hippocampal formation. *Journal of Neuroscience, 16*, 5233–5255.

Roozendaal, B., Portillo Marquez, G., & McGaugh, J.L. (1996). Basolateral amygdala lesions block glucocorticoid-induced modulation of memory for spatial learning. *Behavioral Neuroscience, 110*, 1074–1083.

Russell, W.R. (1971). *The traumatic amnesias*. Oxford: Oxford University Press.

Sapolsky, R.M. (1994). *Why zebras don't get ulcers*. New York: Freeman.

Sapolsky, R.M. (1996a). Why stress is bad for your brain. *Science, 273*, 749–750.

Sapolsky, R.M. (1996b). Stress, glucocorticoids, and damage to the nervous system: The current state of confusion. *Stress, 1*, 1–19.

Sapolsky, R.M., Uno, H., Rebert, C.S., & Finch, C.E. (1990). Hippocampal damage associated with prolonged glucocorticoid exposure in primates. *Journal of Neuroscience, 10*, 2897–2902.

Schacter, D.L., Koutstaal, W., & Norman, K.A. (1996). Can cognitive neuroscience illuminate the nature of traumatic childhood memories? *Current Opinion in Neurobiology, 6*, 207–214.

Schmidtke, K., & Vollmer, H. (1997). Retrograde amnesia: A study of its relation to anterograde amnesia and semantic memory deficits. *Neuropsychologia, 35*, 505–518.

Selye, H. (1956). *The stress of life*. New York: McGraw-Hill.

Semon, R. (1904). *Die Mneme als erhaltendes Prinzip im Wechsel des organischen Geschehens*. Leipzig: Wilhelm Engelmann.

Shallice, T., Fletcher, P., Frith, C.D., Grasby, P., Frackowiak, R.S.J., & Dolan, R.J. (1994). Brain regions associated with acquisition and retrieval of verbal episodic memory. *Nature, 368*, 633–635.

Shin, L.M., Kosslyn, S.M., McNally, R.J., Alpert, N.M., Thompson, W.L., Rauch, S.L., Macklin, M.L., & Pitman, R.K. (1997). Visual imagery and perception in posttraumatic stress disorder. *Archives of General Psychiatry, 54,* 233–241.

Silove, D., Sinnerbrink, I., Field, A., Manicavasagar, V., & Steel, Z. (1997). Anxiety, depression and PTSD in asylum-seekers: Association with pre-migration trauma and post-migration stressors. *British Journal of Psychiatry, 170,* 351–357.

Skodol, A.E., Schwartz, S., Dohrenwend, B.P., Levav, I., Shrout, P.E., & Reiff, M. (1996). PTSD symptoms and comorbid mental disorders in Israeli war veterans. *British Journal of Psychiatry, 169,* 717–725.

Southwick, S.M., Krystal, J.H., Morgan, C.A., Johnson, D., Nagy, L.M., Nicolaou, A., Heninger, G.R., Charney, D.S. (1993). Abnormal noradrenergic function in posttraumatic stress disorder. *Archives of General Psychiatry, 50,* 266–274.

Southwick, S. M., Morgan A. III, Nicolaou, A.L., & Charney, D.S. (1997). Consistency of memory for combat-related traumatic events in veterans of operation desert storm. *American Journal of Psychiatry, 154,* 173–177.

Starkstein, S.E., Fedoroff, P., Berthier, M.L., & Robinson, R.G. (1991). Manic-depressive and pure manic states after brain lesions. *Biological Psychiatry, 29,* 149–158.

Stracciari, A., Ghidoni, E., Guarino, M., Poletti, M., & Pazzaglia, P. (1994). Post-traumatic retrograde amnesia with selective impairment of autobiographical memory. *Cortex 30,* 459–468.

Stuss, D.T., Alexander, M.P., Palumbo, C.L., Buckle, L., Sayer, L., & Pogue, J. (1994). Organizational strategies of patients with unilateral or bilateral frontal lobe injury in word list learning tasks. *Neuropsychology, 8,* 355–373.

Sutker, P.B., Winstead, D.K., Galina, Z.H., & Allain, A.N. (1991). Cognitive deficits and psychopathology among former prisoners of war and combat veterans of the Korean conflict. *American Journal of Psychiatry, 148,* 67–72.

Teicher, M.H., Glod, C.A., Surrey, J., & Swett, C. (1993). Early childhood abuse and limbic system ratings in adult psychiatric outpatients. *Journal of Neuropsychiatry and Clinical Neurosciences, 5,* 301–306.

Tulving, E. (1983). *Elements of episodic memory.* Oxford: Clarendon Press.

Tulving, E. (1995). Organization of memory: Quo vadis. In M.S. Gazzaniga (Ed.), *The cognitive neurosciences* (pp. 839–847). Cambridge, MA: MIT Press.

Tulving, E., Kapur, S., Craik, F.I., Moscovitch, M., & Houle, S. (1994a). Hemispheric encoding/ retrieval asymmetry in episodic memory: Positron emission tomography findings. *Proceedings of the National Academy of Sciences of the USA, 91,* 2016–2020.

Tulving, E., Kapur, S. Markowitsch, H.J., Craik, G., Habib, R. & Houle, S. (1994b). Neuroanatomical correlates of retrieval in episodic memory. Auditory sentence recognition. *Proceedings of the National Academy of Sciences of the USA, 91,* 2012–2015.

Tulving, E., & Markowitsch, H.J. (1998). Episodic and declarative memory: Role of the hippocampus. *Hippocampus, 8,* 198–204.

Van der Kolk, B.A. (1994). The body keeps the score: Memory and the evolving psychobiology of posttraumatic stress. *Harvard Review of Psychiatry, 1,* 253–265.

Vidal, C., Jordan, W., & Zieglgänsberger, W. (1986). Corticosterone reduces the excitability of hippocampal pyramidal cells in vitro. *Brain Research, 383,* 54–59.

Wechsler, A.F. (1973). The effect of organic brain disease on recall of emotionally charged versus neutral narrative texts. *Neurology, 23,* 130–135.

White, P.D., & Moorey, S. (1997). Psychosomatic illnesses are not "all in the mind". *Journal of Psychosomatic Research, 42,* 329–332.

Xu, L., Anwyl, R., & Rowan, M.J. (1997). Behavioural stress facilitates the induction of long-term depression in the hippocampus. *Nature, 387,* 497–500.

Young, E.A., Haskett, R.F., Murphy-Weinberg, V., Watson, S.J., & Akil, H. (1991). Loss of glucocorticoid fast feedback in depression. *Archives of General Psychiatry, 48,* 693–699.

MEMORY, 1999, 7 (5/6), 585–597

Imaging Episodic Memory:
Implications for Cognitive Theories and Phenomena

Lars Nyberg

Umeå University, Sweden

Functional neuroimaging studies are beginning to identify neuroanatomical correlates of various cognitive functions. This paper presents results relevant to several theories and phenomena of episodic memory, including component processes of episodic retrieval, encoding specificity, inhibition, item versus source memory, encoding–retrieval overlap, and the picture-superiority effect. Overall, by revealing specific activation patterns, the results provide support for existing theoretical views and they add some unique information which may be important to consider in future attempts to develop cognitive theories of episodic memory.

INTRODUCTION

In the present paper, I will discuss functional neuroimaging results that are of relevance to cognitive theories and phenomena of episodic memory. The focus will be on results generated at the PET (positron emission tomography) centre in Toronto, and hence the primary neuroimaging technique that will be considered is PET. PET has been used in humans in many different ways, including measurement of brain blood flow, metabolism of glucose and oxygen, receptor pharmacology, and transmitter metabolism (see Raichle, 1994). Here, the focus will be on using PET to measure brain blood flow in cognitive studies.

In brief, PET measures brain activity by monitoring blood flow changes in the brain that take place while subjects are engaged in some kind of cognitive task. It is standard practice to do multiple PET scans in the same subject, measuring blood flow associated with different cognitive tasks during different scans. By comparing the activation pattern associated with different conditions it

Requests for reprints should be sent to Dr Lars Nyberg, Department of Psychology, University of Umeå, S-901 87 Umeå, Sweden. Email: Lars.Nyberg@psy.umu.se

Several studies discussed in this brief review were done in collaboration with the PET group at the Rotman Research Institute and at the Clarke Institute of Psychiatry in Toronto, Canada. Special thanks to Dr A.R. McIntosh for valuable comments on this paper. I would also like to thank Dr J.K. Foster and two anonymous reviewers for helpful suggestions. LN's work is supported by HSFR, Sweden.

is possible to identify brain regions showing differential response in relation to a specific cognitive challenge. There exist many procedures for assessing differential responses between conditions, and new statistical applications for brain blood flow data are continuously being developed. The results to be reported here were for most part generated by using *statistical parametric mapping* (SPM) developed by Friston and colleagues (e.g. Friston et al., 1995) and a *partial-least-squares* (PLS) application introduced by McIntosh and co-workers (e.g. McIntosh, Bookstein, Haxby, & Crady, 1996). Differential responses may have to do with relative changes in brain activity between conditions. Such responses may also refer to the way brain regions interact with each other within different conditions. Both these types of differential responses will be considered in the present paper.

RETRIEVAL MODE, ECPHORY, AND ENCODING SPECIFICITY

In a study published in 1995 we attempted to identify neural correlates of theoretical component processes of episodic memory retrieval (Nyberg et al., 1995). Following Tulving (1983), we focused on two component processes (or *elements*) of retrieval of episodic memories: namely *retrieval mode* and *ecphory*. Retrieval mode refers to processes generally involved in episodic retrieval, and can be thought of in terms of a "mental set". It is assumed that one will engaged in a retrieval mode when given instruction for a test of episodic memory, and these processes help maintain attention on a particular time and place in the past. Such retrieval processes will be operating regardless of whether or not one actually retrieves stored information. By contrast, ecphory refers to the process when a retrieval cue interacts with memory representations (*engrams*) to give rise to actual recovery of stored information.

In brief, the design of the study was as follows: prior to scanning, subjects were given two incidental encoding tasks. One task fostered shallow processing of study words, whereas the other task involved deeper processing of the items. During subsequent PET scanning, subjects were given three different kinds of yes/no recognition memory tests. All of these tests required the subjects to indicate whether they recognised test words from any of the two study lists. The only difference between the tests had to do with the types of words that were shown during the critical scanning interval: (i) words from the shallow study task, (ii) words from the study task involving deeper processing, and (iii) non-studied words. The brain activation pattern associated with each of these retrieval tasks was compared with that of a reference condition involving silent reading of non-studied words.

We reasoned that in all three retrieval conditions subjects would have to be engaged in a retrieval mode—regardless of how/if they had acquired the information at study and how many words were actually recognised as old. We therefore looked for a common pattern of activation in all three retrieval conditions relative to the reference condition. Furthermore, we reasoned that different brain regions may be related to recovery/ecphory depending on the particular nature of the encoding operations (cf. Squire, Knowlton, & Musen, 1993). To address this issue we compared the activation pattern associated with (a) recognition following shallow processing, and (b) recognition following semantic processing with the pattern associated with recognition judgement of non-studied words.

Starting with retrieval mode, we found that all retrieval tasks activated to a similar extent a common set of brain regions, including a right prefrontal cortical area (peak activity in Brodmann area 45 with the activation extending anteriorly into Brodmann area 10). The consistent pattern of increased activity across retrieval tasks was seen as providing support for the notion that subjects were engaged in a retrieval mode in all conditions (Tulving, (1983). Converging evidence that right prefrontal brain regions subserve a general role in episodic retrieval was provided by another study which manipulated the number of targets across retrieval conditions (Kapur et al., 1995). More generally, the findings of our study, pointing to a role of right prefrontal brain regions in episodic memory retrieval, were in agreement with the results of prior PET studies which had also found evidence for prefrontal involvement in episodic memory retrieval (e.g. Grasby et al., 1993a; Shallice et al., 1994; Squire et al., 1992). With regard to ecphory, striking differences in the activation pattern associated with recognition were observed following more shallow (mainly right hemisphere activations) versus deeper (mainly left hemisphere activations) processing of the materials at study. The strong differences in activation pattern during retrieval depending on type of encoding task were discussed in relation to the *encoding specificity principle* (Tulving & Thomson, 1973). I will return to the issue of encoding-retrieval overlap in activation patterns later.

INHIBITION OF TASK-IRRELEVANT PROCESSING

PET studies provide information not only on regions showing increased levels of activity during the experimental condition relative to the reference condition, but also on regions showing relative *decreased* activity. It has been stressed that decreases in activity may be as crucial for adequate task performance as increased activity (e.g. Buckner & Tulving, 1995). Decreased activity associated with episodic memory retrieval has been reported in several studies (see e.g. Nyberg, 1998), and it has been suggested that such decreases may reflect *inhibition* of irrelevant processes (see e.g. Andreasen et al., 1995; Fletcher et al., 1995). This is in line with proposals that an inhibitory modulation of auditory and superior temporal cortices by the left prefrontal cortex is the basis of word generation (Frith, Friston, Liddle, & Frackowiak, 1991).

In the aforementioned study (Nyberg et al., 1995), in addition to the regions showing increased activity, decreased activity was observed in several regions. In line with prior studies, these regions included bilateral lateral temporal regions. To more formally test the idea that regional decreases in activity may result from inhibitory influences, we analysed the covariance pattern between regions showing relative increased and decreased activity (Nyberg et al., 1996a). This was done by means of structural equation modelling (see McIntosh & Gonzalez-Lima, 1994). We found that the influence of regions showing increased activity, including the right prefrontal region, on regions showing decreased activity was generally more negative during retrieval than during reading. This outcome was seen as supporting the hypothesis that inhibition of task-irrelevant processes during episodic retrieval is critical for successful task performance, and more generally it was argued that looking at the total pattern of brain regions showing differential activation and their mutual influences is essential for understanding the neural basis of human episodic memory.

ITEM AND SOURCE MEMORY

To summarise so far, our analyses indicated that episodic memory, as measured by yes/no word recognition, is generally mediated by a set of brain regions showing increased and decreased activity. This form of episodic memory has been labelled item memory, as a contrast to source memory. Whereas the former type of memory involves remembering of what happened, the latter type emphasises remembering of contextual information such as where or when information was encountered. The observed consistent involvement of (right) frontal brain regions in item memory is particularly interesting in the context of item and source memory. This is because it has been assumed that source memory is especially dependent on the integrity of the frontal lobes (see e.g. Schacter, 1987).

We conducted a PET study in which we compared brain activity patterns associated with retrieval conditions that differentially stressed remembering of item versus source information (Nyberg et al., 1996b). Specifically, in the item memory condition subjects were shown single words one at a time and were asked to try to remember as many words as possible for a subsequent test. The words were presented in two different study lists and they were shown on the left or right side of a computer screen, but subjects were told that they did not have to pay attention to this. At test, subjects were presented with single words and asked to indicate whether or not they recognised the words from the study list (i.e. yes/no recognition). Furthermore the design included two measures of source memory. One source memory condition involved asking subjects at study to try to remember the words as well as whether they were part of the first or the second study list. The other source memory condition involved trying to remember the words as well as their spatial location (left/right). At test, in both source memory conditions subjects were informed that all of the to-be-presented words had been part of the study list and their task was to try to remember (i) in which list they had been shown (first/second), and (ii) on which side of the screen they had been presented.

An overall multivariate analysis (McIntosh et al., 1996) revealed that retrieval of item as well as source information involved increased activity in similar regions, including right prefrontal and midbrain regions. This outcome suggested that retrieval of different types of event information share a common neuroanatomical basis. However, in line with the notion that source memory may be especially sensitive to frontal-lobe damage, source memory was found to differentially engage specific frontal regions. That is, trying to retrieve spatial information activated a dorsal region in the left frontal lobe (Brodmann area 8), whereas trying to remember in which list the words had been presented activated a region in the anterior cingulate gyrus (Brodmann area 24/32). By contrast, item retrieval differentially activated a right inferior prefrontal region (Brodmann area 47) and an anterior temporal region (Brodmann area 21) in the right hemisphere. Subsequent studies have confirmed that remembering item and contextual information activates different brain regions (Cabeza et al., 1997). The latter study used different measures of item and temporal memory, and the observed differences did not closely overlap with those observed by Nyberg et al. (1996b). For example, an important extension of the Cabeza et al. study is that it provided evidence that activation of the anterior cingulate cortex may be related to task difficulty. Nevertheless, the two studies converge in pointing to a selective role of temporal-lobe regions in item memory and a selective role of dorsal prefrontal regions in remembering contextual information.

Taken together, an important outcome of the studies of item and source memory is the finding that remembering different types of event information seem to share a common neuroanatomical basis including right prefrontal brain regions. In line with the previous discussion of retrieval mode, this may reflect common task demands such as having to think back to a specific study episode. When additional details of the study event had to be retrieved, notably spatial information, left prefrontal regions were differentially activated. This pattern is in line with recent findings from a functional magnetic resonance imaging study of episodic memory (Nolde, Johnson, & D'Esposito, 1998a). In that study, it was found that left prefrontal activity during episodic remembering was related to the amount of episodic detail required at test. More generally, this pattern is consistent with the ''cortical asymmetry of reflective activity'' (CARA) hypothesis (Nolde, Johnson, & Raye, 1998b), which holds that left prefrontal activation is more likely as more reflective processes are required (such as retrieval of additional event information).

CONSCIOUS RECOLLECTION

Up to now we have mostly been concerned with retrieval "in general", without paying much attention to the issue of whether the neural response related to retrieval differs when retrieval is successful as compared to when it is not. To investigate the functional neuroanatomy of retrieval success, we looked at the correlation between individual level of memory performance (number of recognised words) and individual levels of blood flow in the whole brain (Nyberg et al., 1996c). A similar approach had previously been reported by Grasby and colleagues (Grasby et al., 1993b). They found that bilateral hippocampal flow was significantly correlated with a measure of the engagement of long-term memory. Similarly, in two independent data sets, we found that those subjects who correctly recognised many words tended to have higher levels of activity in the left medial temporal lobe (near left hippocampus). These findings led us to conclude that medial temporal activity is related to retrieval success rather than retrieval attempt, and that the increased medial temporal activity may underlie recollective experience or confidence.

A similar conclusion was put forward in a study by Schacter and colleagues (Schacter et al., 1996). In that study, subjects recalled many targets in one condition and few target words in another condition. Comparison of the high-recall condition with the low-recall condition revealed increased activity in bilateral hippocampal regions, and it was concluded that blood-flow increases in the hippocampal formation are specifically associated with the conscious recollection of studied items.

In our analyses of correlations between individual memory performance and regional blood flow (Nyberg et al., 1996c), we furthermore observed a correlation between retrieval success and activity in bilateral inferior frontal regions. This observation is in agreement with findings by Rugg and colleagues (Rugg et al., 1996). They found that conditions involving higher levels of targets were associated with increased blood flow in several bilateral frontal regions compared with conditions involving lower levels of targets. This finding was discussed in relation to the idea that the prefrontal cortex supports processes that operate selectively on the products of retrieval (Shallice, 1988). Specifically, when information is recovered from memory it has to be decided whether the information is valid and relevant to current goals. The prefrontal cortex is believed to subserve such functions.

The data showing that the response of some prefrontal brain regions is sensitive to level of retrieval success can be contrasted with the data reviewed earlier indicating a general involvement of right prefrontal regions in episodic retrieval (Kapur et al., 1995; Nyberg et al., 1995). The issue of whether the role of frontal brain areas, notably right anterior regions, is best described in terms of retrieval attempt/effort/mode or retrieval success continues to be intensively studied (e.g. Buckner et al., 1998a,b). Given the functional heterogeneity of the frontal lobes (e.g. Petrides, 1994), it is likely that both of these functions will turn out to be valid. That is, different parts of the frontal lobes may subserve distinct cognitive functions. Moreover, analyses of functional connectivity have provided suggestive evidence that the functional role of a given brain area may differ depending on which other brain regions it is functionally linked to (McIntosh, Nyberg, Bookstein, & Tulving, 1997). By this latter account, a detailed understanding of the functional significance of activity within a specific brain region can only be gained by examining its interactions with other parts of the brain.

In sum, several PET studies indicate that activity in or near the hippocampal formation is associated with the conscious recollection of studied information. This is in line with studies of brain-damaged patients showing that hippocampal lesions will impair performance on explicit tests of memory, which require conscious recollection, but not on implicit tests (e.g. Mayes, 1995; Squire, 1992). In addition, PET studies have also provided evidence that the response of some prefrontal regions is sensitive to level of retrieval, which may or may not be related to recollective experience.

DOES RETRIEVAL INVOLVE REINSTATEMENT OF ENCODING OPERATIONS?

Cognitive theories have suggested that encoding and retrieval involve similar processes, and hence engage similar brain regions for their operation (see e.g. Craik, Govoni, Naveh-Benjamin, & Anderson, 1997). Although only a few functional neuroimaging findings speak directly to this issue, there are some relevant patterns of results to consider. One such pattern has been summarised in the "hemispheric encoding/retrieval asymmetry" (HERA) model (Tulving et al., 1994; see also Nyberg, Cabeza, & Tulving, 1996). HERA summarises a rather large body of results showing that encoding of episodic information tends to differentially engage left frontal-lobe regions, whereas retrieval of episodic information has consistently been found to differentially engage right frontal regions. As has been noted, the HERA model, as initially formulated, made no reference to specific subregions within left and right frontal lobe, and more specific analysis of distinct prefrontal areas has been called for (Buckner, 1996). Subsequent studies along this line have associated distinct left prefrontal brain regions with specific encoding (e.g. Fletcher, Shallice, & Dolan, 1998a; Kopelman, Stevens, Foli, & Grasby, 1998) and retrieval-related processes (e.g. Fletcher et al., 1998b). Moreover, the asymmetry is not strict in the sense that left prefrontal regions are never activated during retrieval (see e.g. Nolde et al., 1998a) or in the sense that right frontal regions are never activated during encoding (e.g. Kelley et al., 1998). Nevertheless, there is substantial evidence that encoding and retrieval differentially activate certain prefrontal brain regions.

Another intriguing pattern defines the recently proposed "hippocampal encoding/retrieval" (HIPER) model (Lepage, Habib, & Tulving, 1998). The HIPER model suggests a division of memory-related labour between rostral and caudal portions of the hippocampal formation, such that encoding activations are found predominantly in more anterior regions whereas retrieval activations occur predominantly in more posterior regions. This contradicts findings based on functional magnetic resonance imaging reported by Gabrieli, Brewer, Desmond, and Glover (1997), which indicated that encoding of pictures was associated with increased activation in posterior medial temporal regions whereas retrieval was associated with increased activity in a more anterior region. Moreover, a recent review of functional neuroimaging studies of episodic encoding and retrieval has questioned the conclusion that there is a clear separation between anterior and posterior PET activations during encoding and retrieval, respectively (Schacter & Wagner, 1999). Clearly, more work is needed to resolve this issue, but the important point here is that there is tentative evidence to suggest that distinct hippocampal/medial temporal regions make specific contributions to encoding and retrieval.

Taken at face value, the HERA and HIPER models seem to suggest that encoding and retrieval involve non-overlapping processes and brain regions. However, as has been argued (Craik et al., 1997), encoding and retrieval processes may be operating on similar perceptual regions. By this view, the differential involvement of certain brain regions during encoding and retrieval may be reflecting the workings of higher-order control processes that operate within similar perceptual networks. Although more studies are needed to address this issue, some empirical support is existing. One piece of evidence that seems to suggest that encoding and retrieval challenge overlapping posterior brain regions come from our study of retrieval mode and ecphory (Nyberg et al., 1995). As discussed earlier, we found evidence for different activation patterns associated with ecphory depending on how the information had been processed at study. This observation may be interpreted in terms of reinstatement during retrieval of parts of the activation pattern associated with encoding (cf. Rugg et al., 1997). Another piece of evidence comes from the study of item and source memory (Nyberg et al., 1996b). In this study it was found that the strongest effect of the design had to do with the separation between the reading baseline condition and the experimental cognitive conditions (encoding and retrieval). This outcome showed that relative to the reading task, encoding and retrieval activated similar regions. These included bilateral frontal, bilateral insular, and anterior cingulate regions (see Fig. 1).

A final piece of evidence comes from a study of episodic memory for spatial location and object identity (Köhler et al., 1998). Brain blood flow was measured while subjects engaged in perceptual matching of (i) location or (ii) the identity of line drawings of objects. These perceptual matching tasks served as incidental encoding tasks. Subsequently, blood flow was measured when

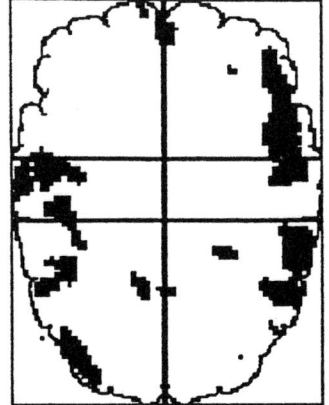 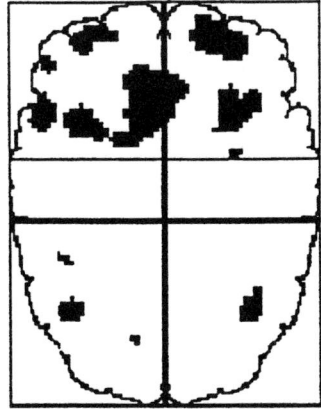

FIG. 1.   Horizontal images displaying brain regions showing increased activity during reading (left) and encoding/retrieval (right). The right image shows those brain regions in which activity was increased relative to baseline/reading during *both* encoding and retrieval. These regions included anterior cingulate, bilateral frontal, and bilateral insular cortices. From Nyberg et al. (1996b).

subjects retrieved information about the location or the identity of the studied objects. The results showed that a common set of brain regions were engaged during perceptual matching of object location and during retrieval of location information. These regions included right middle occipital gyrus, supramarginal gyrus, and superior temporal sulcus. Similarly, a common set of brain regions were engaged during perceptual matching and retrieval of object identity, including bilateral lingual and fusiform gyri. Thus, although additional analyses showed that specific frontal and temporal regions were differentially activated during perceptual matching and retrieval, these findings show that identical regions in dorsal and ventral extrastriate cortex are activated during encoding and retrieval of information about object location and object identity.

In sum, then, there is substantial evidence that certain brain regions are differentially engaged by encoding and retrieval operations, but at the same time there is evidence for a common involvement of specific areas in encoding and retrieval. The latter piece of information indicates that the notion of retrieval involving reinstatement of encoding operations may be true in the sense that similar regions are engaged at both stages.

PICTURE SUPERIORITY

In the context of material-specific activation patterns during encoding and retrieval, it is interesting to note that such activations have been offered as explanation of a basic finding in cognitive psychology; the better retention of pictures over verbal materials (i.e. the picture-superiority effect). In a recent study comparing encoding of verbal and pictorial information it was found that encoding of pictures differentially engaged extrastriate and ventral medial temporal cortices (Grady, McIntosh, Rajah, & Craik, 1998; see also Menard et al., 1996). In the study by Grady et al., pictures were recognised to a higher extent than words, and it was proposed that the ability to remember pictures better than words may be mediated by the stronger engagement of medial temporal and extrastriate cortices during picture encoding. These cortical regions have strong interconnections with one another, allowing for functional interactions to take place. Moreover, other regions were also found to be engaged, such as left ventrolateral prefrontal cortex during intentional encoding. The involvement of frontal regions were largely the same for pictures and words. As such, these findings add to those discussed earlier, showing that some brain regions are generally involved in specific cognitive processes (here intentional encoding) whereas the involvement of other regions is driven by specific factors, such as the to-be-remembered information.

CONCLUSIONS

In this paper, I have discussed PET results that start to define neuroanatomical correlates of various episodic memory phenomena. Overall, the pattern of findings suggests a complex relation between cognitive function and underlying brain function, in that it seems to be necessary to consider relative increases and decreases in activity as well as changes in functional connectivity in order to capture complex brain–cognition relationships. Just as neuropsychological studies of brain-damaged individuals have had a profound impact on theorising in the domain of cognitive psychology, so considering functional neuroimaging results will serve as an important means for constraining cognitive theories. Lesion-based methods and functional-imaging methods can each add unique information, but it is also important to stress that these methods complement each other and that it is important to look for convergent evidence from several different approaches (cf. Nyberg & Tulving, 1996). PET and other functional imaging techniques can be used to address hypotheses derived from lesion studies (e.g. Kopelman et al., 1998), and findings from imaging studies can be used as the basis for exploring brain–cognition relationships in brain-damaged patients (e.g. Buckner et al., 1996). Most likely, "combined" patient-imaging studies will become more common in the near future as will studies combining various imaging techniques (e.g. Düzel et al., 1999).

REFERENCES

Andreasen, N.C., O'Leary, D.D., Arndt, S., Cizaldo, T., Hurtig, R., Rezai, K., Watkins, G.L., Boles Ponto, L.L., & Hichawa, R.D. (1995). Short-term and long-term verbal memory: A positron emission tomography study. *Proceedings of the National Academy of Science, 92*, 5111–5115.

Buckner, R.L. (1996). Beyond HERA: Contributions of specific prefrontal brain areas to long-term memory retrieval. *Psychonomic Bulletin & Review*, *3*, 149–158.

Buckner, R.L., Corbetta, M., Schatz, J., Raichle, M.E., & Petersen, S.E. (1996). Preserved speech abilities and compensation following prefrontal damage. *Proceedings of the National Academy of Science*, *93*, 1249–1253.

Buckner, R.L., Koutsaal, W., Schacter, D.L., Dale, A.M., Rotte, M., & Rosen, B.R. (1998b). Functional-anatomic study of episodic retrieval using fMRI II. Selective averaging of event-related fMRI to test the retrieval success hypothesis. *Neuroimage*, *7*, 163–175.

Buckner, R.L., Koutsaal, W., Schacter, D.L., Wagner, A.D., & Rosen, B.R. (1998a). Functional-anatomic study of episodic retrieval using fMRI I. Retrieval effort versus retrieval success. *Neuroimage*, *7*, 151–162.

Buckner, R.L., & Tulving, E. (1995). Neuroimaging studies of memory: Theory and recent PET results. In F. Boller & J. Grafman (Eds.), *Handbook of neuropsychology* (Vol. 10, pp.439–466). Amsterdam: Elsevier.

Cabeza, R., Mangels, J., Nyberg, L., Habib, R., Houle, S., McIntosh, A.R., & Tulving, E. (1997). Brain regions differentially involved in remembering what and when: a PET study. *Neuron*, *19*, 863–870.

Craik, F.I.M., Govoni, R., Naveh-Benjamin, M., & Anderson, N.D. (1997). The effects of divided attention on encoding and retrieval processes in human memory. *Journal of Experimental Psychology: General*, *125*, 159–180.

Düzel, E., Cabeza, R., Picton, T.W., Yonelinas, A.P., Scheich, H., Heinze, H.-J., & Tulving, E. (1999). Task-and item-related processes in memory retrieval: A combined PET and ERP study. *Proceedings of the National Academy of Science*, *96*, 1794–1799.

Fletcher, P.C., Frith, C.D., Grasby, P.M., Shallice, T., Frackowiak, R.S.J., & Dolan, R.J. (1995). Brain systems for encoding and retrieval of auditory-verbal memory. *Brain*, *118*, 401–416.

Fletcher, P.C., Shallice, T., & Dolan, R.J. (1998a). The functional roles of prefrontal cortex in episodic memory: I. Encoding. *Brain*, *121*, 1239–1248.

Fletcher, P.C., Shallice, T., Frith, C.D., Frackowiak, R.S.J., & Dolan, R.J. (1998b). The functional roles of prefrontal cortex in episodic memory: II. Retrieval. *Brain*, *121*, 1249–1256.

Friston, K.J., Holmes, A.P., Worsley, K.J., Poline, J.B., Frith, C.D., & Frackowiak, R.S.J. (1995). Statistical parametric maps in functional imaging: A general linear approach. *Human Brain Mapping*, *2*, 189–210.

Frith, C.D., Friston, K.J., Liddle, P.F., & Frackowiak, R.S.J. (1991). A PET study of word finding. *Neuropsychologia*, *29*, 1137–1148.

Gabrieli, J.D.E., Brewer, J.B., Desmond, J.E., & Glover, G.H. (1997). Separate neural bases of two fundamental memory processes in the human medial temporal lobe. *Science*, *276*, 264–266.

Grady, C.L., McIntosh, A.R., Rajah, M.N., & Craik, F.I.M. (1998). Neural correlates of episodic encoding of pictures and words. *Proceedings of the National Academy of Science*, *95*, 2703–2708.

Grasby, P.M., Frith, C.D., Friston, K.J., Bench, C., Frackowiak, R.S.J., & Dolan, R.J. (1993a). Functional mapping of brain areas implicated in auditory-verbal memory function. *Brain*, *116*, 1–20.

Grasby, P.M., Frith, C.D., Friston, K.J., Frackowiak, R.S.J., & Dolan, R.J. (1993b). Activation of the human hippocampal formation during auditory-verbal long-term memory function. *Neuroscience Letters*, *163*, 185–188.

Kapur, S., Craik, F.I.M., Jones, C., Brown, G.M., Houle, S., & Tulving, E. (1995). Functional role of the prefrontal cortex in memory retrieval: A PET study. *NeuroReport*, *6*, 1880–1884.

Kelley, W.M., Miezin, F.M., McDermott, K.B., Buckner, R.L., Raichle, M.E., Cohen, N.J., Ollinger, J.M., Akbudak, E., Conturo, T.E., Snyder, A.Z., & Petersen, S.E. (1998). Hemispheric specialization in human dorsal frontal cortex and medial temporal lobe for verbal and nonverbal memory encoding. *Neuron*, *20*, 927–936.

Köhler, S., Moscovitch, M., Winocur, G., Houle, S., & McIntosh, A.R. (1998). Networks of domain-specific and general regions involved in episodic memory for spatial location and object identity. *Neuropsychologia, 36*, 129–142.

Kopelman, M.D., Stevens, T.G., Foli, S., & Grasby, P. (1998). PET activation of medial temporal lobe in learning. *Brain, 121*, 875–887.

Lepage, M., Habib, R., & Tulving, E. (1998). Hippocampal PET activations of memory encoding and retrieval: The HIPER model. *Hippocampus, 8*, 313–322.

Mayes, A.R. (1995). Memory and amnesia. *Behavioural Brain Research, 66*, 29–36.

McIntosh, A.R., Bookstein, F.L., Haxby, J.V., & Crady, C.L. (1996). Spatial pattern analysis of functional brain images using partial least squares. *NeuroImage, 3*, 143–157.

McIntosh, A.R., & Gonzalez-Lime, F. (1994). Structural equation modelling and its application to network analysis in functional brain imaging. *Human Brain Mapping, 2*, 2–22.

McIntosh, A.R., Nyberg, L., Bookstein, F.L., & Tulving, E. (1997). Differential functional connectivity of prefrontal and medial temporal cortices during episodic memory retrieval. *Human Brain Mapping, 5*, 323–327.

Menard, M.T., Kosslyn, S.M., Thompson, W.L., Alpert, N.M., & Rauch, S.L. (1996). Encoding of words and pictures: A positron emission tomography study. *Neuropsychologia, 34*, 185–194.

Nolde, S.F., Johnson, M.K., & D'Esposito, M.G. (1998a). Left prefrontal activation during episodic remembering: An event-related fMRI study. *NeuroReport, 9*, 3509–3514.

Nolde, S.F., Johnson, M.K., & Raye, C.L. (1998b). The role of prefrontal cortex during tests of episodic memory. *Trends in Cognitive Sciences, 2*, 399–406.

Nyberg, L. (1998). Mapping episodic memory. *Behavioural Brain Research, 90*, 107–114.

Nyberg, L., Cabeza, R., & Tulving, E. (1996). PET studies of encoding and retrieval: The HERA model. *Psychonomic Bulletin & Review, 3*, 135–148.

Nyberg, L., McIntosh, A.R., Cabeza, R., Habib, R., Houle, S., & Tulving, E. (1996b). General and specific brain regions involved in encoding and retrieval of events: What, where, and when. *Proceedings of the National Academy of Science, 93*, 11280–11285.

Nyberg, L., McIntosh, A.R., Cabeza, R., Nilsson, L.-G., Houle, S., Habib, R., & Tulving, E. (1996a). Network analysis of positron emission tomography regional cerebral blood flow data: Ensemble inhibition during episodic memory retrieval. *The Journal of Neuroscience, 16*, 3753–3759.

Nyberg, L., McIntosh, A.R., Houle, S., Nilsson, L.-G., & Tulving, E. (1996c). Activation of medial temporal structures during episodic memory retrieval. *Nature, 380* (25 April), 715–717.

Nyberg, L., & Tulving, E. (1996). Classifying human long-term memory: Evidence from converging dissociations. *European Journal of Cognitive Psychology, 8*, 163–183.

Nyberg, L., Tulving, E., Habib, R., Nilsson, L.-G., Kapur, S., Houle, S., & McIntosh, A.R. (1995). Functional brain maps of retrieval mode and recovery of retrieval of episodic information. *NeuroReport, 7*, 249–252.

Petrides, M. (1994). Frontal lobes and working memory: Evidence from investigations of the effects of cortical excisions in nonhuman primates. In F. Boller & J. Grafman (Eds.), *Handbook of neuropsychology* (Vol. 9, pp.59–82). Amsterdam: Elsevier.

Raichle, M.E. (1994). Images of the mind: Studies with modern imaging techniques. *Annual Review of Psychology, 45*, 333–356.

Rugg, M.D., Fletcher, P.C., Frith, C.D., Frackowiak, R.S.J., & Dolan, R.J. (1996). Differential activation of the prefrontal cortex in successful and unsuccessful memory retrieval. *Brain, 119*, 2073–2083.

Rugg, M.D., Fletcher, P.C., Frith, C.D., Frackowiak, R.S.J., & Dolan, R.J. (1997). Brain regions supporting intentional and incidental memory: A PET study. *NeuroReport, 8*, 1283–1287.

Schacter, D.L. (1987). Memory, amnesia, and frontal lobe dysfunction. *Psychobiology, 15*, 21–36.

Schacter, D.L., Alpert, N.M., Savage, C.R., Rauch, S.L., & Albert, M.S. (1996). Conscious recollection and the human hippocampal formation. Evidence from positron emission tomography. *Proceedings of the National Academy of Science, 93*, 321–325.

Schacter, D.L., & Wagner, A.D. (1999). Medial temporal lobe activations in FMRI and PET studies of episodic encoding and retrieval. *Hippocampus, 9*, 7–24.

Shallice, T. (1988). *From neuropsychology to mental structure.* Cambridge: Cambridge University Press.

Shallice, T., Fletcher, P., Frith, C.D., Grasby, P., Frackowiak, R.S.J., & Dolan, R.J. (1994). Brain regions associated with acquisition and retrieval of verbal episodic memory. *Nature, 368*, 633–635.

Squire, L.R. (1992). Memory and the hippocampus: A synthesis from findings with rats, monkeys, and humans. *Psychological Review, 99*, 195–231.

Squire, L.R., Knowlton, B., & Musen, G. (1993). The structure and organization of memory. *Annual Review of Psychology, 44*, 453–495.

Squire, L.R., Ojemann, J.G., Miezin, F.M., Petersen, S.E., Videen, T.O., & Raichle, M.E. (1992). Activation of the hippocampus in normal humans: A functional anatomic study of memory. *Proceedings of the National Academy of Science, 89*, 1837–1841.

Tulving, E. (1983). *Elements of episodic memory.* New York: Oxford University Press.

Tulving, E., Kapur, S., Craik, F.I.M., Moscovitch, M., & Houle, S. (1994). Hemispheric encoding/retrieval asymmetry in episodic memory: Positron emission tomography findings. *Proceedings of the National Academy of Science, 91*, 2016–2020.

Tulving, E., & Thompson, D.M. (1973). Encoding specificity and retrieval processes in episodic memory. *Psychological Review, 76*, 559–573.

MEMORY, 1999, 7 (5/6), 599–612

FDG-PET Analysis and Findings in Amnesia Resulting From Hypoxia

L.J. Reed, P. Marsden, D. Lasserson, N. Sheldon, P. Lewis,
N. Stanhope, E. Guinan, and M.D. Kopelman

St Thomas's Hospital, and King's College, London, UK

The assumptions underlying neuroimaging, and problems in its analysis and interpretation, are commonly underestimated in neuropsychology. The ways in which fluoro-deoxy-glucose (FDG) positron emission tomography (PET) data can be analysed are discussed. PET findings from four patients who had suffered severe amnesia, following episodes of acute hypoxia, are presented. These patients had shown evidence of medial temporal (hippocampal and parahippocampal) atrophy on MRI brain scans. The PET data were analysed in several different ways. The converging findings were that the patients showed bilateral thalamic hypometabolism, and there was also evidence of retrosplenial hypometabolism bilaterally. Cognitively, these patients performed most like other patients with medial temporal lesions, but the results indicate that structural lesions can have distal metabolic effects on structures elsewhere. These findings are interpreted in the light of neuroanatomical observations concerning parallel projections between medial temporal lobe structures and the thalamus, some of which pass via the retrosplenium.

INTRODUCTION

Neuroimaging is increasingly being used in neuropsychological investigations. In many studies, non-quantitative results are reported. In other studies, it is common to use only one form of data analysis. From such information, a ''lesion'' is commonly identified to which a critical cognitive deficit is then attributed in either a single-or double-dissociation. Although this method has served neuropsychology well, particularly in animal studies (Weiskrantz, 1968) or in patients with large focal lesions (Jones, 1983; Shallice, 1988), it becomes more tendentious in patients with more subtle pathology, giving rise to conflicts

Requests for reprints should be sent to M.D. Kopelman, Division of Psychiatry and Psychology, St Thomas's Hospital, London SE1 7EH, UK.

This research was funded by a Wellcome Trust project grant to Drs M.D. Kopelman, J. Wade, and B. Kendall.

over the interpretation, for example, of so-called "isolated retrograde amnesia" (Kopelman, in press).

It is a clinical truism that patients with very large lesions, particularly if of early onset (e.g. congenital hydrocephalus, porencephalic cysts), can show little, if any, cognitive impairment (Lonton, 1979), whereas other patients may show a severe cognitive impairment (e.g. of memory) in the absence of any clear-cut visible alteration on MRI or PET scanning (e.g. Guinan et al., 1998). Moreover, it is common to find abnormalities on one form of neuroimaging that are not evident on another. For example, demyelination is better seen on MRI than CT imaging, whereas calcified lesions are better seen on CT than MRI images. Creutzfeldt-Jakob disease can produce grossly abnormal EEGs in the presence of a normal or near-normal CT or MRI brain scan. It is common in our experience to see abnormalities reported on single-photon emission computerised tomography (SPECT), which are not necessarily replicated on PET scanning, e.g. the case of a patient who was reported to show "typical changes" of myalgic encephalopathy (ME) on SPECT according to one research group, who showed no abnormalities whatsoever on a PET scan conducted by ourselves.

The situation is further complicated when quantified investigations are introduced. Radio-labelled fluoro-deoxy-glucose (^{18}FDG) is widely employed as a measure of metabolism. It has a prolonged half-life and it is insensitive to differences in regional cerebral blood flow (rCBF); whereas ^{15}O labelled water has a brief half-life (two minutes approximately) and is used to measure changes in rCBF in cognitive activation studies. PET findings can be reported in terms of region-of-interest (ROI) results, in which significant differences within the regions of interest are sought across subject groups. These can be expressed as:

(i) FDG-uptake (raw counts) expressed as a ratio to the uptake in a "reference" brain region (for example, temporal lobe counts ÷ occipital values),

(ii) standardised uptake values (SUV), giving a simple correction for injected dose, body weight, and blood glucose, or

(iii) regional cerebral metabolic rate for glucose (rCMRglc) or "absolute metabolism" (after an input function correction for radiotracer delivery).

Alternatively, a statistical parametric mapping (SPM) method is commonly employed (Friston, Frith, Liddle, & Frackowiak, 1991), in which the brain is "warped" to a standard template. Significant differences across voxels are identified, and then the location of the significantly different voxels is sought. Again, this can be done for raw uptake counts as a ratio to a reference region (commonly whole brain metabolism but sometimes cerebellar or occipital metabolism), standardised uptake values, or absolute metabolism. The SPM method has been widely used in functional activation studies (e.g. Fletcher et al., 1995; Grasby et al., 1993), but it can also be used in comparison of groups composed of subjects who are assumed to have a common underlying pathology.

The advantage of ROI analysis is that it does not require any "warping" of the brain, which could conceivably produce important distortion in patients with certain types of pathology. A disadvantage is that it requires a certain amount of operator judgement in evaluating the precise location of the ROIs in some subjects; and only a proportion of the data available in a PET image is usually sampled. By contrast, the SPM programme is semi-automated, and thereby minimises the problem of subjective operator judgements. On the other hand, the effect of warping the brain is often unknown. Moreover, covarying for whole-brain metabolism (using the ANCOVA procedure with SPM) in, for example, Alzheimer patients may draw attention to regions of especially low metabolism, while omitting consideration of other regions of abnormality elsewhere, and hence may not be justified.

There is a dearth of studies comparing the findings from different forms of analysis. Yet understanding of the potential artefacts is crucial before confident interpretation can be made from individual case-studies, particularly where disorders such as psychogenic amnesia are being studied, and also in group studies, where the simple assumption that "normal metabolism = normal function" and "abnormal metabolism = abnormal function" needs to be critically evaluated. Just because a particular cognitive function is considered "modular" on a neuropsychological basis does *not* mean that it necessarily occupies a unique and invariable brain location. A site of focal hypometabolism may represent (i) the critical site for a cognitive function, or (ii) specific node within a network, or (iii) it may be spurious. It can be interpreted only after examining the results of different forms of image analysis and individual findings within the group, as well as in the context of wider neuroanatomical, neuroimaging, and cognitive considerations.

The present investigation is the first of a series of studies examining patients with organic amnesia. In these studies, we have carried out our analyses in a number of different ways in order to seek convergence or discrepancies between them. Detailed cognitive investigations have been carried out, and are being reported in a number of different publications (e.g. Kopelman & Stanhope, 1997; Kopelman, Stanhope, & Kingsley, 1997; Kopelman, Stanhope & Guinan, 1998; Stanhope, Guinan, & Kopelman, 1998). Detailed quantitative MRI findings are being reported elsewhere (Kopelman et al., 1999), but the critical observations in connection with the present subject groups will be mentioned here. We will be reporting the findings in a small group of patients with amnesia resulting from hypoxia.

Since the Zola-Morgan, Squire, and Amaral (1986) and Press, Amaral, and Squire (1989) studies, it has generally been assumed in the neuropsychological literature that amnesia following episodes of hypoxia results from hippocampal damage, particularly to the CAI region, in which there is a marked loss of pyramidal cells. However, Kuwert et al. (1993) have reported thalamic hypometabolism in three patients, medial temporal hypometabolism in two patients, and involvement of the caudate nucleus and cerebellum in one case each. Somewhat similarly, Markowitsch, Weber-Luxenburger, Ewald, Kessler, and Heiss (1997) have reported altered metabolism in the thalami, medial and lateral temporal lobes, and in the occipito-parietal regions bilaterally in a case of cardiac arrest, in whom MRI revealed atrophy without "specific brain damage". Fazio et al. (1992) studied 11 amnesic patients with a variety of underlying pathologies, and they reported that there was a significant reduction of metabolism throughout limbic-diencephalic circuits on fluoro-deoxy-glucose (FDG) PET whatever the site of underlying structural pathology—however, they did not report the individual findings from their different patient groups. In the present study, we were concerned to see (i) whether metabolic changes were confined to the medial temporal regions; or (ii) whether there was wider involvement within the limbic-diencephalic circuits; or (iii) whether there would be widespread hypometabolism across the cerebral cortex.

SUBJECT GROUPS

There were four patients with hypoxic brain damage. One of these patients became hypoxic following a heroin overdose and a period of prolonged unconsciousness: his CT scan showed enlargement of the temporal horns of the ventricles bilaterally, indicating medial temporal lobe atrophy. The second patient had attempted to hang himself, and his initial CT scan showed a moderately large area of infarction in the left temporal lobe. By the time of his research MRI scan, some months later, this infarction was no longer evident, but the patient remained severely amnesic. The third patient had a left temporo-parietal infarction on his CT scan, following a respiratory arrest. The fourth patient developed profound amnesia after a prolonged period of unconsciousness of uncertain aetiology.

The healthy controls were a group of 10 volunteers from a larger group of 20 healthy subjects, employed in the cognitive studies (e.g. Kopelman & Stanhope, 1997; Stanhope et al., 1998). Table 1 reports background cognitive scores in the two groups. The hypoxic patients showed profound impairment in general and delayed memory function. They also showed moderately impaired scores on FAS verbal fluency and card-sorting tasks although, in these small groups, only the cognitive estimates result reached statistical significance.

On quantitative MRI brain scans, using T1, T2, and proton density (PD) images obtained in 3-dimensional acquisitions with segmentation of brain structures by means of a Graphical User Interface (Griffin, Colchester, Roell, & Stuldholme, 1994), the hypoxic patients differed significantly from the healthy controls in terms of right hippocampal ($t = 2.65$, $P < .025$), total hippocampal ($t = 2.17$, $P = .055$), and left parahippocampal volume ($t = 2.48$, $P < .05$) (Kopelman et al., 1999). They did not differ significantly from healthy controls in terms of measures of whole brain, frontal, or total temporal lobe volume, nor in terms of a proton-density measurement of thalamic area (Kopelman et al., 1999).

TABLE 1
Demographic and Basic Neuropsychological Evaluations

Variable	Controls (n = 10)		Hypoxic Patients (n = 4)		Significance (unpaired t)
	mean	sd	mean	sd	
Age	39.00	13.3	37.0	17.4	n.s.
NART[1]	104.7	14.0	107.3	4.0	n.s.
FSIQ[2]	102.1	15.3	92.3	11.0	n.s.
GMQ WMS[3]	104.2	17.2	70.0	17.3	$P<.002$
DMQ WMS[4]	106.2	22.4	63.3	15.7	$P<.0005$
FAS[5]	43.9	15.1	28.0	13.3	n.s.
CARD-SORTING					
Categories achieved[6]	5.2	1.5	3.8	2.2	n.s.
% Perseverative errors[6]	10.1	9.6	17.3	20.6	n.s.
CET[7]	4.2	3.5	7.3	2.8	$P<.05$

[1]Nelson & Willison (1991)
[2]Wechsler (1981)
[3]Wechsler (1987): general memory quotient
[4]Wechsler (1987): delayed recall quotient
[5]Benton (1968)
[6]Nelson (1976)
[7]Shallice & Evans (1978)

METHOD

[18]FDG-PET Image Acquisition

Images of the cerebral distribution of positron emission from [18]FDG were acquired using a CTI ECAT 951R PET camera (CTI/Siemens, Knoxville, Tenn., USA) at Guy's and St Thomas's Hospital Clinical PET Centre. Thirty minutes after injection of about 185MBq of [18]FDG, uptake images were acquired over a 30-minute period under resting state conditions. All subjects were scanned lying supine in a darkened room with their eyes closed. Arterialised-venous sampling was also conducted for nine control subjects and three of the hypoxic patients, and an input function for FDG was obtained for these subjects. This allowed calibration of uptake values of rCMRglc (true metabolic rate) in these subjects by the method of Phelps et al. (1979) and Huang et al. (1980).

[18]FDG-PET Image Analysis

The scans obtained were analysed using two distinct approaches: a region of interest (ROI) based analysis, and a statistical parametric mapping (SPM) approach.

Region of Interest Analysis.   All image transformations and analyses were performed on a Sun SPARC workstation (Sun Computers Europe Inc., Surrey, UK) using proprietary image analysis software (CTI/Siemens, Knoxville, Tenn., USA). Reconstructed images were aligned to the AC–PC plane using an interactive alignment program, resliced, smoothed using a 6mm Gaussian filter, and adjacent planes were summed to give 15 planes approximately aligned to the Talairach Atlas. The resulting images were sampled using regions of interest (ROI) which were placed with reference to the Talairach Atlas, and moved individually to the site of maximal activity of the structure concerned. Measurements ("absolute metabolism") were expressed in terms of regional metabolic rate for glucose rCMRglc (where the input function was available) in units of μmol/100g/min. ROI analysis of the raw FDG-uptake counts was performed in a variety of ways: (i) after normalisation for injected dose of FDG, body weight and blood glucose (SUVs); (ii) as a ratio to cerebellar uptake; (iii) as a ratio to occipital uptake; and (iv) as a ratio to global cerebral uptake. The preferred choice of occipital cortex as a reference region was based on a comparison of the findings in healthy controls (see Results), and on the observation that no significant difference in occipital metabolism was obtained in subjects for whom absolute metabolic values were available. Expression of values as a ratio to a reference region, or to global uptake, is a strategy recognised to reduce inter-individual variation in quantitative imaging (see also Results).

ROIs were sampled by two raters, A and B. Rater A sampled 172 ROIs from a "metabolic image" to determine rCMRglc, and her values are given later. Rater B sampled 208 ROIs in terms of raw FDG uptake counts, and his results are given for this. The intra-class inter-rater reliability between the two raters was 0.86.

Statistical Parametric Imaging.   Images were further analysed using the statistical parametric mapping programs, SPM95 and SPM96, developed at the Wellcome Department of Cognitive Neurology, London UK, implemented in Matlab 4.2c (Mathworks Inc., Sherborn, Mass., USA). This method allows automated semiquantitative and non-hypothesis-dependent comparison of FDG-PET scans of the amnesic subjects with the control subjects in a procedure directly analgous to that conventionally performed in the analysis of cerebral blood flow in functional paradigms. Each subject's scan was transformed into standard stereotactic space using a 12-parameter linear transformation, and a 6-parameter quadratic deformation and a fluid non-linear 3D deformation on a slice by slice basis (Friston et al., 1995a). This allowed inter-subject averaging and comparisons. The stereotactically normalised scans contained 26 planes with a voxel size of $2 \times 2 \times 4$mm corresponding to the brain Atlas of Talairach and Tournoux. Normalisation of each subject's image to standard space was performed using SPM95 and checked individually to ensure accurate transformation. Smoothing was performed on all scans using an isotropic Gaussian kernel of 18mm FWHM (full width half maximum) in order to allow for differences in gyral anatomy between individuals and to increase signal-to-noise ratio. The effect of inter-individual variance in scans resulting from differing injected doses, body weights, etc., was removed by using a voxel-by-voxel analysis of covariance (ANCOVA) with values for mean occipital cortex signal as the covariate, obtained from the preceding ROI analysis. In separate analyses, cerebellar values and global cerebral activity were also used as covariates, but these will not be reported here as the findings were broadly consistent with those in which the occipital signal was the covariate. Group comparisons were made by definition of the appropriate linear contrasts within the SPM96 program, generating SPM{t} maps of voxel-by-voxel t statistics which were subsequently transformed into SPM{Z} maps (Friston et al., 1995b). The exact level of significance of volumes of activation was characterised by peak amplitude or "height" and spatial extent (Friston et al., 1995b). Clusters of voxels that had a peak Z score of > 3.09 (threshold $P < .001$) were considered to show significant differences.

RESULTS

Table 2 shows the means and coefficients of variation (percentage standard deviations) in healthy controls for a range of brain regions according to normalisation method. From this, it can be seen that both standardised uptake values (SUVs) (normalising for injected dose, body weight, and blood glucose) and rCMRglc (using the arterialised-venous input function for FDG) show high inter-individual variability of the order of 15–20%. Use of reference region methods comparing regional uptake to cerebellar, occipital cortex, and global cerebral uptake showed progressively improved inter-individual variability ranging from 8%, 6%, to 4% respectively (table 2). The high variability in SUV and rCMRglc values may reflect a real difference between individuals but, alternatively, it could have been introduced by errors in the correction procedure, which is supported by the fact that variability was reduced when a reference region was employed. The use of global activity as a covariate, or reference region, has to be employed cautiously however, given the possibility of widespread changes in cerebral metabolism induced by hypoxia (or any other brain pathology, for that matter). Hence, in our subsequent analyses, we used occipital metabolism as our covariate or reference region.

Table 3 shows rCMRglc values in healthy controls and hypoxic patients in μmol/100g/min. It will be seen that the hypoxic patients showed significant reduction in anterior and posterior thalamic metabolism, compared with healthy controls. On the other hand, there were no differences in the temporal lobe regions, the posterior cingulate region, or elsewhere in the brain. In particular, there were no differences in occipital rCMRglc between patients and controls,

TABLE 2
Control Group Analysis

Normalisation Method Brain Region	Standardised Uptake Values mean (SD) %SD	rCMRglc or "Absolute Metabolism" (n = 9) mean (SD) %SD	Ratio to Cerebellum mean (SD) %SD	Ratio to Occipital Cortex mean (SD) %SD	Ratio to Global Activity mean (SD) %SD
Frontal Cortex	5.97 (1.27) 21.22	39.12 (6.69) 17.11	1.13 (0.10) 8.5	1.00 (0.05) 5.07	1.05 (0.02) 2.15
Temporal Cortex	5.11 (1.08) 21.22	33.68 (5.27) 15.64	0.96 (0.08) 8.14	0.85 (0.04) 4.21	0.90 (0.02) 1.86
Occipital Cortex	6.03 (1.38) 22.88	38.68 (5.31) 13.73	1.13 (0.10) 8.50	—	1.06 (0.04) 3.74
Cerebellum	5.35 (1.23) 23.06	35.79 (4.77) 13.33	—	0.89 (0.07) 8.39	0.94 (0.07) 7.41
Thalamus	5.37 (1.10) 20.54	41.90 (5.00) 11.93	1.01 (0.07) 6.45	0.90 (0.05) 6.11	0.95 (0.04) 4.63
Caudate Nucleus	5.75 (1.26) 21.95	42.28 (6.40) 15.14	1.08 (0.07) 6.57	0.96 (0.06) 6.32	1.01 (0.04) 4.03

Means and percentage standard deviations according to normalisation method for the FDG-PET scan analysis of the control group (n = 10).

TABLE 3
FDG-PET Measures of rCMRglc: "Absolute metabolism"

Region of Interest	Controls (n = 9)		Hypoxic Patients (n = 3)		Significance (unpaired t)
	mean	sd	mean	sd	
Dorsolateral frontal cortex	38.8	6.4	39.4	7.7	n.s.
Orbitomedial frontal cortex	38.6	7.0	42.9	6.8	n.s.
Anterior cingulate cortex	41.3	7.7	42.8	10.3	n.s.
Posterior cingulate cortex	44.5	7.4	40.5	10.3	n.s.
Medial temporal cortex	30.0	4.4	30.7	4.3	n.s.
Temporal pole	25.7	5.0	26.4	3.3	n.s.
Inferior temporal cortex	33.4	5.1	35.1	3.5	n.s.
Lateral temporal cortex	36.9	5.9	38.4	5.7	n.s.
Left anterior thalamus	42.8	4.4	29.7	9.3	$P<.01$
Right anterior thalamus	43.5	6.6	29.2	9.8	$P<.02$
Left posterior thalamus	40.3	5.9	28.8	9.1	$P<.05$
Right posterior thalamus	40.2	4.8	28.9	8.3	$P<.02$
Occipital cortex	38.6	5.3	38.8	8.3	n.s.
Caudate	42.3	6.4	43.6	7.0	n.s.
Cerebellum	35.8	4.8	36.2	5.3	n.s.

justifying the use of occipital uptake as a reference region (covariate) in subsequent analyses. Findings were consistent across the left and right hemisphere with only minimal differences between them.

Table 4 shows regional FDG-uptake relative to occipital uptake in control subjects and the total group of four hypoxic patients. There was significant thalamic hypometabolism bilaterally in the hypoxic group. Again, there was no evidence of temporal lobe hypometabolism. In this case, there was also evidence of significant hypometabolism in posterior cingulate (retrosplenial) uptake relative to the occipital cortex. Again, the findings were consistent across the left and right hemisphere with only minimal differences between them.

Analysis of the individual results for the hypoxic group showed that there was reduced thalamic metabolism in each subject, whether the analysis was in terms of rCMRglc or values normalised relative to occipital metabolism. Values in the fourth patient (where the underlying aetiology was somewhat uncertain) were virtually identical to the other three.

Plates 5 and 6 show the results of SPM comparisons of the hypoxic group with the healthy controls with occipital uptake as reference covariate, rendered on to a reference T1 weighted MRI shown in three planes. There was evidence of two abnormalities—reduced uptake bilaterally in the thalamus and in the retrospenial region of the posterior-cingulate gyrus. Table 5 shows the Z values corresponding to the voxels located within each structure, derived by

TABLE 4
Ratio of regional FDG-uptake to Occipital Cortex Uptake

Region of Interest	Controls (n = 9)		Hypoxic Patients (n = 3)		Significance (unpaired t)
	mean	sd	mean	sd	
Dorsolateral frontal cortex	1.03	0.05	1.03	0.05	n.s.
Orbitomedial frontal cortex	0.91	0.06	0.83	0.13	n.s.
Anterior cingulate cortex	1.01	0.07	1.00	0.08	n.s.
Posterior cingulate cortex	1.15	0.05	1.02	0.11	P<.025
Medial temporal cortex	0.76	0.04	0.81	0.05	n.s.
Temporal pole	0.83	0.04	0.88	0.08	n.s.
Inferior temporal cortex	0.86	0.05	0.91	0.08	n.s.
Lateral temporal cortex	0.92	0.03	0.96	0.05	n.s.
Left anterior thalamus	0.94	0.07	0.75	0.06	P<.001
Right anterior thalamus	0.94	0.07	0.77	0.05	P<.001
Left posterior thalamus	0.92	0.05	0.79	0.08	P<.005
Right posterior thalamus	0.90	0.07	0.79	0.05	P<.025
Caudate	0.96	0.06	0.94	0.05	n.s.
Cerebellum	0.89	0.07	0.97	0.09	n.s.

TABLE 5
Contrast Between Control and Hypoxic Groups

Brain Region	Talairach Coordinates (x, y, z)	Z Value
Left posterior cingulate (BA 31)	−5, −42, 32	3.19
Right posterior cingulate (BA 31)	+5, −42, 32	3.15
Left thalamus	−16, −16, 8	3.27
Right thalamus	+16, −16, 8	3.17

SPM96 Analysis of contrast between control subjects (n = 10) and the hypoxic group (n = 4) FDG-uptake images with occipital uptake as confounding covariate, height threshold Z > 3.09, P < .001, showing brain regions (with Brodmann Areas as applicable), Talairach coordinates, and corresponding Z values for voxels at those coordinates.

interrogating the SPM{Z} shown in Plates 5 and 6. (As mentioned in the Methods section, the findings were consistent when either cerebellar uptake or global cerebral uptake were used as the reference covariate.)

DISCUSSION

The present findings illustrate an interesting double-dissociation. The hypoxic group showed MRI evidence of medial temporal lobe atrophy, but metabolism values were not affected in the temporal lobes. On the other hand, our estimates of thalamic volume in this group were entirely normal, whereas they showed consistent evidence of thalamic hypometabolism on PET scan, which was evident across each of our analyses. There was also evidence of posterior cingulate (retrosplenial) hypometabolism on the analyses of FDG-uptake, although this was not statistically significant for rCMRglc (in which variability was greater).

The finding of thalamic hypometabolism in this group is not entirely surprising: altered signal in deep grey matter structures is occasionally seen on MRI or even CT scans following acute episodes of hypoxia. Moreover, Kuwert et al. (1993) described thalamic hypometabolism in three out of seven subjects investigated, and Fazio et al. (1992) reported widespread limbic-diencephalic changes, including the thalamus, in 11 amnesic patients, of whom 5 had an hypoxic aetiology. Markowitsch et al. (1997) have also reported widespread metabolism changes in a patient resuscitated after a cardiac arrest.

What is perhaps more surprising is the fact that structural abnormalities can be reported in one location, whereas metabolic abnormalities are found elsewhere. Aggleton and Saunders (1997) have described three parallel projections between medial temporal structures and the thalamus. Hippocampal projections, originating in the subiculum, travel through the fornix to the anterior thalamic nuclei and (via the mammillo-thalamic tract) to the mammillary bodies. Second, there is a dense projection from the entorhinal cortex to the lateral dorsal nucleus of the thalamus, and lighter projections to the anterior and medial dorsal nuclei of the thalamus. The projection into the lateral dorsal nucleus does not course through the fornix but by other routes, some of which pass in close proximity to the mammillo-thalamic tract. Third, there is a projection from the perirhinal cortex to the medial dorsal nuclei of the thalamus, but not to the lateral dorsal nucleus. Valenstein et al. (1987) described a retrosplenial lesion producing severe amnesia, and these authors argued that such a lesion disrupted non-fornical pathways from the hippocampus to the anterior thalamus via the retrosplenial cortex *as well as* input from the anterior and lateral dorsal thalamic nuclei to the retrosplenial cortex and medial temporal lobe, thereby causing a disconnection syndrome. In a subsequent study in this patient, Heilman et al. (1990) found FDG-PET hypometabolism in the thalamus and posterior cingulate (retrosplenium) but not the medial temporal regions (very similar findings to our own), which they interpreted in terms of disruption to this circuit. In brief, there are a number of routes whereby structural pathology in the medial temporal region might produce secondary metabolic effects "upstream" or "downstream" in the thalamic nuclei, and some of these routes implicate the retrosplenial cortex. It should be noted, however, that herpes encephalitis patients with severe medial temporal lobe damage did not necessarily show secondary effects in the thalamus (Reed and others, in preparation), and this may relate to how far back the pathology extended in the herpes patients.

With respect to cognitive findings, our hypoxic patients performed more like other patients with temporal lobe lesions (e.g. herpes encephalitis) than patients with diencephalic pathology (as determined by quantitative MRI in the Korsakoff patients), where cognitive differences existed. This was particularly true in terms of subjective memory evaluations, where hypoxic and herpes encephalitis patients performed closely similarly (with relative preservation of "insight"), and differently from Korsakoff patients or patients who had had irradiation to the diencephalon (Kopelman et al., 1998). It was also true of measures of spatial and temporal context memory, where their performance was closely similar to herpes encephalitis patients, and they did better than Korsakoff patients on temporal context memory, but worse than Korsakoff patients on spatial context memory (Kopelman et al., 1997). On rates of forgetting (Kopelman & Stanhope, 1997), frequency judgements (Stanhope et al., 1998), and recall versus recognition memory (Kopelman & Stanhope, 1998), there was very little difference across any of the diencephalic and temporal lobe groups. In brief, where cognitive differences existed, the hypoxic group performed more like other patients who have medial temporal lesions than like patients who show thalamic dysfunction. Nevertheless, the putative contribution of their thalamic hypometabolism cannot be entirely discounted.

In conclusion, this paper indicates that metabolic changes may exist at sites distal to the location of structural abnormality in patients with cognitive impairment. We have analysed our data in a number of different ways in order to prevent artefactual or chance findings, and we would argue that such a procedure should be employed more widely in quantitative neuroimaging investigations. The finding of thalamic and retrosplenial hypometabolism in patients with medial temporal structural damage is consistent with the existence of parallel interconnections between these brain structures, some passing via the fornix and others via the retrosplenium. Although our patients' cognitive performance was more like that of patients with medial temporal damage than those with thalamic pathology, the findings warn against the over-hasty attribution of cognitive impairments to "naked eye" neuroimaging "lesions".

REFERENCES

Aggleton, J.P., & Saunders, R.C. (1997). The relationships between temporal lobe and diencephalic structures implicated in anterograde amnesia. *Memory, 5*, 49–71.

Benton, A.L. (1968). Differential behavioral effects of frontal lobe disease. *Neuropsychologia, 6*, 53–60.

Fazio, F., Perani, D., Gilardi, M.C., Colombo, F., Cappa., S.F., Vallar, G., Bettinardi, V., Paulesu, E., Alberoni, M., Bressi, S., Franceschi, M., & Lenzi, G.L. (1992). Metabolic impairment in human amnesia: A PET study of memory networks. *Journal of Cerebral Blood Flow and Metabolism, 12* 353–358.

Fletcher, P.C., Frith, C.D., Grasby, P.M., Shallice, T., Frackowiak, R.S., & Dolan, R.J. (1995). Brain systems for encoding and retrieval of auditory–verbal memory. An in vivo study in humans. *Brain, 118,* 401–416.

Friston, K.J., Ashburner, J., Frith, C.D., Poline, J-B., Heather, J.D., & Frackowiak, R.S.J. (1995a). Spatial registration and normalization of images. *Human Brain Mapping, 3,* 165–188.

Friston, K.J., Frith, C.D., Liddle, P.F., & Frackowiak, R.S.J. (1991). Comparing functional (PET) images: The assessment of significant change. *Journal of Cerebral Blood Flow and Metabolism, 11,* 690–699.

Friston, K.J., Holmes, A.P., Worsley, K.J., Poline, J-B., Frith, C.D., & Frackowiak, R.S.J. (1995b). Statistical parametric maps in functional imaging: A general linear approach. *Human Brain Mapping, 2,* 189–210.

Grasby, P.M., Frith, C.D., Friston, K.J., Bench, C., Frackowiak, R.S., & Dolan, R.J. (1993). Functional mapping of brain areas implicated in auditory–gerbal memory function. *Brain, 116,* 1–20.

Griffin, L.D., Colchester, A.C.F., Roell, S.A., & Stuldholme, C.S. (1994). Hierarchical segmentation satisfying constraints. In E.R. Hancock (Ed.), *Proceedings of the British Machine Vision Conference* (pp.135–144). Sheffield, UK: BMVA Press.

Guinan, E.M., Lowy, C., Lewis, P.D.R., Stanhope, N., & Kopelman, M.D. (1998). The cognitive effects of pituitary adenomas and their treatments: Two case studies and an investigation of 90 patients. *Journal of Neurology, Neurosurgery and Psychiatry,* in press.

Heilman, K.M., Bowers, D., Watson, R.T., Day, A., Valenstein, E., Hammond, E., & Duara, R. (1990). Frontal hypermetabolism and thalamic hypometabolism in a patient with abnormal orienting and retrosplenial amnesia. *Neuropsychologia, 28,* 161–169.

Huang, S.C., Phelps, M.E., Hoffman, E.J., Sideria, K., Selin, C.J., & Kuhl, D.E. (1980). Non-invasive determination of local cerebral metabolic rate of glucose in man. *American Journal of Physiology, 238,* E69–82.

Jones, G.V. (1983). On double dissociation of function. *Neuropsychologia, 21,* 397–400.

Kopelman, M.D. (in press). Focal retrograde amnesia and the attribution of causality: An exceptionally critical review. *Cognitive Neuropsychology.*

Kopelman, M.D., Colchester, A., Lasserson, D., Bello, F., Stanhope, N., Rush, C., Stevens, T., Goodman, G., Kendall, B., & Kingsley, D. (1999). *Structural MRI volumetric analysis in patients with organic amnesia: Methods and findings.* Manuscript submitted for publication.

Kopelman, M.D., & Stanhope, N. (1997). Rates of forgetting in organic amnesia following temporal lobe, diencephalic, or frontal lobe lesions. *Neuropsychology, 11,* 343–356.

Kopelman, M.D., & Stanhope, N. (1998). Recall and recognition memory in patients with focal frontal, temporal lobe and diencephalic lesions. *Neuropsychologia, 36,* 785–796.

Kopelman, M.D., Stanhope, N., & Guinan, E. (1998). Subjective memory evaluations in patients with focal frontal, diencephalic, and temporal lobe lesion. *Cortex, 34,* 191–207.

Kopelman, M.D., Stanhope, N., & Kingsley, D. (1997). Temporal and spatial memory in patients with focal frontal, temporal lobe, and diencephalic lesions. *Neuropsychologia, 35,* 1533–1545.

Kuwert, T., Homberg, V., Steinmetz, H., Unverhau, S., Langen, K.J., Herzog, H., & Feinendegen, L.E. (1993). Posthypoxic amnesia: Regional cerebral glucose consumption measured by positron emission tomography. *Journal of the Neurological Sciences, 118,* 10–6.

Lonton, A.P. (1979). The relationship between intellectual skills and the C.A.T.s of children with spina bifida and hydrocephalus. *Zeitschrift für Kinderchirugerie und Grenzgebiete, 28,* 368–374.

Markowitsch, H.J., Weber-Luxenburger, G., Ewald, K., Kessler, J., & Heiss, E.-D. (1997). Patients with heart attacks are not valid models for medial temporal lobe amnesia. A neuropsychological and FDG-PET study with consequences for memory research. *European Journal of Neurology, 4,* 178–184.

Nelson, H.E. (1976). A modified card-sorting test sensitive to frontal lobe deficits. *Cortex, 12,* 313–324.

Nelson, H.E., & Willison, F.R. (1991). *The National Adult Reading Test* (2nd Ed.). Windsor, UK: NFER-Nelson.

Phelps, M.E., Huang, S.C., Hoffman, E.J., Selin, C.J., Sokoloff, L., & Kuhl, D.E. (1979). Tomographic measurement of local cerebral glucose metabolic rate in humans with (F-18)-2-fluoro-2-deoxy-D-glucose: Validation of method. *Annals of Neurology, 6*, 371–388.

Press, G.A., Amaral, D.G., & Squire, L.R. (1989). Hippocampal abnormalities in amnesic patients revealed by high resolution magnetic resonance imaging. *Nature, 341*, 54–57.

Shallice, T. (1988). *From neuropsychology to mental structure.* Cambridge: Cambridge University Press.

Shallice, T., & Evans, M.E. (1978). The involvement of the frontal lobes in cognitive estimates. *Cortex, 14*, 294–303.

Stanhope, N., Guinan, E., & Kopelman, M.D. (1998). Frequency judgements of abstract designs by patients with diencephalic, temporal lobe or frontal lobe lesions. *Neuropsychologia, 36*, 1387–1396.

Valenstein, E., Bowers, D., Verfaellie, M., Heilman, K.M., Day, A., & Watson, R.T. (1987). Retrosplenial amnesia. *Brain, 110*, 1631–1646.

Wechsler, D. (1981). *Wechsler Adult Intelligence Scale—Revised.* London and New York: Psychological Corporation.

Wechsler, D. (1987). *Wechsler Memory Scale—Revised.* London: Psychological Corporation.

Weiskrantz, L. (Ed.). (1968). *Analysis of behavioral change.* New York: Harper & Row.

Zola-Morgan, S., Squire, L.R., & Amaral, D.G. (1986). Human amnesia and the medial temporal region: Enduring memory impairment following a bilateral lesion limited to field CA1 of the hippocampus. *Journal of Neuroscience, 6*, 2950–2967.

MEMORY, 1999, 7 (5/6), 613–659

The Neuroimaging of Long-term Memory Encoding Processes

Andrew R. Mayes and Daniela Montaldi

University of Sheffield, UK

There needs to be more crosstalk between the lesion and functional neuroimaging memory literatures. This is illustrated by a discussion of episode and fact encoding. The lesion literature suggests several hypotheses about which brain regions underlie the storage of episode and fact information, which can be explored by functional neuroimaging. These hypotheses have been underexplored because neuroimaging studies of encoding have been insufficiently hypothesis-driven and have not controlled encoding-related processes sufficiently well to allow clear interpretations of results to be made. Nevertheless, there is good evidence that certain kinds of associative encoding and/or consolidation are sufficient to activate the medial temporal lobes, and preliminary evidence that some kinds of associative priming may reduce activation of this region. It remains to be proved that attentional orienting to certain kinds of novel information activates the medial temporal lobes. Evidence is growing that the HERA model, developed from neuroimaging rather than lesion data, requires modification and that frontal cortex encoding activations are probably caused by executive processes that are important in effortful memory processing. Neuroimaging studies allow the detection of encoding-related activations in previously unexpected brain regions (e.g. parietal lobes) and, in turn, these findings can be explored with lesion studies.

INTRODUCTION

Long-term episodic and semantic memory processes can be investigated not only by examining the effects of selective brain lesions, but also by functional neuroimaging in normal and brain-damaged people. It is, therefore, possible to follow a convergent operations approach in which the findings from neuroimaging have to agree with those from lesioning studies before one can be confident about any conclusions reached. At present, the lesion literature is used to direct what is expected to be found in neuroimaging studies rather than vice-versa, although this will no doubt change as the neuroimaging literature

---

Requests for reprints should be sent to Andrew R. Mayes, Department of Clinical Neurology, Royal Hallamshire Hospital, University of Sheffield, Glossop Road, Sheffield S10 2JF, UK.

expands. When conflicts occur between the two literatures, however, it becomes essential to explain them in a way that modifies our understanding of one or both literatures.

An example of such a conflict arose when nearly all early neuroactivation studies of episodic encoding failed to find evidence of medial temporal lobe (MTL) activation (Demonet et al., 1992; Fletcher et al., 1995; Frith et al., 1991; Grasby et al., 1994; Kapur et al., 1994; Petersen et al., 1988; Raichle et al., 1994; Shallice et al., 1994; Tulving et al., 1994a). As damage to the MTL severely disrupts episodic memory, the lesion literature might yield the expectation that this region should be active during encoding of episodic information (defined as the processing and representation of episodic information at input). Potential explanations have been advanced to resolve the tension between the two literatures although later studies have found MTL activation during encoding (e.g. Dolan & Fletcher, 1997; Montaldi et al., 1998a). These potential explanations have focused on modifying our understanding of what is going on during neuroactivation. Thus, it has been suggested that the MTL is indeed involved with encoding operations, but that very few MTL neurons are activated during any specific encoding operation (''sparse encoding''). Indeed, connectionist modelling has typically been conducted using sparse hippocampal representations (e.g. Foster et al., 1997; Rolls, 1996). If encoding is sparse, the number of neurons activated may often be insufficient to produce detectable blood flow or blood oxygenation changes (Fletcher, Frith, & Rugg, 997). Similarly, it has been suggested that the MTL is continuously engaged in encoding and other memory operations so that any explicitly imposed encoding task only marginally increases its activity level. As with the previous explanation, the effect of this may again be that any changes are undetectable (Fletcher et al., 1997.)

An alternative way of resolving the tension is to modify our understanding of the implications of the lesion literature. Thus, one could argue that MTL lesions do not disrupt encoding and storage of episodic information, but selectively impair retrieval, in which case one would expect episodic retrieval, but not encoding, to activate the MTL. The early neuroimaging studies, however, also usually failed to find MTL activation with episodic retrieval (e.g. Shallice et al., 1994) although some did (Schacter et al., 1995; Squire et al., 1992). In addition, Grasby et al. (1993) found MTL activation in a study that confounded encoding and retrieval so a full interpretation cannot be given. It is, of course, possible that tension resolution requires a modification in our understanding of both neuroimaging and lesion literatures. In other words, it might be true that the MTL is a more or less continuously active ''sparse'' processing system, not concerned with episodic encoding, but instead with the initial consolidation of episodic information that is triggered by encoding, so that it only becomes marginally more active fairly late in and after the window of time designated for scanning encoding.

In our view, the convergent operations approach needs to be followed much more rigorously by functional neuroimaging investigators of long-term episodic and semantic memory. In order to do this it is important to use a hypothesis-driven approach. At present, most of the hypotheses about long-term episodic and semantic memory have been derived from lesion work and so neuroactivation research should be more focused on testing these hypotheses. As the anatomical precision of the hypotheses has increased in the past few years, developments have become more dependent on animal studies because it is now possible to produce very focal lesions in animals using appropriate neurotoxins (see Murray, in press). It is often very difficult to test whether these hypotheses that are based mainly on animal lesion evidence apply equally to humans because testing their predictions requires access to the very rare patients who have highly selective lesions. Probably no human case with relatively selective damage to a structure, such as the hippocampus, has a lesion that approaches in focality what is now achievable in animals that are given neurotoxic lesions. In some cases, the situation may be even more serious as there are no cases where even *relatively* focal damage has been reported. For example, lesions to the human perirhinal cortex (a region of great interest in memory hypotheses largely derived from animal research) appear always to be accompanied by damage to other structures important for memory. Thus, testing hypotheses about episodic and semantic memory has become increasingly difficult in human patients, so the desirability of supplementing lesion work with neuroimaging work is clear. If neuroimaging can achieve sufficient spatial resolution, it should be relatively easy to test the key predictions of the more anatomically specific hypotheses about episodic and semantic memory.

EVIDENCE FROM LESION STUDIES ABOUT THE NEURAL MECHANISMS UNDERLYING THE ENCODING OF FACTS AND EPISODES INTO LONG-TERM MEMORY

Evidence from Medial Temporal Lobe Lesions

Although, as indicated in the Introduction, the early neuroactivation of episodic encoding studies failed to find MTL activation, such activations have commonly been found in more recent studies. Fletcher et al. (1997) pointed out that recent studies have more often found MTL activation with the encoding of visuospatial materials, such as complex visual scenes, rather than with verbal materials. One possible explanation of this is that the visuospatial materials are typically more complex so that subjects are engaged in more complicated encoding processes. However, the precise processes that produce MTL activation during encoding operations still need to be conclusively identified.

Three hypotheses about the psychological processes that produce MTL encoding-related activations are feasible on the basis of lesion studies. The first hypothesis is that the MTL mediates the encoding and/or consolidation into long-term memory of certain kinds of information. The second hypothesis is that the MTL mediates an attentional orienting response triggered by the detection of certain kinds of novelty and so often becomes active when these kinds of novelty are detected. Novelty detection should be inhibited by the retrieval of familiar (non-novel) information, so can be inaccurate as well as accurate depending on the correctness of memory. Activation of attention (which might be operationally defined in terms of autonomic indices) triggered by accurate or inaccurate novelty detection would only have indirect effects on long-term memory through the elaborative encoding that may result when attention is applied to novel information. This elaborative encoding would depend on a different mechanism. The third hypothesis is that the MTL stores certain kinds of information such that when it retrieves (and consequently re-encodes) this information, it is less activated than it would have been when initially exposed to the same information. This effect fits a plausible operational definition of priming or information-specific implicit memory (ISIM) which is that priming is present when a representation is reactivated more completely and efficiently from an encoded cue than it would otherwise have been as a result of being stored in memory. It is generally assumed that such a memory-based increase in processing efficiency is not sufficient to produce aware or explicit memory. Reduced activation would be expected assuming that more efficient processing depends on more economic representation involving fewer neurons (see Wiggs & Martin, 1998). This kind of hypothesis nevertheless implies that the MTL stores certain kinds of information and that it mediates both explicit and implicit memory for these kinds of information, which means that MTL lesions should disrupt both these kinds of memory. The MTL is not, however, responsible for ISIM for those kinds of information (such as words) for which priming is preserved in amnesia (e.g. Schacter & Graf, 1986; and see Shimamura, 1993, for a review).

The MTL comprises not only the hippocampus and amygdala, but also the underlying parahippocampal, perirhinal, and entorhinal cortices. Although the amygdala is believed to play a different role in memory, there is currently controversy about whether lesions of the remaining MTL regions disrupt different psychological processes or whether they disrupt the same process(es) although possibly to different degrees (see Aggleton & Brown, 1999). Aggleton and Shaw (1996) argued, on the basis of a meta-analysis, that lesions of the hippocampus and other structures in Papez circuit including the fornix, the mammillary bodies, and the anterior nucleus of the thalamus, disrupt free recall as much as more global MTL lesions, but have a minimal disruptive effect on item recognition. More recently, Vargha-Khadem et al. (1997) reported that three young patients with early, fairly selective, hippocampal lesions were normal on item recognition, but impaired both on tests of free recall and the associative recognition of face–voice and object–location pairs. The patients were, however, unimpaired at the associative recognition of word–word, nonword–nonword, and face–face pairs. The authors also argued that their patients showed relatively normal memory for facts to which they had been repeatedly exposed over many years.

In unpublished data, we have found fairly similar results with a patient who suffered selective bilateral damage to the hippocampus in adulthood. This patient was impaired at recognition not only of recently studied object–location and face–voice associations (whereas she performed completely normally at object and face recognition tasks, which normal subjects found as hard as the associative tasks), but also at recognition of recently studied intra-list temporal order, animal picture–named occupation associations, and picture–sound associations. Every one of these recognition tasks tapped memory for associations between different kinds of information. In addition, however, the patient was impaired at recognition of word–meaning associations and also at memory for facts to which she had been repeatedly exposed over many years. These findings imply that semantic as well as episodic memory is impaired by hippocampal lesions when different kinds of information have to be linked in memory, which is inconsistent with the view of Vharga-Khadem and her colleagues.

One interpretation of these results, which is a common view of hippocampal and Papez circuit lesion effects (see Mayes & Downes, 1997), is that hippocampal damage only disrupts the consolidation into long-term memory of those factual and episodic associations, the components of which are represented in different neocortical regions (see Mishkin, Vargha-Khadem, & Gadian, 1998). The empirical support for this interpretation should be regarded as preliminary, and future lesion research may well show that the characterisation of the kinds of associative memory hippocampal lesions disrupt, needs to be changed. There is, for example, evidence from human lesion studies that lesions to the parahippocampal cortex, but not the left or right hippocampus, disrupt performance on a spatial memory task designed to be a human equivalent of the Morris water maze (Bohbot et al., 1997). This conflicts with other evidence about the effects of selective hippocampal lesions on spatial memory in both humans and animals (e.g. Parkinson, Murray, & Mishkin, 1988). Bohbot et al.'s hippocampal patients, however, had mainly suffered anterior damage and it has been argued that it is the posterior hippocampus that is specialised in spatial memory in humans (Moser & Moser, 1998). This may explain why these particular hippocampal patients did not show a spatial memory deficit. Although more work clearly needs to be done before the exact roles of the parahippocampal cortex and different regions of the hippocampus in spatial memory can be confidently identified, two comments are warranted. First, if Moser and Moser are correct, only the posterior hippocampus should activate when encoding certain kinds of spatial information, although encoding other kinds of associative information may activate more anterior hippocampal regions. Second, the parahippocampal cortex may primarily be activated by encoding spatial information, as damage to it seems to have a much larger effect on visual object-location association memory than visual object memory in monkeys (Parkinson et al., 1988).

Although the hippocampus might be concerned with storing certain kinds of association, the precise nature of which remains controversial, the mnemonic functions of other MTL structures may be different. It has been accepted for some time that amygdala damage does not cause a general deficit in long-term memory for fact and event information. There is evidence, however, that such damage disrupts emotional memory under some conditions. Phelps et al. (1998) have argued that such damage only impairs the beneficial effects of emotion on memory that relate to increased arousal. This would be consistent with the amygdala modulating the activity of other MTL structures involved in consolidating fact and episodic information into long-term memory (see Cahill & McGaugh, 1998). This kind of modulation should increase the strength of memory storage as may be seen in phenomena like flashbulb memory. If the account is true, then the amygdala's level of activation during encoding should correlate with the strength of subsequent memory for emotional stimuli, but not for neutral stimuli as has indeed been claimed in a positron emission tomography (PET) activation study (Cahill et al., 1996). Phelps and her colleagues argued that it is such stronger consolidation into long-term memory, triggered by the modulatory activity of the amygdala, that produces better memory rather than richer encoding of the emotionally arousing information. Determination of this in both lesion and neuroimaging studies would require that encoding is either controlled or carefully monitored and effects on subsequent memory for emotional and neutral materials carefully assessed.

There is some evidence from animal studies that hippocampal and perirhinal cortex lesions doubly dissociate in their disruptive effects on memory (for example, Ennaceur, Neave, & Aggleton, 1996). Lesion studies with animals show that perirhinal cortex damage disrupts item recognition whereas hippocampal damage does not. In contrast, hippocampal damage disrupts spatial memory whereas perirhinal cortex damage does not, at least when the location of specific objects does not have to be remembered (see Murray, in press). So, the perirhinal cortex may be primarily concerned with storing intra-item associations, i.e. associations between the components that constitute an item and which are vital for item memory. It may also be involved in storing item–item associations when the associated items are of the same kind and are, therefore, represented in the same neocortical region (see Aggleton & Brown, 1999). Although the perirhinal cortex may not be concerned with linking components represented in different neocortical regions, damage to it may still disrupt some of these forms of memory because it supplies the hippocampus, where such memories may be consolidated, with critical information (for example, about items).

Not everyone believes that the MTL is functionally heterogeneous. For example, Reed and Squire (1997) have reported that six patients, who they argued had selective hippocampal lesions, were very impaired at item recognition when a wide range of item recognition tests were used. If they were correct, this would imply that both the hippocampus and perirhinal cortex are equally involved in storing item information, which must include intra-item associations. They have provided no evidence, however, that perirhinal cortex lesions disrupt the same kind of inter-item associative memories that are disrupted by selective hippocampal lesions. All episodic and semantic memory is probably associative in the sense that forming such memories involves strengthening the links between components that are either items, parts of items, or relationships between items or their parts. On the view of Reed and Squire, the hippocampus and perirhinal cortex are equally involved in storing both intra- and inter-item associations (of all kinds) whereas the view that we considered earlier suggests that the hippocampus is mainly concerned with memory for cross-regional associations whereas the perirhinal cortex is concerned with memory for intra-regional associations either between items of the same kind or components of single items. Resolution of which view is correct depends on clarifying whether or not selective hippocampal damage causes item recognition deficits. At present, some patients, described as selectively damaged, show preserved item recognition whereas others, such as the patients of Reed and Squire (1997), are clearly impaired. The difference may reflect undetected damage to other structures related to item recognition memory that occurs in the impaired patients, but not in patients with normal or nearly normal item recognition. This possibility can be tested by measuring controlled resting state cerebral blood flow (CBF) in patients using Positron Emission Tomography (PET) or Single Photon Emission Computed Tomography (SPECT) techniques in order to determine whether any structures, apparently normal when examined with structural magnetic resonance imaging (MRI), display functional abnormalities. If Reed and Squire are correct, then ''hippocampal'' patients with and without item recognition deficits will not differ with respect to amount of reduced blood flow in extra-hippocampal brain regions. If Aggleton and Brown are correct, then patients with worse recognition deficits will show additional regions of reduced blood flow.

Several issues related to these theoretical ideas need to be clarified. First, no reason has been given to suggest that amnesics have a problem with consolidation rather than with encoding or retrieval. Such evidence does, however, exist. Many amnesics show preserved intelligence. It is, therefore, difficult to believe that they encode complex information more slowly and less richly so that encoding deficits underlie their memory failures. Mayes et al. (1993) have also shown that amnesics can answer spatial, semantic and other kinds of questions about recently encoded pictures as well as their controls when performance relies primarily on their intact short-term memories. There is also direct evidence that initial consolidation failure underlies amnesia in so far as amnesics with either MTL or midline diencephalic lesions show accelerated loss of free recall of organised word lists and stories, but not of item recognition (Isaac & Mayes, in press a, b). Free recall depends more than item recognition on retrieving inter-item associations and the memory deficit for these associations would be expected to get worse as normal memory performance depends increasingly on consolidated long-term storage with the passage of time.

Second, it may seem implausible to argue that the perirhinal cortex and hippocampus have different psychological functions. This is because the perirhinal and parahippocampal cortices provide about two thirds of the cortical projections received by the entorhinal cortex, which in turn provides most of the cortical input into the hippocampus, and the hippocampus backprojects to these cortical regions. The perirhinal cortex does, however, also project to the dorsomedial nucleus of the thalamus and it could be that this circuit mediates the ability to store intra-item associations and other intra-regional associations whereas projections from other perirhinal cortex neurons to the hippocampus provide the cross-regional inter-item associative information that it stores. This would be compatible with a double dissociation between perirhinal cortex and hippocampal lesion effects. On the other hand, if key associative information is projected to the hippocampus via the perirhinal cortex, then only a single dissociation would be expected. In this dissociation, lesions to the perirhinal cortex, but not the hippocampus, should disrupt item memory whereas both kinds of lesions should disrupt inter-item associative memory.

Third, it is widely believed that whatever information the hippocampus stores, it does so only temporarily because over time through processes of explicit as well as unintentional rehearsal the memory trace is reorganised so that the information comes to be stored in association neocortical sites (Squire & Alvarez, 1995.) One implication of this hypothesis is that the hippocampus should not be involved with retrieval after reorganisation has occurred. This hypothesis does not go unchallenged, however as, for example, Moscovitch and Nadel (1997) have argued that the relevant memories remain stored in the hippocampus indefinitely.

The lesion evidence considered so far supports the view that the hippocampus directly mediates the storage of factual and episodic information. However, Gray (1982) argued that the hippocampus is not directly involved in memory at all. Rather, he argued, that if it and other Papez circuit structures detect either novelty (a mismatch between actual and predicted events) or aversiveness, they switch on a behavioural inhibition system (that underlies anxiety). In addition to the inhibition of behaviour, the Papez circuit structures switch on increased arousal and attention that is particularly directed at the aspects of the environment that are regarded as novel. This should clearly have at least indirect beneficial effects on subsequent memory for these environmental events. It could be, of course, that believers in the direct role of the MTL are correct and Gray is only partially correct because although the MTL is involved in attentional orienting to novelty, which has an indirect boosting effect on memory, it is also directly involved with storing certain kinds of association.

Some recent lesion evidence supports part of Gray's hypothesis because it implies that MTL damage disrupts the making of orienting reactions to certain kinds of novelty. Thus, Knight (1996) reported that patients with MTL lesions extending beyond the hippocampus showed reduced event related potential (ERP) and autonomic responses to novel stimuli. In his study, he used an oddball task, but was able to interpret his data as showing a problem with novelty orienting because he used both familiar and novel items as the rare events, and the patients only showed ERP signs of deficient attentional orienting to the novel items. There is some evidence from rats that more selective hippocampal lesions do not disrupt novelty responding to items, but do disrupt the expression of novelty responding to new cross-modal associations between items (Honey, Watt, & Good, 1998).

Parker, Wilding, and Akerman (1998) also found support for this last conclusion. They showed that monkeys with bilateral lesions of the amygdala and fornix showed a normal von Restorff effect with coloured fractal stimuli, but that monkeys with lesions disconnecting prefrontal cortex from either perirhinal cortex or the magnocellular mediodorsal thalamus showed no such effect. The study raises the question of what ''novelty'' means. Several senses of novelty have been suggested which include: (a) information that has never been encountered before, (b) information that has not been encountered before in this context, or (c) a context that has not been encountered before (see Martin, 1999). In each case, it can be asked ''Does the information need to be objectively novel in the defined sense or is it subjective novelty (i.e. the information is believed to be novel even when it is not) that matters?'' The von Restorff effect involves detecting that a novel item is different from other novel items in a study set because it belongs to a different class from the other items. For example, the target is a blue shape and the distractors are red shapes. In other words, the item stands out because it is unexpected. If this is regarded as novelty, it is most similar to (b) provided this includes both items that are novel in a context and kinds of item that are novel in a context because all other items are of a different kind. Given the pattern of Parker et al.'s results, it could be, therefore, that the hippocampal system triggers attention to associations between different kinds of information that are deemed worthy of attention whereas the perirhinal cortex system triggers attention to items, deemed so worthy. The information could be worthy of attention because it is novel in any of the aforementioned senses or aversive (see Gray, 1982). Activation of this orienting system results in better memory (the von Restorff effect), which probably results from more elaborative encoding although better memory could also result from more efficient consolidation of the attended inputs. Future work needs to establish to what degree detecting these different things, and the additional attentional, encoding, and possibly consolidational processes that may be triggered, activate the same or different brain structures.

The postulated orienting systems involving the MTL require that mechanism(s) exist for detecting whether specified kinds of informational input are worthy of attention, a mechanism for triggering an attentional orienting response associated with autonomic and EEG markers, and possibly a mechanism for engaging the encoding of additional information (or even more effective consolidation of encoded information). The major issue to be resolved is what brain regions underlie these different mechanisms. It remains unresolved whether detection of novelty in the different senses indicated earlier depends on the same brain mechanisms. It also remains unresolved whether novelty detection and the triggering of attentional orienting depend on distinct brain mechanisms. The detection of novelty must require that novel information is encoded sufficiently thoroughly so that retrieval processes can be mounted in order to decide that the information is not in memory and is appropriately novel. Current lesion evidence does not show directly that the MTL is involved with these processes. For example, Knight (1996) found that MTL lesions disrupted the autonomic and ERP markers of attentional orienting to novelty. Both he and Honey et al. (1998) have only shown that MTL lesions disrupt components of the orienting reaction to novelty, and not the detection of novelty itself. Indeed, it is unclear that MTL damage impairs the ability to identify all forms of novelty because most amnesics are very ready to declare that information is not in their memory, i.e. is novel.

The relationship between detecting novelty and the attentional orienting functions, the elaborative encoding functions, and possibly the consolidation functions that this may trigger, have been little explored. If novelty detection often triggers the other processes, it is likely that all these processes will not be statistically independent of each other. If MTL structures are involved in mediating both attentional orienting to novelty and certain kinds of associative encoding or storage, then it will need to be determined whether these two kinds of processes are mediated by the same MTL structures or different ones. It is obvious that neuroimaging studies have the potential to address this issue as well as the issue of whether novelty detection without attentional orienting is sufficient to activate certain parts of the MTL or whether it activates other brain regions.

It may also be the case that repeatedly encoding exactly the same information may progressively reduce the degree of MTL activation found so that initial encoding of the information should produce the biggest MTL activation. This reduced activation may be linked to a diminished impact of the encoding processes on episodic memory for the encoded information. If reduced MTL activation occurs, it could also possibly reflect the priming of the kinds of information that are stored in the MTL. Martin (1999) has suggested that MTL activation may reduce when stimuli and encoding operations are repeated even when MTL lesions do not seem to disrupt priming for the information in question. This is clearly possible and would mean that the MTL is not critically involved in the studied kind of priming. Care should be taken before reaching this conclusion, however, because the MTL deactivation may relate to priming of different information that is not tapped intentionally by the priming task, performance on which is unaffected by MTL lesions. The unmeasured kind of priming may depend critically on the MTL.

Although amnesics with MTL lesions often show deficits in their priming of information that had been novel prior to study, it is unclear whether this indicates a deficit in ISIM for novel item and novel associative information or whether it arises because normal subjects make use of their superior effortful explicit memory processes to aid their performance (see Schacter & Buckner, 1998a). The one exception to this generalisation is a study by Chun and Phelps (1998). This involved visual search of complex arrays of shapes, some of which were repeated. Although normal subjects showed no recognition of repeated arrays, their search speed increased. Amnesics did not show this speed-up effect. The array comprised the kind of item–spatial location associations likely to be stored in the MTL. The results are, therefore, consistent with the view that MTL structures are involved with ISIM for certain kinds of novel association. This view is plausible if one accepts: (1) that explicit and implicit memory for the same information is stored in the same neurons, and (2) that associations between different kinds of information are stored in the hippocampus.

If it is also assumed that when stored information is re-encoded in the same way as it was when novel, the representing brain regions will show less activation than during the initial encoding, then the hippocampus should be less activated when certain kinds of inter-item association are re-encoded. This third assumption is directly supported by neuroimaging studies of perceptual and semantic kinds of repetition priming, nearly all of which have found reduced activation on repetition of the same encoding operation on a repeated item in the neocortical regions that are likely to represent the information that is being re-encoded (for example, Buckner et al., 1998; Demb et al., 1995; Martin et al., 1995). It is also supported by single-unit recording work in animals (see Aggleton and Brown, 1999; Wiggs & Martin, 1998), which shows that some neurons probably concerned with stimulus representation show reduced firing rates with stimulus repetition. Wiggs and Martin (1998) have plausibly suggested that these changes arise because information is more sharply and efficiently coded by fewer neurons in the representing region. Those neurons showing reduced activity on stimulus repetition may be being "tuned out" from representing the stimulus so that representation comes to involve a reduced set of neurons that are more intensely activated. Neuroimaging studies would probably find a reduction in activation in the representing regions because many fewer neurons would be activated following repetition although they would be more intensely activated. The smaller neural pool involved should also lead to enhanced speed and accuracy of responding (such enhanced processing is the defining characteristic of priming or ISIM). In other words, the sharpened neural coding should lead to behavioural priming or ISIM.

Although two ERP studies have shown that priming is associated with reduced amplitude of parts of the waveform (see Wiggs & Martin, 1998), Rugg et al. (1998) found equivalent enhanced positivity of the ERP 300 to 500ms following word presentation at parietal electrode sites for previously studied words whether or not they were recognised. This indicates that unaware memory, and hence presumably a kind of priming, was sufficient to produce short latency enhanced positivity of the ERP at specific electrode sites. The enhanced positivity could be driven by increased synchronisation of neural activity in the representing region. Wiggs and Martin should be able to accommodate such synchronisation within their model if they postulate that the smaller neural pool can sometimes work synchronously when it represents the primed information, and that a reduction in blood flow or blood oxygenation in the brain area that includes the neuronal pool probably occurs whether the neurons fire synchronously or asynchronously.

It is possible, therefore, that MTL and perhaps hippocampal activation is produced by either or both of: (1) the encoding or consolidation into long-term memory of various kinds of information, the nature of which depends on the MTL regions involved, and (2) the production of attentional orienting to the same kinds of information that are deemed worthy of attention or possibly even the mere detection of novelty (or other kinds of feature such as aversiveness or surprisingness that trigger orienting). Involvement of the MTL in novelty detection alone seems somewhat implausible, however, because *inter alia* it implies that patients with hippocampal or MTL damage cannot identify whether certain pieces of associative information come from their remotely pre-morbid associative memories or are novel. This is contrary to the majority view that remote pre-morbid memory is relatively preserved in such patients. In other words, where patients' memory is normal, it would be surprising if their novelty detection were not as well.

There is also another possible source of MTL activation if re-encoding the same associative information (a kind of operational definition of priming or ISIM for associations) activates the MTL region less than the first encoding of that information. The implication is that associative encoding leads to a maximal MTL activation when it is first performed and that this effect has nothing to do with attentional orienting towards novelty or any other kind of detected feature. Thereafter, repetition of the encoding will lead to progressively decreasing activation of the MTL so that any effects on long-term memory may also decline. It is even possible that prolonged repetition may ultimately cause an inhibition of the MTL.

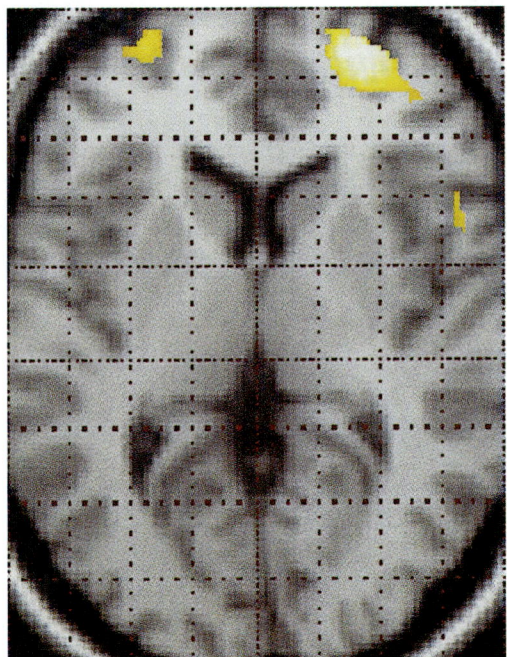

PLATE 1 (Van der Linden et al.). Brain activation observed when the short-term memory task is subtracted from the updating task. Regions with significant rCBF increase are superimposed on a transverse T1-weighted magnetic resonance imaging slice normalised into a standard stereotactical space (Talairach & Tournoux, 1988). Left hemisphere is on the right. Section is located 4mm above the reference plane.

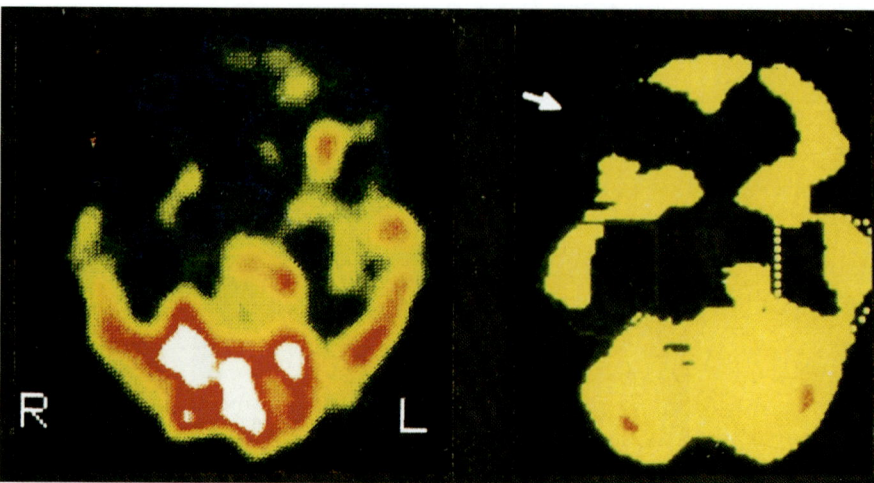

PLATE 2 (Markowitsch). Horizontal SPECT-images through the brains of two patients with selective retrograde amnesia for autobiographical information. The section on the left is from a patient with a probable organically based amnesia (herpes simplex encephalitis; Calabrese et al., 1996). It was done three years post-infection and demonstrates the area of hypoperfusion in the right temporo-frontal region. The section on the right shows the brain of a patient with probable psychogenic amnesia (Markowitsch et al., 1997a). Again, a significant metabolic reduction is visible in the right temporo-frontal junction zone (after Calabrese et al., 1996, and Markowitsch et al., 1997a).

PLATE 3 (opposite, top: Fletcher & Dolan). Regions of PFC showing a significant activity in association with the presentation of *wholly familiar* compared to *wholly novel* material. A statistical parametric map rendered onto sections of a stereotactically normalised structural mri is shown. The sections were chosen (coordinates [Talairach & Tournoux, 1988] X, Y, Z = 48, 12, 12) to show area of prefrontal activation. In the bottom right panel is shown the plot of parameter estimates for this voxel (48, 12, 12) for conditions 1 (wholly novel material), 2 (partially familiar), and 3 (wholly familiar). It can be seen that the level of activity in the region is highest in association with the presentation of wholly familiar material, with the partially familiar condition showing an intermediate level of activity.

PLATE 4 (opposite, bottom: Fletcher & Dolan). Regions of PFC showing a significant activity in association with the presentation of *partially familiar* compared to *wholly novel* material. A statistical parametric map rendered onto sections of a stereotactically normalised structural mri is shown. The sections were chosen (coordinates [Talairach & Tournoux, 1988] X, Y, Z = 44, 20, 26) show a more dorsal region of right PFC. In the bottom right panel is shown the plot of parameter estimates for this voxel for conditions 1 (wholly novel material), 2 (partially familiar), and 3 (wholly familiar). It can be seen that the level of activity in the region is highest in association with the presentation of partially familiar material, with the wholly familiar condition reflected in an intermediate level of activity.

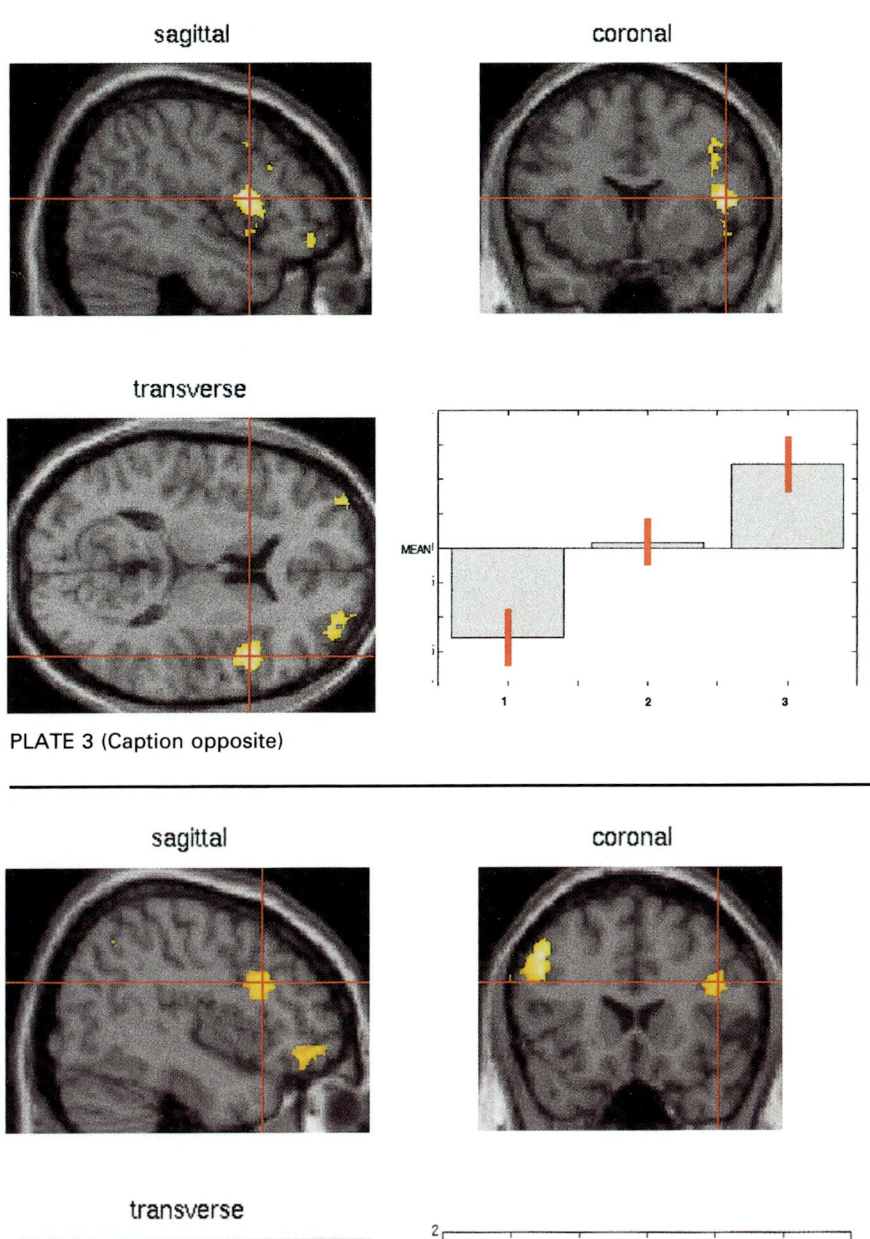

sagittal

coronal

transverse

PLATE 3 (Caption opposite)

sagittal

coronal

transverse

PLATE 4 (Caption opposite)

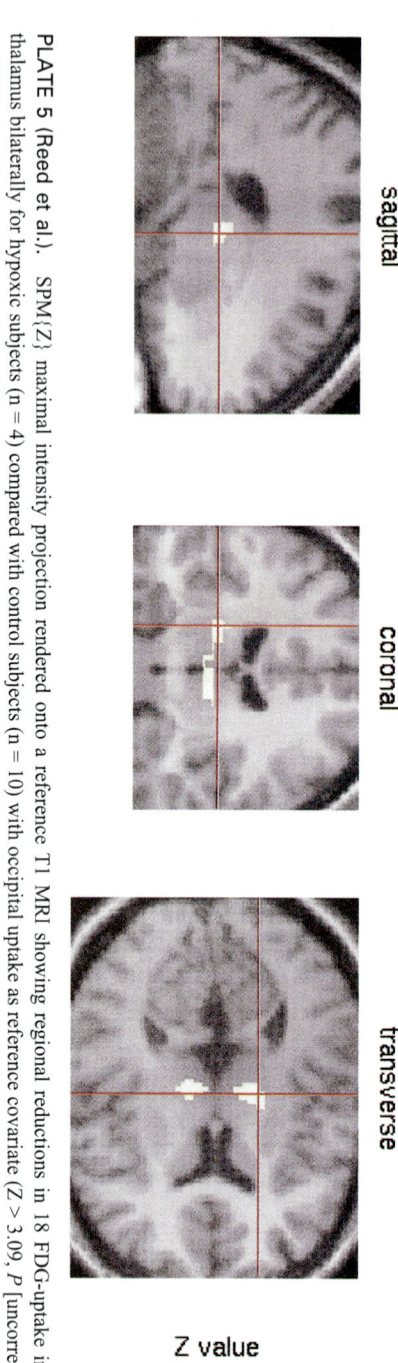

sagittal　　　coronal　　　transverse

PLATE 5 (Reed et al.). SPM{Z} maximal intensity projection rendered onto a reference T1 MRI showing regional reductions in 18 FDG-uptake in the thalamus bilaterally for hypoxic subjects (n = 4) compared with control subjects (n = 10) with occipital uptake as reference covariate (Z > 3.09, P [uncorrected] < .001).

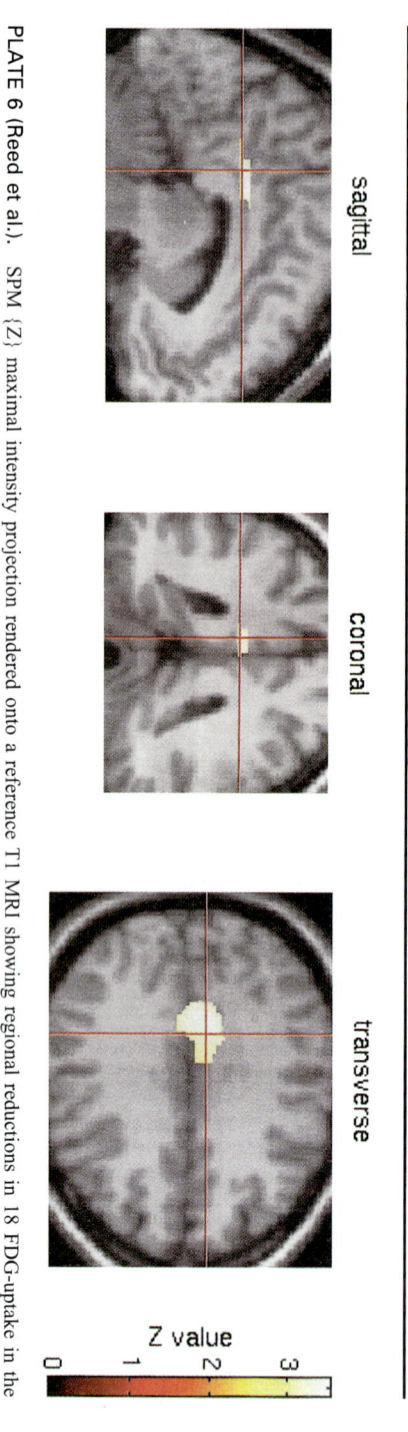

sagittal　　　coronal　　　transverse

PLATE 6 (Reed et al.). SPM {Z} maximal intensity projection rendered onto a reference T1 MRI showing regional reductions in 18 FDG-uptake in the retrosplenial posterior cingulate cortex bilaterally for hypoxic subjects (n = 4) compared with control subjects (n = 10) with occipital uptake as reference covariate (Z > 3.09), P [uncorrected] < .001).

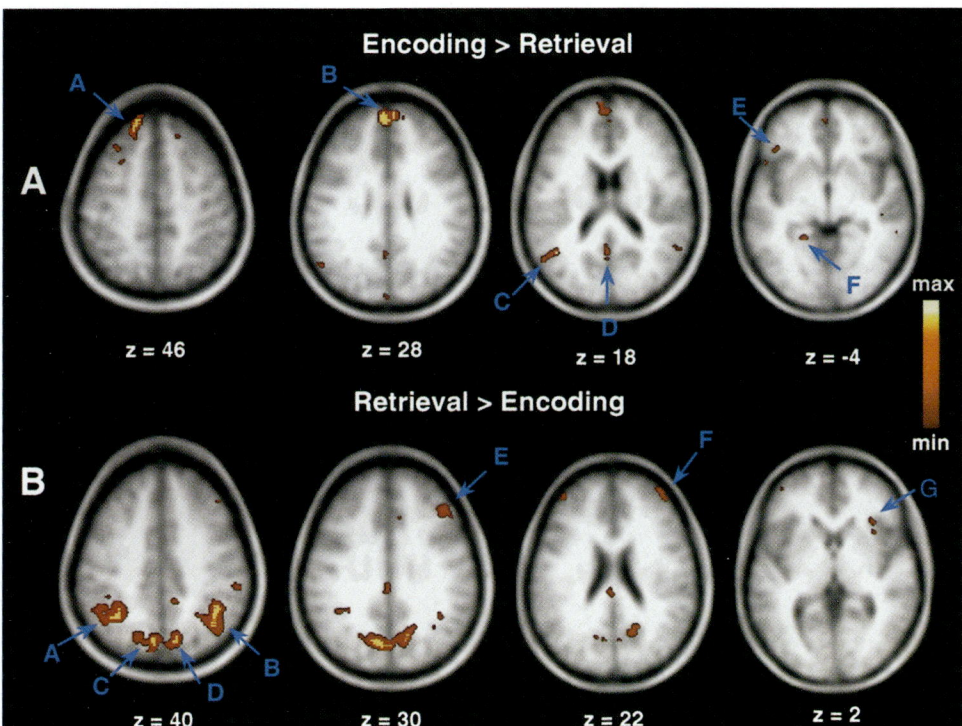

PLATE 7 (McDermott et al.). Regions differentially active in encoding and retrieval. Coloured pixels exceeded the statistical threshold and were superimposed on the corresponding anatomical images (averaged for eight subjects, and warped into atlas space). The colour scale represents the significance level for activations from red (lowest) to yellow (highest). The left side of the images correspond to the left side of the brain. Panel A. Regions more active in encoding than retrieval. Peak activations included left superior frontal cortex (A); medial frontal cortex (B); left superior temporal cortex (C); posterior cingulate (D); left inferior frontal cortex (E); and left parahippocampal gyrus (F). Panel B. Regions more active in retrieval than encoding. Peak activations included bilateral inferior parietal cortex (A, B); bilateral precuneus (C, D); right dorsolateral prefrontal cortex (E); right frontal polar cortex (F); and right inferior frontal/insular cortex (G).

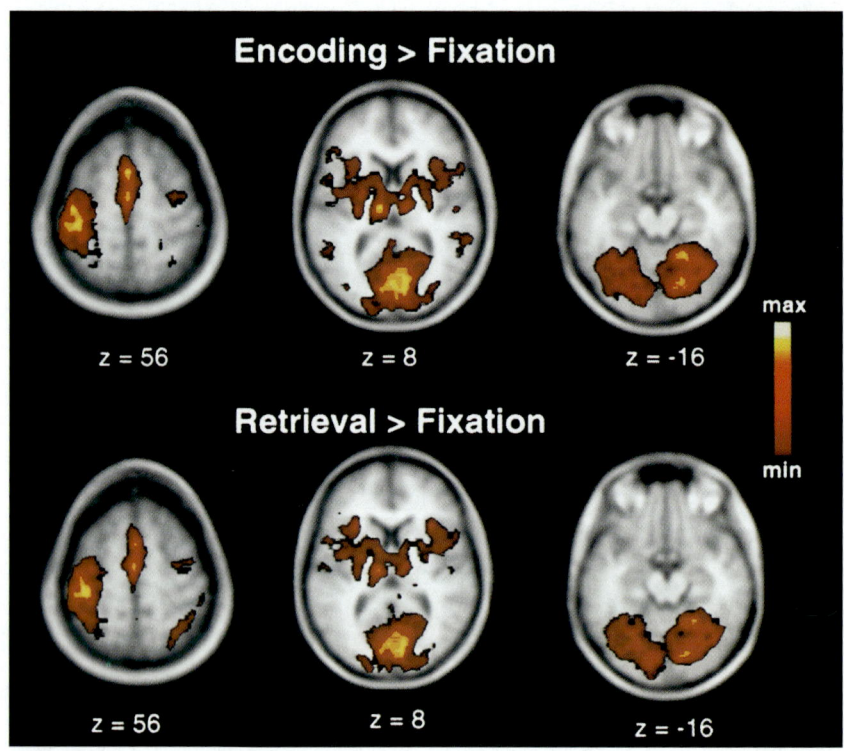

PLATE 8 (McDermott et al.).   Similarity of activation observed in encoding and retrieval runs can be seen in these slices. The most superior slice (z = 56) demonstrates SMA and motor cortex. The middle slice (z = 8) shows activations in bilateral frontal opercula, bilateral thalamus (L>R), bilateral putamen, and visual cortex. The most inferior slice shows cerebellar activation.

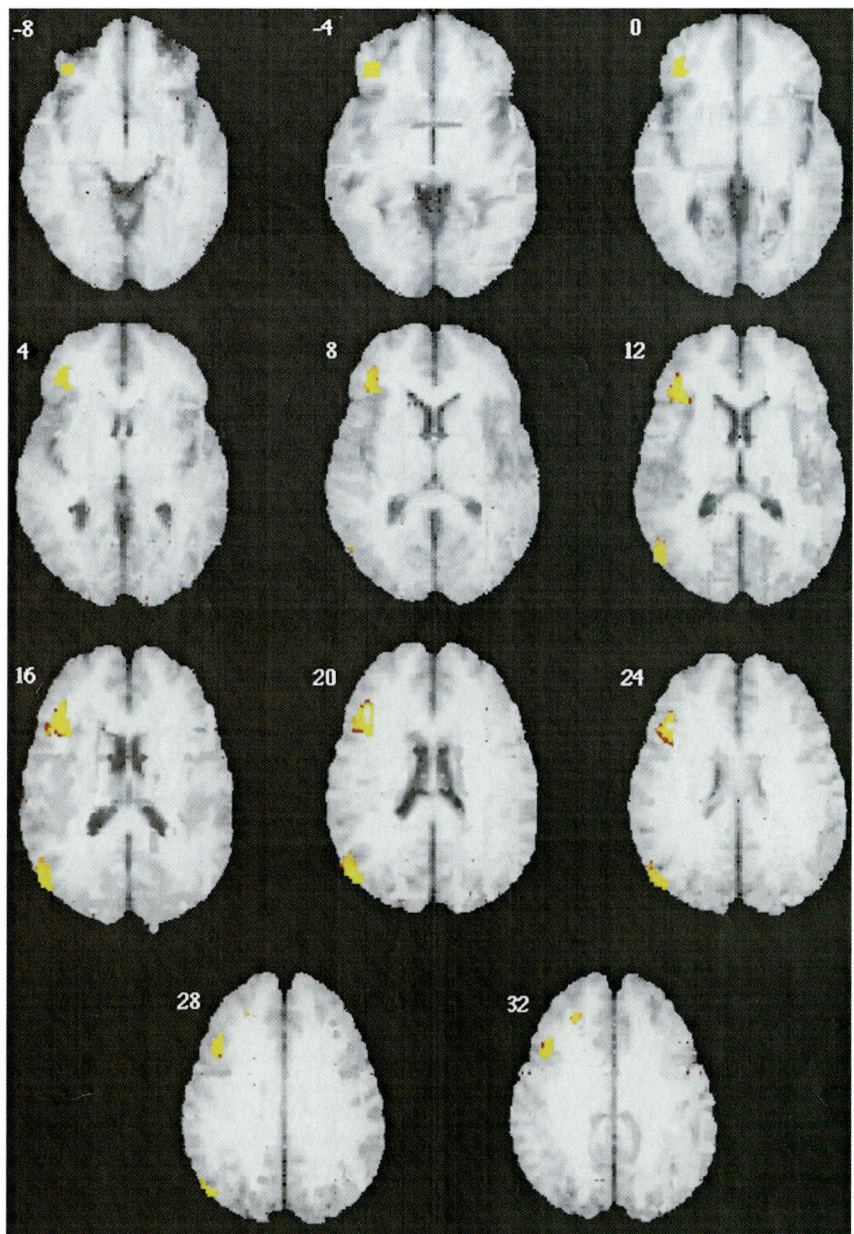

PLATE 9 (Conway et al.). Areas of functional activation during AM relative to PA. SPM-generated foci are overlaid onto the co-registered summed MRI derived from all study participants' data.

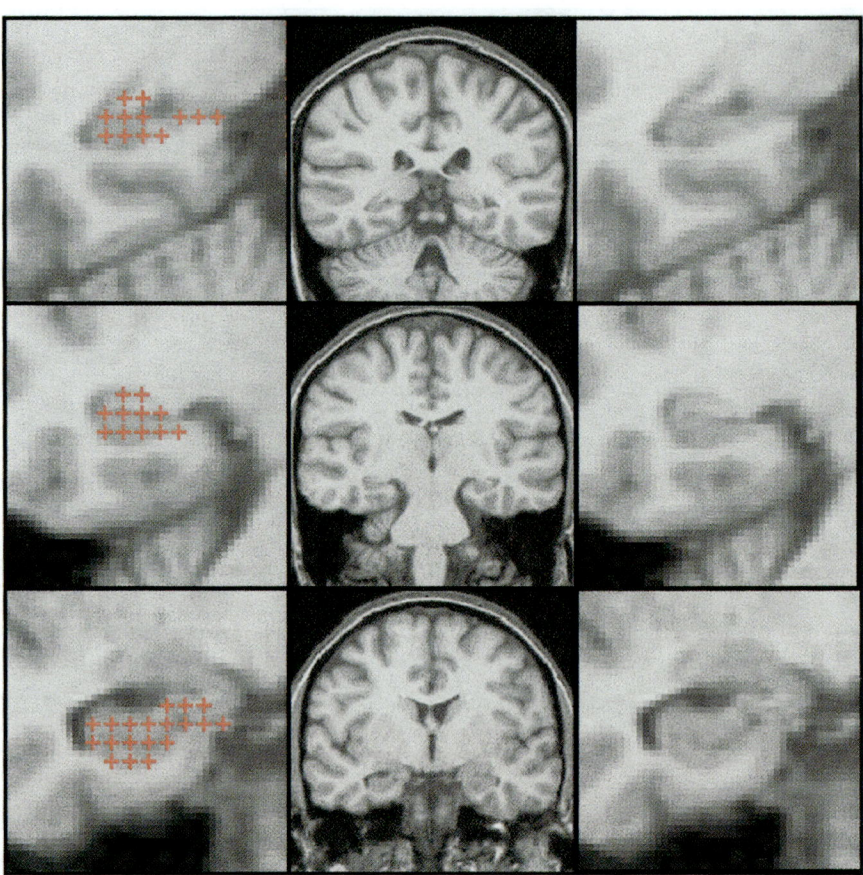

PLATE 10 (Foster et al.). Stereological estimation of hippocampal volume. Three sets of sections through the tail, body, and head are shown (rows 1, 2, and 3 respectively). These sections illustrate the hippocampus overlain with the stereological grid (mag ×2; column 1), slice location (column 2), and magnified (×2) view of the temporal lobe (column 3). Row 1 shows the posterior limit of the hippocampus, and in row 3 the alveus delineates the hippocampus from the amygdala.

Evidence from Frontal Lobe Lesions

The MTL is not the only brain region involved in mediating long-term memory for facts and personally experienced episodes. It is well known that frontal association cortex lesions also disrupt encoding and retrieval of long-term memory. Lesions in this brain region have been reported typically to impair free recall more than recognition, disrupt temporal order and source memory, increase susceptibility to interference, and cause certain kinds of metamemory failure (see Mayes, 1988). The reason for these impairments is most likely to be that prefrontal association cortex damage disrupts the executive processes that are important in effortful encoding and retrieval. Encoding very often requires a person to relate the components of experienced information together as well as to other information that must be retrieved in an organised fashion from the person's long-term memory. Similarly, retrieval often requires a person to search for appropriate retrieval cues that form part of the target memory and are capable of automatically eliciting it. Also, it requires the retriever to check whether any retrieved memories satisfy the criteria for being targets. Although the memory deficits produced by frontal and MTL lesions sometimes appear to be similar, it is proposed that whereas frontal lesions disrupt memory because they disturb effortful and plan-dependent encoding and/or retrieval processes, this is not true of MTL lesions which disrupt storage or consolidation processes, leaving effortful encoding and retrieval unaffected.

One possible exception to this generalisation is that orbitofrontal cortex lesions may disrupt long-term recognition memory in much the same way as perirhinal cortex lesions (e.g. Meunier, Bachevalier, & Mishkin, 1997). This would follow if Aggleton and Brown (1999) are correct in arguing that perirhinal cortex forms a serial processing system with the dorsomedial nucleus of the thalamus and the orbitofrontal cortex. If this is correct, then the orbitofrontal cortex should activate whenever the perirhinal cortex is activated by an encoding challenge task. In contrast, other frontal cortex regions such as the dorsolateral pre-frontal cortex should activate only when certain kinds of effortful encoding or retrieval operations are engaged. Neuroimaging should provide a powerful method of determining which kinds of executive processes are engaged during long-term memory encoding. Such imaging may also be valuable in identifying whether there are other brain regions, not previously highlighted by lesion studies, that are prominently activated during the encoding of some or all kinds of fact/episode information. If essentially involved in encoding, selective damage to these regions, when formally investigated, should be found to cause appropriate kinds of memory failure. Appropriate analysis of neuroimaging studies should help determine to what extent the MTL, pre-frontal regions, and other brain regions are coherently activated during the various kinds of encoding-related processes.

DESIDERATA FOR SHOWING WHAT PROCESSES UNDERLIE MTL AND OTHER KINDS OF ENCODING-RELATED NEUROACTIVATION

Identifying the Causes of MTL Effects

At present, neuroimaging research has shown that the MTL is activated sometimes during encoding, but has not specifically confirmed whether activations or deactivations result from the encoding/consolidation into memory of certain information, processes connected to novelty detection, the priming of information of certain kinds, or some combination of these processes. More is perhaps known about the different MTL activations produced by encoding different kinds of information such as verbal and spatial materials.

In order to show that MTL activation results from a certain kind of associative encoding, it is possible to use the standard subtraction or conjunction techniques (Friston, 1997), matching the stimuli across conditions for the relevant kinds of novelty and ensuring that the conditions differ solely with respect to the critical kind of associative encoding. This requires that subjects are not allowed to engage in spontaneous encoding, but encode only in specified ways. After scanning, some information can be gained about whether subjects engaged in equivalent degrees of novelty detection across conditions by debriefing them appropriately. This may be important because doing some kinds of demanding encoding tasks may reduce the likelihood of detecting novelty. It should not be assumed that because novel materials are presented, their novelty is detected by subjects. It is important to ask people appropriately about the extent to which they detected that materials were novel actually at the time these materials were being processed. Detecting that information is novel in the study context may produce different activations in the MTL from detecting that it is novel in a context-free sense, so it is also necessary to identify which kind of novelty subjects have detected if one wishes to pursue this question. Of course, post-scan debriefing is likely to lead to relatively inaccurate reporting which can only identify broad trends. An alternative is to get subjects' reports on novelty detection during the scan itself. Although clearly more accurate, this may prevent other important measures being taken during the scanning session.

As lesion work suggests that item encoding will activate the perirhinal cortex, it will be important to show that single item encoding activates this structure in contrast to associative encoding of the appropriate kinds which should activate the hippocampus. Lesion work with monkeys also suggests that parahippo-campal activation may be found when spatial information is encoded, but to a much smaller and probably undetectable level when items are encoded (see Parkinson et al., 1988). However, although neuroimaging indicates that encoding allocentric spatial information does activate the parahippocampal cortex (Maguire et al., 1998a), encoding words has been reported to do so as well (e.g. Wagner et al., 1998b). Either there is a functional difference between human and monkey parahippocampus, the item encoding studies have been misinterpreted (associative encoding may also be occurring incidentally), or there is an unexplained mismatch between lesion and neuroimaging literatures, which requires resolution.

The procedures suggested earlier do not, however, distinguish between encoding (defined as the processing and representation of specific kinds of information) and the consolidation of this information into long-term memory. If one wishes to determine whether the hippocampus is involved with the consolidation, but not the encoding of cross-regional inter-item associations, one might use one or more of three approaches. First, one could functionally neuroimage amnesics who have apparently intact hippocampal regions, but damage to structures such as the fornix. If, as is likely (Mayes et al., 1993), these patients can be shown to have encoded the associative information normally, but memory for it is impaired, and hippocampal activation reflects consolidation but not encoding, then these patients, unlike normal subjects, should not show MTL activation.

Second, one could correlate degree of neuroactivation produced by an associative encoding task with the level of performance on a subsequent associative memory test. In other words, one could examine whether those subjects who show more activation in specific regions also tend to show better memory for the encoded information. If there is a strong positive correlation, this suggests that it is consolidation rather than the initial encoding that activates the hippocampus. This interpretation would, however, only be strongly supported if one controlled encoding very tightly in order that there was little variation across subjects, so that any correlations between subjects' level of activation in specific structures and their associative memory could not plausibly be explained as results of richer encoding producing more activation and better memory.

A third and related approach, which has several advantages over this cross-subject correlational method, is only possible with event-related functional MRI (fMRI). Emission tomography and earlier fMRI methods required that different conditions were presented in different scanning blocks. In event-related fMRI procedures, however, different types of psychological event can be intermixed randomly and activations produced by the different kinds of event can be analysed separately in a manner similar to ERPs (see Josephs, Turner, & Friston, 1997). This procedure prevents subjects adopting different strategy sets for the different kinds of event, which is a risk with block design procedures. Event-related fMRI can, therefore, be used to show that subsequently remembered associations produce more activation in hippocampal or other MTL sites than unremembered associations despite the fact that encoding across items has been closely matched (e.g. Brewer et al., 1998; Wagner et al., 1998b). Unlike the correlational method, intra-subject activations can be related directly to whether or not encoded items are later remembered. Selection of appropriate trial lengths with such event-related fMRI might also enable one to identify the time course of the MTL activation.

These three kinds of procedure could also be used to determine whether it is the encoding or the consolidation into long-term memory of item information that activates the perirhinal cortex. The only difference apart from the need to control item rather than associative encoding is that, for the first procedure, patients with selective damage to the projections from the perirhinal cortex would need to be functionally neuroimaged. For example, patients with fairly selective dorsomedial thalamic lesions could be scanned. The procedures should also enable one to determine whether encoding of associations between different kinds of information activates more than one neocortical region, as was suggested in the previous section for those forms of associative memory that are disrupted by hippocampal lesions (see Mishkin et al., 1998). These encoding-related neocortical activations should be the same whether or not encoded information is later remembered. Demonstrating them clearly requires the choice of an appropriate comparison baseline.

It is much harder to determine whether an MTL effect results from one or more processes connected with the detection of novelty (such as attentional orienting) or to an effect that is operationally equivalent to priming or ISIM of certain kinds of information such as the re-encoding of information stored in the MTL. If one uses the standard subtraction procedure, matches the kind of encoding performed across conditions, and varies the degree of novelty of the stimuli in different conditions, then any observed MTL novelty activation could reflect either the attentional orienting resulting from the detection of novelty, the detection of certain kinds of novelty alone, or the reduced MTL activation produced when the same encoding operation is repeated.

With respect to novelty-related MTL activations, it is important to remember that these may only be triggered by the switching on of an attentional orienting response when novelty of the right kind is detected. But it is also important to determine whether the detection of the right kind of novelty alone is sufficient to trigger MTL activation. As we stressed earlier, it needs to be identified whether subjects have detected the right kinds of novelty, and, if they have, whether this has produced an attentional orienting response, or, for that matter, more elaborative encoding. Novelty detection might be assessed crudely by a later debriefing of subjects, or, if event-related fMRI is available, they might be asked to indicate whether they have detected novelty while information is presented during scanning. Similarly, subjects could rate the level of their attention to information during scanning so as to determine whether more attention is given to novel than to similar, but familiar information. Alternatively, their attentional response to novelty could be measured indirectly by measuring autonomic or ERP indices. With event-related fMRI, one might be able to average separately those activations to novel stimuli that do not elicit detection of novelty, those where novelty is detected but this does not lead to attentional orienting (whether defined behaviourally or in terms of autonomic/ERP measures), and those that are detected as novel and are attended to more strongly as a result.

Provided that encoding is controlled and similar across the stimuli so that varying levels of associative encoding cannot explain any MTL activation differences, such event-related fMRI studies can provide a powerful means of assessing whether there is an MTL role in producing attentional orienting to novel stimuli. They can also provide evidence for or against the possibility that detection of certain kinds of novelty alone, relative to the failure to detect such novelty in similar objectively new stimuli, can activate the MTL. For this last procedure to work subjects must fail to detect that some objectively novel stimuli are new when familiar and novel stimuli are mixed together in an event-related fMRI design and the subjects have to determine novelty event by event. We do have evidence with a blocked design procedure that subjects may not be aware that information is novel at the time that it is presented when they have to perform complex encoding operations. This is plausible because when subjects are required to encode information in complex ways, there is little capacity free with which to detect novelty. It may, therefore, be possible to achieve appreciable failure of novelty detection in an event-related fMRI procedure if subjects are required to report whether information is or is not novel and then immediately perform a complex encoding operation on it. With this design, there is also a good chance that when novelty is detected on many occasions it will not trigger attentional orienting, so appreciable numbers of the following categories of event should be achievable with objectively novel materials: novelty detected and attention triggered; novelty detected but attention not triggered; novelty not detected. As all three kinds of event involve only objectively novel materials, any novelty activations cannot be confounded with priming effects.

Two other possible confounds cannot be so readily excluded, however. First, if failure to detect that information is novel corresponds to making a false alarm, then it is possible that this false recognition is causing an MTL activation. It has been shown that false recognition found in an adaptation of Deese's (1959) false memory paradigm, which was designed to produce high levels of false alarms, produced similar levels of MTL activation to true recognition (Schacter et al., 1997). There would be a risk that a false memory MTL effect could conceal a novelty detection-related effect if two things are true: (a) false memory in standard tasks outside the false memory paradigm also produces appreciable MTL activation relative to correctly rejecting new items; and (b) failing to detect novelty is equivalent to falsely recognising something. It is perhaps unlikely that either of these things is true, but this needs to be shown properly. Second, even if encoding is matched across events whether or not the novelty of to-be-encoded information is detected, memory may be better when novelty is detected, particularly if attentional orienting is triggered. There is direct evidence that even when encoding is reasonably matched, that which leads to better memory produces more MTL activation (e.g. Brewer et al., 1998; Wagner et al., 1998b). If this confound is not to be serious, therefore, it must be shown that memory is equivalent following encoding whether or not novelty is detected (or attention triggered) with new items.

Even if attentional orienting triggered by novelty detection increases kinds of associative encoding and/or consolidation that themselves activate the MTL, novelty of input information need not be an essential condition for associative encoding to activate the MTL. The point needs to be tested appropriately. To do this, there is a need to distinguish between the novelty of an input at encoding and the novelty of the specific information that is encoded when an input is presented. These two forms of novelty or their absence are usually confounded. For example, the same information may be repeatedly presented and encoded in the same way. This is often the case with priming procedures. The two forms of novelty can be separated, however, by getting subjects to encode in a specific way input information that has been familiarised by previously getting them to perform *different* encoding operations on the input. Using such procedures with event-related fMRI, it should be possible to compare activations associated with any combination of psychological events. Thus, both forms of novelty might be present, both absent, or either one alone might be present. The effects of multiple repetitions might also be explored as there is evidence that priming effects may increase as repetitions are increased and fluency presumably increases (see Wiggs & Martin, 1998). We wish to stress that distinguishing between the nominal stimulus and what is actually encoded (and later remembered) may be critical for the sensible interpretation of neuroimaging memory studies.

The best way of determining whether effects arise because of the increased fluency of reactivating remembered representations is to use a parametric design. In this procedure, one would compare the effect of encoding the same stimuli in the same way repeatedly so as to achieve different levels of fluency of the encoding process. If repeatedly encoding already familiar stimuli in the same way results in progressively less MTL activation, then the effect cannot arise from novelty-related effects because novelty is not present. As indicated in the previous paragraph, the effect could instead reflect enhanced fluency, i.e. ISIM, because there is evidence that multiple repetitions of the same encoding operation on the same information produces graded effects not only on behavioural fluency, but also on neurophysiological responses (see Kopelman et al., 1998; Wiggs & Martin, 1998). To be convincing, however, enhanced fluency should be shown behaviourally.

There is one other potential problem with interpreting the progressive MTL activation reduction as an effect of priming or enhanced fluency. Subjects are likely to recognise the inputs and their encoding, so MTL effects may be related to aware memory retrieval (see Schacter & Buckner, 1998b) and its repetition rather than to the enhanced fluency process *per se* which does not on its own produce aware memory. This kind of possible confound can only be removed if enhanced fluency and aware memory retrieval effects influence different MTL regions or only one repetition is used, so that subjects can show enhanced fluency both with and without aware memory for different events. The latter manoeuvre reintroduces the problem of comparing novel and already exposed inputs or encodings.

As we have argued, the reduced activation produced by the re-encoding of familiar relative to initial encoding of novel stimuli could result from either priming or the detection of certain kinds of novelty and/or the triggering of an attentional response. It is important to note that current neuroimaging studies of perceptual and semantic priming or ISIM do not eliminate the possibility that the observed effects are caused by a novelty detection response rather than decreased activation related to enhanced fluency. One way of addressing this problem would use an event-related fMRI procedure and separately average cases where subjects failed to detect novelty when it was present, cases where novelty was detected and responded to (as assessed by behavioural and autonomic/ERP measures), cases where familiar information was neither recognised, nor associated with any sign of enhanced fluency at re-encoding, and cases where familiar information was re-encoded in a more fluent manner although not recognised. If unrecognised, fluently processed, repeated information produces less MTL activation than less fluently processed, unrecognised, repeated information, this would be consistent with a priming interpretation.

Comparison of fluently processed, unrecognised repeated information with less fluently processed objectively novel information would be less convincing as a demonstration of priming because novelty-related effects could also be operating if novelty detection does not need to be an aware process. This problem arises in a study by Elliot and Dolan (1998) in which the right parahippocampal cortex was reported to be more activated by objectively novel Kanji ideograms than by ideograms that were previously shown in a subliminal fashion so that subjects were never aware of having seen them. Precisely what caused the MTL activation cannot be identified in the study because the key processes were neither monitored nor controlled. The study also needs replication because another study by Beauregard et al. (1998), in which activation to objectively novel words and words that had been previously exposed subliminally was compared, found *more* MTL activation in a right anterior hippocampal region with the subliminally exposed words. The two studies did show effects in probably distinct MTL regions, but, nevertheless, what is going on clearly must be clarified. As has been suggested, these studies need to monitor novelty detection, attentional levels, what is encoded, subsequent memory, and processing efficiency (to tap any priming). Variations in any of these factors could explain the different results. It should also be noted that what unaware novelty detection means is unclear. That the brain discriminates between new and old materials without the subject's awareness may not be sufficient because novelty detection involves the further knowledge of why the materials differ (a kind of meta-judgement).

Event-related fMRI could also be used to compare old items that were recognised, but not more fluently re-encoded with old items that were unrecognised, but were more fluently re-encoded. This would allow the identification of any differences between aware (recognition) and unaware (ISIM) memory for the same or, at least, very similar, information. If event-related fMRI procedures are not available, it would still be possible to use a correlational approach to see whether activation or deactivation effect sizes related more strongly to autonomic/ERP measures of attention or to measures of degree of ISIM.

Baseline and Spatial Resolution Issues

One of the things that requires more investigation with MTL effects at encoding is the use of different baseline comparisons. This is important for at least two reasons. The first reason is that direct comparisons of encoding and retrieval of broadly the same kinds of information have suggested that the two processes may activate at least partially non-overlapping structures (see Tulving & Markowitsch, 1997) and a meta-analysis of PET studies has even suggested the two processes may activate distinct MTL regions (Lepage, Habib, & Tulving, 1998). However, it also often seems that encoding produces greater MTL activation than does retrieval (Tulving et al., 1996). It needs to be determined whether this is an ISIM-related phenomenon or whether a different explanation is required.

The second reason relates to the possibility that it is hard "to switch the hippocampus off". It is often assumed that there is more chance of finding hippocampal activation effects when the comparison condition is a low-level one such as fairly passive processing of disorganised material or fixating a cross-hair. However, it needs to be shown that comparing an encoding task of interest with such a low-level baseline leads to a greater MTL activation than does comparing it with an apparently more closely matched encoding task. This is partly because repeatedly performing the same encoding operation may not only reduce activation of the MTL, but inhibit it relative to a condition that apparently involves no associative encoding or consolidation into long-term memory and which should not, therefore, have any effect on MTL activation. For example, Bellgowan et al. (1998) found that the making of indoor/outdoor judgements with novel pictures produced more MTL activation than repeatedly making the same judgements with the same pictures, but not than looking at cross-hairs. This suggests that repeated encoding judgements produced slightly, if insignificantly, less activation in the MTL than a supposedly low-level task.

As some of the evidence derived largely from the lesion literature suggests that different processes may activate hippocampus, amygdala, parahippocampal cortex, and perirhinal cortex differentially, it is important that neuroimaging research should be able to discriminate whether an activation is of one or more of these structures. At present, the selectivity of MTL activations is probably exaggerated in reports of encoding studies, particularly those based on PET. These studies often describe an activation as involving the hippocampus or other MTL regions when it is unclear that they are justified in doing so. For example, Klingberg, Roland, and Kawashima (1994) claim that the entorhinal cortex is activated in associative memory. The claims are unjustified because although spatial resolution with PET is very good, most forms of data analysis require stages of smoothing and warping which greatly decrease spatial resolution so that it probably lies between 1 and 2cm. Although fMRI has finer spatial resolution, particularly when systems with more powerful magnets and better signal to noise ratios can be used, even here it is difficult to know whether an activation involves the parahippocampal cortex or a hippocampal region with a comparable anterior–posterior co-ordinate. There is an urgent need to improve the spatial resolution with which studies can be done so as to be able to address theoretical issues related to the possible functional fractionation of the MTL.

Identifying the Causes of Frontal Lobe Effects

Frontal lobe involvement with encoding processes needs to be assessed with respect to the kind of information being encoded and the kinds of effortful or automatic processes that are applied to the encoding in question. It must also be borne in mind that there should be considerable overlap between activations associated with encoding and with retrieval because there must surely be many processes in common between the two activities. The HERA (hemispheric encoding/retrieval asymmetry) view, advanced by Tulving and his colleagues (Nyberg, Cabeza, & Tulving, et al., 1996; Tulving et al., 1994a), has suggested, however, that encoding and retrieval may produce dissociable activations in the frontal association cortices. HERA, which is really more a summary of the literature at a particular time than an explanatory hypothesis, states that encoding of episodic information, regardless of whether it is verbal or non-verbal in nature, activates certain left frontal cortex regions more than right-sided regions, whereas episodic retrieval produces greater activation of the right frontal cortex. According to HERA, episodic encoding requires semantic information retrieval so that this is, at least in part, responsible for the material-independent activation of the left frontal cortex produced by encoding.

Neuroimaging studies of any frontal cortex activations produced by encoding must, therefore, be very careful to monitor and control the kinds of information that are being encoded, and the degree of effort involved in such encoding. This clearly needs to be done when comparing verbal with non-verbal encoding or other finer-grained encoding comparisons. Such comparisons provide a test of HERA's claim that the laterality of frontal encoding activations is uninfluenced by whether verbal or non-verbal information is being encoded. As HERA also implies that left frontal encoding activations relate to the retrieval of semantic information, it is important to compare encoding focused on the meaning of inputs with encoding focused on the perceptual features of inputs. All such comparisons should monitor levels of effort to clarify whether frontal activations depend on degree of effort in encoding. Two comments are warranted. First, it would be interesting to determine whether the frontal cortex and the MTL are most activated by encoding the same kinds of information (e.g. associations between different kinds of information). If this is found, it would also be interesting to see whether frontal activation, like MTL activation, is greater for encoding that leads to memory. Second, it is important to determine whether different frontal sites within each hemisphere are activated when different information is encoded and/or different executive processes are involved.

If the kind of information encoding is controlled or monitored, then the aim should be to vary the degree of effort required and/or the kinds of executive processes that are involved in the effortful encoding. Degree of effort can probably be varied suitably by comparing the activations produced by repeating the same encoding operation again and again with those produced by the same kinds of encoding when made for the first time. It will be harder to vary the kind of executive process involved with particular kinds of encoding, but it seems likely, for example, that encoding in a different way than previously (in other words, inhibiting a dominant response tendency) will activate different frontal regions from those activated by relating current information to what is already in memory in an organised fashion.

Future work will need to identify the relationship between encoding activations produced in different brain regions such as the frontal cortex and MTL. Dissociations may be expected as the MTL should be activated even when the frontal cortex is not, provided the appropriate kinds of association have been encoded in a relatively automatic fashion. On the other hand, the frontal and MTL regions must often engage in encoding and consolidation processes in concert, so neuroimaging procedures need to be used to identify what the effective connectivity actually is. For example, assessment of effective connectivity could be used to assess Tulving et al.'s (1996) claim that encoding novel information activates a coherent MTL–frontal lobe system. The same kind of assessment is obviously appropriate for identifying effective connectivity involving any other brain sites that activate during encoding, particularly when this is unexpected on the basis of lesion studies. If event-related fMRI can be developed to constrain the localisation of the sources that generate ERP components, then it will become possible to determine not only the functional systems underlying encoding, but also the latencies of activation shown by components of such systems in the millisecond range. Such knowledge will greatly increase the power of any neural network models devised to explain how the systems mediate the functions that neuroimaging and lesion studies have identified.

WHAT HAVE NEUROIMAGING STUDIES OF ENCODING REVEALED SO FAR?

Encoding and Consolidation-related MTL Effects

When a subtraction procedure is used to show that associative encoding and/or consolidation activates parts of the MTL, it is important to match novelty, control encoding, and test associative memory. It may also be useful to debrief subjects afterwards to identify crudely how much novelty detection and associative encoding has been engaged. All these things have rarely been done in encoding studies that have found MTL effects so it is hard to be sure that the activations observed resulted from encoding, let alone the encoding and/or consolidation of associations. Table 1 summarises some recent encoding studies that have yielded MTL activations, and indicates whether they have matched novelty of materials and kind of encoding across condition, and controlled encoding. Many of the studies that have shown MTL activations did not match stimulus novelty across the two conditions being compared or try to control what was encoded, so it is unclear whether effects were due to orienting attention to novelty, re-encoding or ISIM deactivations, or encoding and/or consolidation (Dolan & Fletcher, 1997; Tulving et al., 1996; Stern et al., 1996).

A partial exception to this pattern was a PET study by Grady et al. (1995) which did match novelty of the encoded information across two compared conditions. These workers showed that more right-sided posterior MTL activation was produced when young subjects attempted to remember novel faces compared to when they tried to perceptually match similar novel face pictures. Although subjects were not debriefed, it is unlikely that novelty contributed to this activation which was related to relatively better face recognition memory. The MTL activation, therefore, may well be related to encoding and/or consolidation, but because encoding was spontaneous it is not possible to specify with confidence what information was encoded beyond the obvious statement that it must have been related to faces in some way.

Other studies have tried to control encoding, but not novelty of encoded stimuli. For example, in an fMRI study, Gabrieli et al. (1997) found that more right-sided posterior MTL activation was produced by judging whether novel pictures represented indoor or outdoor scenes compared to making the same judgement with two familiar pictures repeatedly. As the study did not control novelty of the pictures, however, one cannot be sure that the MTL effects observed resulted from associative encoding of the pictures, attentional orienting to pictorial novelty, or the reduced activations produced by repeating the same encoding operation, i.e. ISIM or priming.

We have tried to control both novelty and encoding of pictures in a two-condition SPECT neuroimaging study of encoding (Montaldi et al., 1998a). Ten subjects were required either to encode the themes of novel pictures by determining the relationships between the components of each picture or to

TABLE 1
Summary of Encoding Studies

(a) Author	(b) Stimulus Materials	(c) Proposed Isolated Cognitive Process	(d) Encoding Controlled	(e) Encoding Matched	(f) Novelty Level Matched	(g) Left MTL Activation	(h) Right MTL Activation
Tulving et al. 1994b	Complex scenes	Novelty	✗	✗	✗	✗	✓
Grady et al. 1995	Faces	Face Encoding	✗	✗	✓	✗	✓
Gabrieli et al. 1997	Complex scenes	Novelty-related Encoding	✓	✗	✗	✓	✓
Kapur et al. 1996	Unrelated word pairs	Associative Encoding	✓	✗	✓	✓	✗
Stern et al. 1996	Complex scenes	Novelty-related Encoding	✗	✗	✗	✓	✓
Dolan et al. 1997	Related word pairs	Associative Encoding	✓	✗	✗	✗	✗
	Related word pairs	Novelty of Associations	✓	✗	✗	✓	✗
Martin et al. 1997	Object/Words	Encoding Meaning	✗	✗	✓	✓	✓
	Objects/Words	Encoding Form	✗	✗	✓	✗	✓
	Objects/Words	Context Novelty	✗	✓	✗	✗	✓
Henke et al. 1997	House scenes/Faces	Associative Encoding	✓	✗	✓	✗	✓
Mayes et al. 1997	Unrelated word triplets	Associative Encoding	✓	✗	✓	✓	✗
	Unrelated word triplets	Novel Encoding	✓	✗	✗	✓	✗
Montaldi et al. 1998a	Complex scenes	Associative Encoding	✓	✗	✓	✓	✗
Montaldi et al. 1998b	Complex scenes	Associative Encoding	✓	✗	✓	✓	✗
	Complex scenes	Item Novelty	✓	✓	✗	✗	✗
Fernandez et al. 1998	Word lists	Encoding	✗	✗	✓	✓	✓

Study	Stimuli (c)	Cognitive process (c)	(d)	(e)	(f)	
Bellgowan et al. 1998	Complex scenes	Configural Encoding	✓	✗	✓	✓
	Complex scenes	Novelty	✓	✗	✓	✓
Kopelman et al. 1998	Word lists	Novelty	✗	✗	✗	✗
	Word Lists	Incremental Learning	✗	✗	✓	✗
Wagner et al. 1998	Words (Event-related)	Encoding/Memory formation	✓	✗	✓	✗
Brewer et al. 1998	Scenes (Event-related)	Encoding/Memory formation	✓	✗	✓	✗
Fernandez et al. 1999	Words Lists	Encoding/Memory formation	✓	✗	✓	✓

Summary of recent encoding studies that have produced MTL activations, illustrating whether study designs controlled for novelty and/or encoding. Column (c) of the Table describes the cognitive process hypothesised by the authors to be isolated within their particular experimental design. If a cognitive process has been isolated, it must not be matched across conditions and therefore reference to a process being "matched" (either novelty or encoding) implies that it was not isolated by the experiment. Similarly, the interpretation of results requires knowledge of what was encoded and so controlling encoding becomes crucial. Therefore, "encoding controlled" means that how the stimuli were encoded was specified and, preferably, that this was somehow ensured and confirmed. It is important to note that the cognitive process identified in column (c) determines the interpretation of the information in columns (d), (e), and (f). Thus, where novelty is identified in (c), the forms of encoding referred to in (d) and (e) will be the same. However, when an encoding-related process is specified in (c), then the distinction between the forms of encoding referred to in (d) and (e) becomes crucial. In this case, the encoding in (d) refers to experiment-dependent encoding determined by the study design, while the encoding referred to in (d) and isolated cognitive process. For example, Gabrieli et al. controlled associative encoding (d) by using a specific orienting task, but did not match novelty-related encoding (e) as this was their selected cognitive process of interest. The interpretation of column (f) is also dependent on the cognitive process identified in column (c). Unless otherwise specified, novelty in both columns (c) and (f) refers to novelty of the stimuli within the experimental context. If instead, a specific form of novelty is specified in (c) (e.g. context novelty), then this is also the form of novelty referred to in column (f).

perform a perceptual matching task with novel pictures (similar to that used by Grady et al. 1995 with faces). Analysis with statistical parametric mapping (SPM) showed a significant anterior MTL activation on the left with encoding, and a regions of interest analysis confirmed this, and also suggested that there might have been a weaker activation at a corresponding site in the right MTL. Debriefing showed that subjects had performed the tasks properly and memory testing indicated that the associative encoding task had led to better associative recall of the components of the pictures.

In a follow-up study, published in abstract form (Montaldi et al., 1998b) we used a four-condition comparison with SPECT to manipulate picture novelty as well as encoding. This time we compared a slightly different form of associative encoding with perceptual matching. As far as possible, as in the previous experiment, we matched the associative and matching tasks for difficulty. Each task was performed with novel pictures, and, in two further conditions, with familiarised pictures. The pictures were familiarised by getting subjects to point quickly to the centre of action of each depicted scene. This was done eight minutes before scanning, and piloting showed that item (picture) recognition at over 90% correct was produced. Debriefing after each scan indicated that subjects had performed the encoding and matching operations as instructed and that equivalent amounts of novelty detection were reported for the perceptual and encoding tasks with novel pictures. Pilot work also indicated that these tasks occupied subjects' attention during nearly all of the six seconds that were allowed for completing the tasks. Memory testing showed that associative memory for the pictures was clearly superior following the associative encoding task.

A conjunction analysis with SPM showed that the associative encoding task produced more left posterior MTL activation than the perceptual task with both novel and familiar pictures. Interestingly, the same conjunction analysis failed to show a right MTL activation, although a single subtraction analysis with SPM showed a right-sided posterior MTL activation when associative encoding and perceptual matching was compared for the familiar pictures only. The study clearly shows that this kind of associative encoding is sufficient to activate the MTL region regardless of whether the encoded information is novel or familiar. Unlike the earlier Montaldi et al. (1998a) study, all the activations in the second study were in the posterior MTL. This is of interest because the encoding conditions of the two studies seemed similar, and yet, if the studies are replicable, these small changes are sufficient to shift activation from anterior to posterior MTL regions.

In the second study, subjects' recognition memory for associations between items in the same pictures was tapped (for example, did a pig and a church tower appear together in one picture?). Foils comprised recombinations of objects from different pictures that had been shown. There were inter-subject correlations between this kind of associative recognition memory and not only level of activation in the right MTL, but also level of activation in precuneus bilaterally, left inferolateral parietal cortex, and left prefrontal neocortex. As encoding was controlled, it is likely that these encoding-related activations reflected processes that build long-term memories for these pictorial associations.

Fernandez et al. (1998) have used an intra-subject correlational procedure with fMRI to demonstrate that "episodic" verbal encoding activates the posterior MTL. They examined correlations between encoding activations and subsequent free recall of different sets of five encoded words for each scanned subject. During multiple scanning blocks, 13 subjects spent 15 seconds encoding five sequentially presented words in a supposedly rote fashion, 15 seconds doing a distraction task which required same–different judgements to be made with pairs of signs, and then 45 seconds recalling the words. The authors implied that the specific aim of their study was to separate the MTL activating effects of encoding and "novelty assessment". What they found was that 11 of their 13 subjects showed a statistically significant positive correlation between the size of posterior, but not anterior, MTL blood oxygen level dependent (BOLD) signals bilaterally during encoding and level of recall. They argued that this activation included the posterior hippocampus.

Fernandez and his colleagues proposed that their study showed that successful encoding, but not other processes such as attention, elaboration, or emotional arousal, produced bilateral hippocampal activation. There was, however, no attempt either to control or to monitor whether novelty detection and attentional orienting, elaboration, and emotional arousal were greater during encoding of those word lists for which subsequent recall was better. One needs to try and control these processes, and certainly monitor them in order to determine what processes are responsible for subsequent memory. It seems particularly likely that better memory would be related to those occasions when subjects did not manage to encode in a rote manner as this makes forming associations between words unlikely. It is almost impossible to prevent subjects from doing certain things unless their time is occupied by a task that prevents their attention wandering in the undesired direction.

Two event-related fMRI studies (Brewer et al., 1998; Wagner et al., 1998b) have provided somewhat better control of encoding processes that lead to memory while at the same time separating encoding activations that lead to memory from those that do not. Wagner et al. (1998b) initially showed, using a blocked design, that semantic encoding produced *inter alia* more left posterior MTL activation than low-level encoding which produced worse memory. Then, in an event-related fMRI study, they showed that when words (that were novel in the study context) were encoded using a concrete/abstract judgement task, those words that were later confidently recognised were encoded with more left posterior MTL activation than less confidently recognised words, which in turn were encoded with more activation in this region than unrecognised words. They also presented evidence that makes it unlikely that this effect related strongly to the speed with which these judgements were made. In a similar study, Brewer et al. (1998) showed that when novel pictures were encoded as either representing indoor or outdoor scenes, greater right posterior MTL activation was found at encoding with pictures that were later recognised and remembered than those that subjects merely knew they had seen before, and that, in turn, "known" pictures were associated with more activation than unrecognised pictures. As the studies matched item novelty across the different trial categories, this could not be a factor in any activations found.

Neither of these studies claimed that the hippocampus had been activated when encoded words or pictures were later recognised, but they did show that encoding-related posterior MTL activations (probably of the parahippocampal cortex) were critically related to the production of aware memory rather than merely the representation of specific information at input. The studies did not address whether encoding-related MTL activations (in relation to an appropriate baseline task) were found with unrecognised items for which there was evidence of priming or ISIM, or indeed, whether such encoding-related activations were found even with items for which there was later neither aware nor unaware memory. Wagner et al. (1998b) did show, however, that comparing studied but later unrecognised words with the fixation baseline condition revealed a smaller left posterior MTL activation than that found for later recognised words. This provides initial evidence that the same MTL region is activated during encoding both when aware and unaware memory is later present, although the activation is greater when aware memory is produced. The study did not measure priming so it remains unresolved whether encoding items for which neither aware nor unaware memory is later shown produces any MTL activation. It is important to measure priming in order to determine whether encoding activates the same brain region although to differing extents when it leads to aware and unaware memory respectively. This is particularly important when evidence suggests that MTL lesions disrupt the unaware memory (priming) in question (e.g. Chun & Phelps, 1998).

It remains unclear what exactly was being remembered by the subjects. Remembering involves retrieving specific item–context associations whereas even knowing involves more general associations of the same kind. Similarly, it could be that confident recognition involves stronger kinds of associative memory. So, it remains uncertain to what extent the kinds of memory that testing showed encoding had produced reflect item memory rather than associative memory. Several studies do indicate that encoding specific kinds of association activates the MTL more than does encoding the same kind of items individually. Thus, Cohen et al. (1994) found this effect with associations between faces, occupations, and names, Henke et al. (1997) found it with associations between houses and faces, Kapur et al. (1996) found it with word pairs, and Mayes et al. (in press) found it with unrelated word triplets. Unlike the Brewer et al. (1998) and the Wagner et al. (1998b) studies, these four studies did not demonstrate that the encoding-related activations directly related to the production of long-term memory. Only the two event-related fMRI studies indicate that transient activation changes in the posterior MTL predict later memory.

In a second study, Fernandez et al. (1999) extended their original procedure to examine not free recall of words, but cued recall using cues comprising the opening three letters of studied words. In this study, they argued that the levels of bilateral entorhinal cortex activations in five of the six subjects correlated significantly with their cued recall performance. The entorhinal cortex activation was tonically present from prior to the first word presentation, continued throughout presentation of the entire set, and for over 13 seconds after this, during which time subjects looked at a central fixation cross. The authors argued that cued recall performance depended on this slowly modulated entorhinal cortex activation. They raise the point that MTL activations that predict later memory following encoding could either involve relatively tonic activations or more transient activations related to individual encoding events of the kind identified by event-related fMRI encoding studies (e.g. Wagner et al., 1998b and Brewer et al., 1998). The lack of claimed hippocampal activation in the cued recall study and its claimed presence in the free recall study currently have no clear explanation. It is possible, however, that whereas free recall involves the hippocampus (see Aggleton & Brown, 1999), the form of cued recall that was used resembles item recognition and does not involve the hippocampus.

There is other evidence that not all activations related to encoding and later memory are transient and may persist for many seconds. Thus, Kato et al. (1997) also reported that MTL BOLD activation may well persist for some time following the apparent completion of encoding. In this study, encoding of six animal words was followed by a period of mild distraction and the shape of the BOLD response was analysed. The authors claimed that it took the MTL BOLD response, which they described as hippocampal, between one and two minutes to return to baseline levels following the encoding of the words. Although it might be argued that the prolonged time taken by the BOLD response to return to baseline reflects a peculiarity of the BOLD response in this region, rather than prolonged neural activity, this is unlikely because transient activations have also been reported in event-related fMRI studies (e.g. Wagner et al., 1998b). Such prolonged activations are, therefore, consistent with a role for the MTL in the development of consolidation into long-term memory.

Several of the aforementioned studies claim to find encoding-related activations in specific regions of the MTL such as the posterior hippocampus (Fernandez et al., 1998) or the entorhinal cortex (Fernandez et al., 1999). It is unclear whether these claims can be easily sustained although they are theoretically important. For example, even though a 3T MRI system was used in the Fernandez et al. (1998) study, it is doubtful whether it can confidently be claimed that activations were in the posterior hippocampus rather than only in the parahippocampal cortex, because the fMRI BOLD signal is associated with susceptibility artefacts in the MTL, which may result in signal displacements and distortions. In other words, although it may be fairly easy to discriminate between anterior and posterior MTL activations, it will probably require special techniques to make discriminations between MTL structures at the same anterior–posterior co-ordinate. This is illustrated by a study of Bookheimer et al. (1998), which used a series of procedures to maximise spatial resolution and accuracy of the BOLD response with a 3T MRI system. They showed that, when they replicated Stern et al.'s (1996) procedure in which spontaneous encoding of novel pictures was compared with the spontaneous encoding of repeated pictures, all subjects showed activations in the parahippocampal gyrus, but only one showed hippocampal activation. This was contrary to the claim of Stern and her associates that they had found hippocampal activation from this task. Resolution of the issue requires spatial resolution at the limits of current fMRI procedures, if not beyond them, as Kirchhoff et al. (1998) have recently reported that they have used a 3T GE MRI system and replicated Stern et al.'s (1996) results. Resolution of the apparent disagreement is important, but it is hard to decide which conclusion is correct.

The claim by Gabrieli et al. (1997) that the activation associated with encoding of novel pictures in their task was in a more posterior MTL region than the activation associated with recognising such pictures may, however, be acceptable. This is because their claim requires far lower levels of spatial resolution and accuracy than do the claims of Stern et al. (1996) and Fernandez et al. (1998). Nevertheless, it is doubtful that Gabrieli and his colleagues were entitled to localise the encoding and retrieval activations to the more posteriorly located parahippocampal cortex and the more anteriorly located subiculum, because this exceeds the spatial precision that their procedure could reliably yield. They are also not entitled to claim that encoding and retrieval of the same information was mediated by partially distinct MTL regions even when they attempted to match the materials used at encoding and retrieval. This is because pictorial recognition may depend on retrieving partially different information from that which was encoded when indoor/outdoor judgements were made about the pictures. For example, it might have been more appropriate to ask subjects to visualise as many pictures as possible that had depicted indoor, then outdoor, scenes as this was specifically the information they were asked to encode. In general, the fact that encoding and recognition relate to the same nominal stimuli does not mean that the same information is encoded as is later retrieved. This is a critical point which has not yet been seriously addressed, although Montaldi et al. (1998b) made an initial attempt to do so.

Even though both PET and fMRI should be capable of confidently discriminating between anterior and posterior MTL activations associated with memory-related processes, there is no established explanation of why some encoding activations are anterior and others are posterior. This problem is highlighted in two recent meta-analyses of PET (Lepage et al., 1998) and both PET and fMRI (Schacter & Wagner, 1999) memory studies. Lepage et al.'s analysis, based on 54 MTL activations that were found in 20 PET studies of encoding and retrieval, found that encoding activations were more frequently found in the anterior MTL whereas retrieval activations tended to cluster more posteriorly. In contrast, Schacter and Wagner's (1999) analysis, based on 31 MTL activations drawn from nine fMRI studies, showed that encoding activations tended to be primarily in the posterior MTL (there were too few retrieval activations to provide a reliable analysis). This second meta-analysis also found that PET encoding activations were more anterior, but noted that the contrast was not as strong as Lepage et al.'s analysis suggested, as some PET encoding activations were more posteriorly located.

Schacter and Wagner (1999) consider and tentatively reject the possibility that the mismatch between PET and fMRI could relate to the loss of sensitivity to the BOLD signal in the anterior MTL that may result from susceptibility artefact. Fernandez et al. (1999) have suggested that because PET has poorer temporal resolution than fMRI, it may be more sensitive to slowly modulated activity whereas fMRI may be more sensitive to transient event-related activities. However, this would only explain the mismatch if slowly modulated activities were located more anteriorly in the MTL than transient activities. Schacter and Wagner (1999) have suggested instead that the mismatch is more likely to relate to subtle differences between the encoding tasks that have been used most often in PET and fMRI studies respectively. The issue remains to be systematically examined. In preliminary work, we have found fMRI picture encoding activations in a very similar anterior MTL region to those reported by Montaldi et al. (1998a) with SPECT. This suggests that at least some of the mismatch is due to the factor favoured by Schacter and Wagner (1999).

Even so, the reason why MTL activation varies between anterior and posterior locations is not explained, and as the Montaldi et al. (1998a) and Montaldi et al. (1998b) studies show, the encoding differences that respectively trigger anterior and posterior MTL activations may be very small. One possibility is that more posterior activations of the hippocampus and of the parahippocampal cortex may relate primarily to spatial kinds of encoding (see Moser & Moser, 1998) whereas encoding other information activates more anterior MTL sites. This is consistent with some lesion studies in both humans (Sullivan et al., 1995) and animals (Laurent-Demir & Jaffard, 1997), which suggest that the posterior MTL and hippocampus, in particular, is more important for certain kinds of associative memory (including spatial) than are the more anterior MTL cortices and hippocampus. However, Amaral (1999) has argued, on the basis of Moser and Moser's (1998) data, that more complex forms of spatial memory require the presence of at least 70% of the hippocampus to be intact, which would imply that encoding complex spatial information probably activates anterior as well as posterior MTL regions.

Evidence from spatial memory activation studies is currently inconclusive about whether effects primarily involve anterior or posterior MTL. Maguire et al. (1998b) conducted an elegant PET study using retrieval of what was probably allocentric spatial information from a virtual reality set-up. They argued that retrieving this spatial information activated either the right hippocampus or the hippocampus bilaterally depending on the baseline used. According to Lepage et al.'s (1998) meta-analysis, one would expect spatial retrieval to activate posterior MTL whereas spatial encoding should be more likely to activate the anterior MTL. However, the data did not strongly support this expectation, as the peak of one of the retrieval activations fell anterior to the arbitrary MTL cut-off point used by Lepage and his colleagues, and the other fell on this cut-off point. In contrast, the Maguire et al. (1998a) PET spatial encoding study found an activation posterior to this MTL cut-off point. These posterior activations are not specific to spatial encoding because non-spatial PET encoding tasks have also found more posterior MTL activations (e.g. Kapur et al., 1996, with word pair associations; Wiggs et al., 1999 with objects).

If the fact that different encoding-related processes activate either anterior or posterior regions of the MTL is not simply a result of encoding non-spatial and spatial information respectively, other factors must be involved. One suggestion is that the encoding of perceptual features primarily activates the anterior MTL. In an fMRI study, Dolan and Fletcher (1999) examined the learning of which four letter strings conformed to a finite state grammar rule. Novel strings were presented repeatedly within study blocks, and there were six blocks each of which contained its own initially novel strings. Compared to a sensorimotor baseline condition, deciding whether strings were grammatical or not activated the anterior MTL most when the strings were first presented and then decreasingly within the block when the strings became more familiar. The effect changed across blocks as subjects learned the grammatical rule. Dolan and Fletcher argued that when the effect was strongest, subjects had not yet learned the rule, so relied on perceptual processing of the items.

This is an interesting suggestion that warrants more systematic examination, but there are several problems with it. First, the argument for it is currently indirect and it needs to be examined directly by comparing controlled perceptual and semantic encoding of similar materials. Second, it is not clear whether it is predicted that semantic encoding is expected to activate more posterior MTL. Third, the authors also reported that a posterior MTL region became more activated within blocks as subjects became more familiar with each of the strings. They viewed this as a retrieval activation. They were aware that the pattern of their data is not typical of that found in Schacter and Wagner's meta-analysis. However, whenever discrepancies exist in the literature it is likely that unidentified factors are playing an important role. For example, Bottini et al. (1994) found an anterior MTL activation when subjects judged sentences for plausibility versus when they made lexical decisions. This suggests that there must be factors other than encoding of perceptual or semantic information that play a key role in determining whether anterior or posterior MTL structures are activated.

What causes encoding-related processes to activate anterior or posterior MTL regions is, therefore, currently not a resolved issue. There is, however, good evidence about whether encoding specific kinds of information activates the left or right MTL, which is well summarised by Martin (1999). This evidence indicates that either incidental or intentional encoding of verbal information typically activates the left MTL whereas either incidental or intentional encoding of visual material typically activates the right MTL or the MTL bilaterally. Kelley et al. (1998b) have provided evidence that these activations are greater when encoding is intentional. Nevertheless, the occurrence of activation with incidental encoding indicates that the MTL is automatically involved in putting information about facts and episodes into memory. Martin, Wiggs, and Weisberg (1997) have provided further evidence that the lateralisation of the MTL encoding-related activation is partly related to whether the input is interpreted in a meaningful manner. For example, encoding real object information activates the MTL bilaterally whereas encoding meaningless objects activates only the anterior right MTL. This suggests that semantic encoding primarily activates the left MTL, probably because it involves using verbal information, whereas perceptual encoding may primarily activate the right MTL.

Identifying which specific MTL subregions are activated by particular kinds of encoding operation when the activations lie at a similar anterior–posterior point in the same hemisphere depends on being able to achieve spatial resolution at or beyond current limits. Full identification will depend critically on improving the spatial resolution of fMRI activations and the accuracy with which they can be localised. For example, both Kapur et al. (1996) and Mayes et al. (in press) found posterior MTL activations. These may well have been of the parahippocampal cortex rather than the hippocampus, which is consistent with the evidence about focal hippocampal lesions (e.g. Vargha-Khadem et al., 1997). However, the lesion evidence also suggests that the hippocampus should be activated when associations between different kinds of information are encoded. These kinds of association were reported in the studies of Cohen et al. (1994) and Henke et al. (1997), but it is unclear whether one can be confident about the MTL subregion activated in these studies. The same unclarity applies to spatial encoding activations, particularly as it is of theoretical interest whether the precise kinds of spatial information encoded lead to activation of distinct MTL subregions. For example, a study by Epstein and Kanwisher (1998) reported that a parahippocampal region was activated as strongly when subjects encoded empty rooms as when they encoded furnished rooms, and more strongly than when they encoded multiple objects without a three-dimensional context. The question of interest is whether any of these encoding tasks activated the hippocampus or only the parahippocampal cortex, and how these activation effects relate to the effects of focal lesions to these structures. Claims of very precise localisation within the MTL should be viewed sceptically unless the authors can provide strong justification for these claims.

In summary, there is evidence that encoding certain kinds of information so that a memory is created activates parts of the MTL. Many issues, related to the lesion evidence, remain unresolved however. These issues include whether encoding different kinds of information into memory activate different MTL subregions, whether encoding of the kinds of information with which the MTL deals, even when it only produces unaware memory, still produces some MTL activation, and whether just the process of representing information at input activates the MTL even when no memory is produced.

Novelty-related MTL Effects

We have indicated that novelty has been used in several different senses and that processes related to each of these senses may include aware or even unaware detection, triggering of attentional orienting, additional encoding processes, and possibly enhanced consolidation. Any of these processes associated with the different senses of novelty may activate MTL structures and other brain regions. Studies that have shown MTL encoding activations when novelty has been matched across conditions (e.g. Montaldi et al., 1998a; Wagner et al., 1998b) show that novelty, or at least a difference in novelty, is not necessary for producing encoding-related MTL activations. Montaldi et al.'s (1998b) study showed that stimuli do not even need to be novel for MTL encoding activations to be produced. In fact, somewhat greater MTL activation was produced when already familiar pictures were encoded in the same way as novel pictures. This study also showed that novelty detection was not sufficient to activate the MTL when encoding processes were matched across novel and familiar picture conditions. Not only did a conjunction analysis that compared novel with familiar pictures, when encoding processes were matched, show no signs of activation in the MTL, it actually showed no activations anywhere in the brain. Piloting and debriefing both indicated that the subjects still recognised that the novel pictures were novel at the time they were presented, but the manipulation probably minimised any additional attentional orienting towards such novel pictures because subjects were so busily engaged in the associative encoding or perceptual matching tasks. Unless unaware novelty detection produces more MTL activation than aware novelty detection, the null finding with novelty detection also makes it very unlikely that Elliot and Dolan's (1998) finding, referred to in the last section, is caused by novelty detection activating the MTL. It is more likely to result from encoding differences directed towards objectively novel ideograms and ones previously presented subliminally.

Current neuroimaging studies have also not proved that the triggering of attention following the detection of either absolute novelty or novelty in context is sufficient to activate the MTL. This is because, although several studies have shown MTL activation is associated with novelty (see Tulving et al., 1996), they have not monitored the processing that may accompany this novelty and have not attempted to control the more elaborative encoding that it may initiate. This means that any MTL activation found could reflect the associative encoding accompanying novel information rather than the process of attentional orientation to novelty. Future work must determine whether this process does activate the MTL, and, if so, whether it activates the same parts as does associative encoding and/or consolidation.

Apart from Montaldi et al. (1998b), neuroimaging studies have not tried to control the encoding that accompanies novelty, so it remains possible that any MTL activation effects found relate to this. Dolan and Fletcher (1999) have argued that novelty is a matter of degree. Thus, the most novel items would be unlike any encountered before, whereas moderately novel items would be like others seen before. Similarity is of course a matter of degree. They then argue that novelty can be related to an item's inherent meaning so that meaningful materials are less novel than meaningless ones. On their view, novelty detection of relatively meaningless materials involves mainly perceptual processing whereas more familiar materials will also receive a considerable degree of semantic processing. They postulate that novelty-related perceptual encoding activates the anterior hippocampus, whereas the more semantic encoding presumably activates other MTL regions. Whether correct or not, this hypothesis (which addresses only a very specific sense of novelty), is proposing that novelty-related MTL activations reflect specific kinds of encoding. This obviously implies that exactly the same MTL activation would be produced when subjects encode familiar materials in terms of the same kinds of perceptual information. Although we agree that any MTL activations associated with novelty detection are likely to be caused by specific kinds of encoding (and perhaps memory creation), we think that the Dolan and Fletcher (1999) view does not reflect the full reality. This is because people strive to make sense of new materials (whatever degree of inherent meaningfulness these possess) by encoding them in strongly semantic ways although there also, of course, needs to be perceptual processing (see Tulving et al., 1996).

The aforementioned senses of novelty relate primarily to the newness of specific items either absolutely or in a context, but Martin (1999) has used novelty to refer to the newness of an environment or a context. He and his colleagues have examined whether processes related to contextual novelty influence the functions of the MTL. PET or fMRI studies provide an excellent chance to examine this issue because for many subjects the scanners initially are completely novel environments (contexts) to which they become moderately used in the course of the experiment. Martin et al. (1997) tested how becoming familiar with the scanning environment influences brain activity in the course of an encoding study. Within one PET session, these workers found that the extent to which the encoding of similar kinds of novel materials produced right-sided MTL activation was less as subjects became familiar with the experimental context. The decrease in right MTL activation was most striking when subjects' first and second visual noise baseline conditions were compared. These occurred first and last in the scanning session, so the opportunity for the effects of familiarity to be manifested was greatest for this contrast. Their finding indicates that order effects should be controlled in neuroimaging studies to avoid artefactual results being generated. It also indicates that the second visual noise baseline provides a more appropriate baseline if the aim is to find a baseline condition that minimally activates the MTL. Martin (1999) interprets the greater right MTL activation found when subjects are less adapted to the scanner as reflective of *tonic* arousal and attention, which may be more controlled by right hemisphere structures.

An alternative interpretation to the one offered by Martin, which needs to be examined, is that MTL activation reduces because subjects become used not to the environment, but to performing specific kinds of encoding operations (e.g. silently naming real objects or even looking at visual noise). One way of testing this possibility would be to scan subjects who were very experienced in the scanner environment on the same procedure as that used by Martin et al. (1997). One related point that should be noted is that Martin et al. used novel items not only in the encoding tasks, but also in the visual noise condition for which the "context novelty" MTL diminution effect was strongest. If, instead, low-level baseline conditions involve repeated presentation of the same stimulus, it might be argued that priming or ISIM explains some or all of the diminished MTL activation, even though it is associated with low-level processing.

Priming or ISIM-related MTL Effects

Is there any evidence that priming or ISIM for certain kinds of association reduces MTL activation? We believe that the Mayes et al. (in press) fMRI verbal associative encoding study provides preliminary evidence for just this. In this study, the activation generated by forming novel sentences to link triplets of previously unrelated concrete words together (the novel association condition) was compared with that resulting from repeatedly producing the same sentence to link a single triplet of once unrelated words (the overlearnt condition). This sentence and its associative components had been overlearnt in the week prior to scanning. The novel association condition produced more activation in the posterior left MTL. The comparison resembles a priming paradigm in which multiple repetitions are used rather than just one. As in a priming paradigm, in the overlearnt condition, subjects repeatedly performed the same encoding operation on the same information and this was compared with the novel association condition where they performed the encoding operation for the first time on novel information. As with priming, performance of the encoding operation in the overlearnt condition involved retrieval. The repeated encoding and repeated retrieval operations were basically the same. Consistent with our findings, Petersson, Elfgren, and Ingvar (1997) have found that repetition of retrieval led to a reduction in MTL activation.

Similar reduced MTL activation effects may be found with repetition of encoding operations. As already indicated, Gabrieli et al. (1997) found that repeatedly performing the same indoor/outdoor encoding operation on the same pictures produced a similar reduction in posterior MTL activation when compared to performing this same operation for the first time on novel pictures. Three other studies of encoding repetition have also found reduced MTL activation with repetition of encoding, but these studies did not control encoding, so the same encoding operation may not have been repeated. First, Stern et al. (1996) observed greater MTL activation comparing first-time encoding of novel pictures with repeated encoding of the same picture. Second, Dolan and Fletcher (1997) found a similar effect when comparing initial and repeated encoding of word pairs. Third, Kopelman et al. (1998) also found MTL activations when the encoding of novel word lists was contrasted with the re-encoding of word lists that had been studied more than once.

Even when encoding is controlled, it might be argued that the effect observed by Mayes et al. (in press) and Gabrieli et al. (1997) could have been caused by orienting to associative novelty in the novel association condition. However, at least with the verbal encoding study (Mayes et al., in press), a simulation showed that subjects were scarcely aware of item and associative novelty, presumably because the encoding task was very demanding, so the postulated attentional orienting is very unlikely to have occurred. It seems likely, therefore, that repeatedly performing the same encoding operation (which also involves retrieval) produces progressively less MTL activation and this process may well be an example of ISIM for novel verbal associative information. We also have some evidence from the Mayes et al. study that repeating the same encoding operation has less effect on resultant episodic memory than does initial encoding.

The evidence that the decreased MTL activation produced by repeated encoding involves ISIM for certain kinds of novel association is only preliminary, because our subjects had explicit memory for the overlearnt sentence and its verbal triplet, but not for anything in the novel association condition. Two studies (described earlier) that circumvented this problem used subliminal presentation of stimuli at study to ensure that there was later no explicit memory for them when presented later (Beauregard et al., 1998; Elliot & Dolan, 1998). Activations in different MTL sites, as was reported in these studies, might reasonably be expected given that the materials used and encoding operations required also differed. One would not, however, expect the effects to be in different directions (i.e. greater activation for objectively novel stimuli vs subjectively novel stimuli and the reverse respectively). The bulk of priming studies have found deactivations for repeated stimuli (e.g. Wiggs & Martin, 1998) so the Beauregard et al. (1998) study is anomalous. If it represents unaware retrieval, finding right MTL activation is also surprising because there is evidence that MTL activations reduce when aware retrieval is less successful (Schacter et al., 1996). Replication is required and replications should take care to show that subliminal priming effects are clearcut in the scanner as these effects are not generally robust. Great care should also be taken to ensure that encoding is very tightly controlled and that explicit memory is tested in a sensitive manner (not by free recall as was done by Beauregard et al.).

Subliminal priming is not the only way to address the possibly confounding effects of explicit memory on MTL activations related to priming of the kinds of associations likely to require MTL memory processing. The visual search task (Chun & Phelps, 1998), referred to earlier, would be able to examine the nature of MTL priming effects with a task disrupted by large MTL lesions in which subjects show no recognition of primed items. The items were not presented subliminally and the priming effect was robust.

Event-related fMRI has already demonstrated deactivations at mid-levels of the neocortical sensory processing hierarchy with an object categorisation priming task (Buckner et al., 1998). This imaging procedure may be adaptable to measuring priming events both associated with and not associated with explicit memory. If MTL deactivation can be demonstrated when studied associations are processed more fluently, it would be interesting to discover what changes occur when there is also aware memory for these associations. One possibility is that when encoding information into memory activates the MTL, subsequent retrieval of this information (whether explicit or implicit) is done more economically and, therefore, causes less MTL activation. If, however, some forms of explicit memory depend on attributions based on the fluency of processing of repeated information (Jacoby, Kelley, & Dywan, 1989), making these attributions could activate additional specific brain regions.

Encoding-related Activations of the Frontal Lobes

Current research examining the frontal lobe activations associated with encoding is leading to modifications in the HERA account (e.g. Kelley, Buckner, & Petersen, 1998a). In particular, the suggestion that encoding and retrieval activations are mainly left and right sided respectively in the frontal lobes may need to be modified. Kelley et al. (1998b) used fMRI to scan subjects while they were encoding visually presented words, line drawings of objects, or face pictures. Relative to a cross-hair fixation baseline condition, verbal encoding produced most activation at a left dorsal frontal lobe site, line drawing encoding produced bilateral frontal lobe activations, and face encoding produced greatest activation in a right frontal lobe site homologous to that activated by verbal encoding.

These results are what would be expected from the lateralisation of verbal and non-verbal forms of memory to the left and right sides of the brain respectively, rather than from the HERA model. Although Nyberg, Cabeza, and Tulving (1998) argued that this finding is an exception to the general HERA-derived rule that encoding any kind of material mainly activates the left prefrontal cortex, there are in fact quite a few exceptions to this rule (e.g. Brewer et al., 1998; Gabrieli et al., 1997; Montaldi et al., 1998a; Wagner et al., 1998a). Furthermore, unlike most studies, that of Kelley et al. compares stimuli likely to be encoded verbally, non-verbally and in both ways in a controlled manner, and finds results suggesting that activations are lateralised not in conformity with HERA, but with material specificity. This procedure makes it unlikely that face encoding does not activate the left prefrontal cortex because stimuli were only presented briefly, preventing elaborative encoding because words and line drawings were presented equally briefly. If the elaborative encoding proposal were correct, then encoding words and line drawings should not produce left prefrontal cortex activation either. It looks increasingly as if prefrontal cortex encoding-related activations lateralise in the same way as do MTL encoding-related activations.

HERA does not specifically focus on the role of the frontally mediated executive processes in memory encoding and retrieval. It seems likely, however, that the frontal regions that activate during memory tasks will depend on the executive processes required. Two studies that have attempted to control the kind of executive process that may be critical for encoding are those of Dolan and Fletcher (1997) and Fletcher, Shallice, and Dolan (1998). The former study ingeniously compared encoding of repeated word pairs like "dog–boxer", novel word pairs, and half changed word pairs like "fighter–boxer" or "dog–corgi". Although MTL activation was greatest for the completely novel pairs, left frontal activation was greatest for the half changed pairs. The reason may well be that subjects had to inhibit a dominant encoding response tendency, which was mediated for verbal materials by the activated left frontal lobe region. This study raises the question of whether a different frontal region is activated when subjects engage a detailed planning strategy when encoding the same kind of material. To some extent, the study of Fletcher et al. (1998) addresses this question because it examined the effects of encoding word lists for which the requirement of semantically organising the lists varied. They found that left frontal cortex activation was least when the words were already organised, whereas it was greatest when subjects had to generate an organisational structure. They confirmed the functional specificity of the activation in this left dorsolateral prefrontal region by combining encoding with a concurrent distraction task known to disrupt organisation, but not other encoding processes. This produced a reduction in activation in the same left dorsolateral prefrontal cortex region only with the encoding task that required maximal organisation. This was the same region activated in the Dolan and Fletcher (1997) encoding study, so it may be that inhibition of dominant tendencies shares processes with the organisation of material that involves the abstraction of relevant semantic attributes (such abstraction may necessarily involve inhibiting dominant tendencies). Most other left frontal cortex encoding-related activations have been more ventral (e.g. Shallice et al., 1994) so presumably reflected different processes associated with encoding.

A retrieval study by Wiggs et al. (1999) has even shown that controlling degree of effort across semantic and episodic retrieval changes the laterality pattern of frontal activations found. The experimenters asked subjects to recall the colour of items from semantic memory (e.g. What colour is the moon? Yellow) or from episodic memory (they were briefly shown drawings showing, for example, a blue sun), and subjects then had to give the colour of the objects shown when presented with colourless drawings of them. On average, subjects only required 1.4 trials per object to achieve the 90% criterion, so it is implausible to suggest that later memory of the colours of the studied objects was dependent on semantic rather than episodic memory. Recall was slightly faster for episodic memory colours, suggesting that this task was, if anything, less effortful than semantic retrieval. There was no evidence that episodic retrieval produced more activation than semantic retrieval at any right frontal lobe sites. This suggests that any frontal lobe laterality activation differences in retrieving episodic and semantic information disappear when factors like effort are controlled. The same may be true of encoding.

A meta-analysis with retrieval (nothing similar has yet been done with encoding) has provided further evidence that the left prefrontal cortex is activated as executive processes are required to a greater degree in order to achieve successful retrieval (Nolde, Johnson, & Raye 1998). Thus, more left-sided activations were associated with Yes/No recognition than with forced choice recognition, and with free recall than with cued recall. Retrieval of more complex information such as the temporal location of items, their specific features, or their source also activated the left prefrontal cortex to a greater extent. All these instances involving greater left-sided activation are likely to require high levels of effort and executive processing, typified by Nolde et al. as reflective activity. One interesting feature of this meta-analysis is that the left-sided shift seems to apply equally to the retrieval of verbal and non-verbal materials. How the operation of different executive processes interacts with different materials during encoding remains to be explored.

Encoding studies frequently find that multiple frontal areas are activated, and future work will need to determine to what extent localisation is driven by the kind of information that is being encoded and to what extent it is driven by the executive processes involved in this encoding. Repetition of an encoding operation so that it becomes progressively automated should mean that less and less left frontal lobe activation is produced because executive processes are increasingly less required. Results from Kopelman et al. (1998) support this suggestion, as the repeated encoding of word lists produced reduced left frontal activation compared to initial encoding. In relation to this, Petersson, Elfgren, and Ingvar (1998) have reported that repeated retrieval that requires the recall of abstract designs produces a similar deactivation of the left dorsolateral prefrontal cortex as well as the middle and lateral orbital frontal cortex relative to initial retrieval. It seems then that as automatisation increases, retrieval and encoding both activate the frontal lobe region less.

Encoding not only activates MTL and frontal cortex regions, but also other posterior association cortex regions. We suspect that these latter activations have often not been reported even when they have been found because they were not predicted. One example of this kind of activation occurred in our second picture encoding SPECT study (Montaldi et al., 1998b), where we not only found MTL and frontal lobe activations with associative encoding, but also activations in parietal association cortex on the left, and the precuneus bilaterally. Similar MTL, bilateral precuneus, and parietal cortex encoding activations were reported by Roland and Gulyas (1995). The extent of the activations we found with associative encoding in the precuneus bilaterally and the left parietal region correlated with the strength of associative memory for the pictures. One would expect, therefore, that, if the activations are obligatory rather than incidental, relatively selective damage to these regions should impair picture memory in human subjects. This possibility needs to be investigated. If the expectation is confirmed, it will change our view of the brain lesions that disrupt fact and event memory in humans.

CONCLUSION

The main message of this review is that neuroimaging studies of encoding should be much more focused on the testing of theories, which are developed primarily from lesion research at present. To achieve this the studies need to be much more carefully controlled than has typically been the case until relatively recently. It should be easier to achieve control of key psychological factors if event-related fMRI is used. There is also clearly an urgent need to improve the accuracy and degree of spatial resolution that can be achieved in order to discriminate between different hypotheses derived from the lesion literature. In the meantime, research should realistically report conclusions based on neuroanatomical localisation, taking into consideration limitations of spatial resolution. Exaggerated claims about spatial localisation of activations could seriously distort the truth and slow the rate of scientific advance. In the longer run, a combination of this improved spatial resolution with the temporal resolution in the millisecond range that can be achieved with ERP procedures may enable us to identify accurately when and where the obligatory processes underlying fact and episode memory occur. Achievement of this goal will depend on being able to use the location of event-related fMRI activations to solve the inverse problem with respect to the sources of ERP signals. This will allow the development of much more powerful neural network models of how these processes are mediated by interlinked networks of neurons.

Two other points are important to make. First, using lesion and functional neuroimaging research together does more than provide two sources of evidence with which to scrutinise hypotheses. Hypotheses can be derived from either lesion or neuroimaging research and then be tested using the other approach. Apparent disagreements may also stimulate research in unpredicted ways, and lead to improved understanding of the limitations of each approach, but also of substantive issues about how the brain mediates memory. Second, there are a number of processes underlying fact and episode memory. Mediating these processes involves interactions between brain structures, which will change depending on the processes that are active. Assessing effective connectivity while different memory-related processes are engaged has so far been little explored (but see Kohler et al., 1998). However, it has to be a central goal of future neuroimaging research on memory.

REFERENCES

Aggleton, J.P., & Brown, M.W. (1999). Episodic memory, amnesia, and the hippocampal-anterior thalamic axis. *Behavioral Brain Sciences, 22*, 425–489.

Aggleton, J., & Shaw, C. (1996). Amnesia and recognition memory: A re-analysis of psychometric data. *Neuropsychologia, 34*, 51–62.

Amaral, D.G. (1999). Introduction: What is where in the medial temporal lobe? *Hippocampus, 9*, 1–6.

Beauregard, M., Gold, D., Evans, A.C., & Chertkow, H. (1998). A role for the hippocampal formation in implicit memory: A 3-D PET study. *Neuroreport, 9*, 1867–1873.

Bellgowan, P.S.F., Binder, J.R., Hammeke, T.A., Frost, J.A., & Possing, E.T. (1998). Configural associations and novelty are necessary for hippocampal-dependent encoding. *Neuroimage, 7*, S51.

Bohbot, V., Kalina, M., Stepankova, K., Spackova, N., Petrides, M., & Nadel, L. (1997). Lesions to the right parahippocampal cortex cause navigational memory deficits in humans. *Neuroimage, 5*, S626.

Bookheimer, S.Y., Zeineh, M.M., Strojwas, M.H., & Hariri, A.R. (1998). Localization of memory-related activation on a picture priming task using fMRI. *Neuroimage, 7*, S824.

Bottini, G., Corcoran, R., Sterzi, R., Paulesu, E., Schenone, P., Scarpa, P., Frackowiak, R.S.J., & Frith, C.D. (1994). The role of the right hemisphere in the interpretation of the figurate aspects of language. *Brain, 117*, 1241–1253.

Brewer, J.B., Zhao, Z., Glover, G.H., & Gabrieli, J.D.E. (1998). Making memories: Brain activity that predicts whether visual experiences will be remembered or forgotten. *Science, 281*, 1185–1187.

Buckner, R.L., Goodman, J., Burock, M., Rotte, M., Koutstaal, W., Schacter, D., Rosen, B. & Dale, A.M. (1998). Functional-anatomic correlates of object priming in humans revealed by rapid presentation event-related fMRI. *Neuron, 20*, 285–296.

Cahill, L., Haier, R.J., Fallon, J., Alkire, M.T., Tang, C., Keator, D., Wu, J., & McGaugh, J.L. (1996).

Amygdala activity at encoding correlated with long-term free recall of emotional information. *Proceedings of the National Academy of Science, USA, 93*, 8016–8021.

Cahill, L., & McGaugh, J.L. (1998). Mechanisms of emotional arousal and lasting declarative memory. *Trends in Neurosciences, 21*, 294–299.

Chun, M., & Phelps, E. (1998). *Amnesia and memory for context*. Presentation at the 10th Memory Disorders Research Society Meeting, October 29–31, Boston.

Cohen, N.J., Ramzy, C., Hut, Z., Tomaso, H., Strupp, J., Erhard, P., Anderson, P., & Ugurbil, K. (1994). Hippocampal activation in fMRI evoked by demand for declarative memory-based bindings of multiple streams of information. *Society for Neuroscience Abstracts, 20*, 1290.

Deese, J. (1959). On the prediction of occurrence of particular verbal intrusions in immediate recall. *Journal of Experimental Psychology, 58*, 17–22.

Demb, J.B., Desmond, J.E., Wagner, A.D., Vaidya, C.J., Glover, G.H., & Gabrieli, J.D.E. (1995). Semantic encoding and retrieval in the left inferior prefrontal cortex: A functional MRI study of task difficulty and process specificity. *The Journal of Neuroscience, 15*, 5870–5878.

Demonet, J.F., Chollet, F., Ramsay, S., Cardebat, D., Nespoulous, J.L., Wise, R., Rascol, A., & Frackowiak, R.S.J. (1992). The anatomy of phonological and semantic processing in normal subjects. *Brain, 115*, 1753–1768.

Dolan, R.J., & Fletcher, P.C. (1997). Dissociating prefrontal and hippocampal function in episodic memory. *Nature, 388*, 582–585.

Dolan, R.J., & Fletcher, P.C. (1999). Encoding and retrieval in human medial temporal lobes: An empirical investigation using functional magnetic resonance imaging (fMRI). *Hippocampus, 9*, 25–34.

Elliot, R., & Dolan, R.J. (1998). Neural response during preference and memory judgments for subliminally presented stimuli: A functional neuroimaging study. *Journal of Neuroscience, 18*, 4697–4704.

Ennaceur, A., Neave, N., & Aggleton, J.P. (1996). Neurotoxic lesions of the perirhinal cortex do not mimic the behavioural effects of fornix transection in the rat. *Behavioural Brain Research, 80*, 9–25.

Epstein, R., & Kanwisher, N. (1998). A cortical representation of the local visual environment. *Nature, 392*, 598–601.

Fernandez, G., Brewer, J.B., Zhao, Z., Glover, G.H., & Gabrieli, J.D.E. (1999). Level of sustained entorhinal activity at study correlates with subsequent cued-recall performance: A functional magnetic resonance imaging study with high acquisition rate. *Hippocampus, 9*, 35–44.

Fernandez, G., Weyerts, H., Schrader-Bolsche, M., Tendolkar, I., Smid, H.G.O.M., Tempelmann, C., Hinrichs, H., Scheich, H., Elger, C.E., Mangun, G.R., & Heinze H-J. (1998). Successful verbal encoding into episodic memory engages the posterior hippocampus: A parametrically analyzed functional magnetic resonance imaging study. *Journal of Neuroscience, 18*, 1841–1847.

Fletcher, P.C., Frith, C.D., Grasby, P.M., Shallice, T., Frackowiak, R.S.J., Dolan, R.J. (1995). Brain systems for encoding and retrieval of auditory-verbal memory: An in vivo study in humans. *Brain, 118*, 401–416.

Fletcher, P.C., Frith, C.D., & Rugg, M.D. (1997). Functional neuroanatomy of episodic memory. *Trends in Neuroscience, 20*, 213–218.

Fletcher, P.C., Shallice, T., & Dolan, R.J. (1998). The functional roles of prefrontal cortex in episodic memory. 1. Encoding. *Brain, 121*, 1239–1248.

Foster, J., Ainsworth, J., Faratin, P., & Shapiro, J. (1997) Investigating the mnemonic functions of the hippocampus: A computational neuroscience perspective. In M. Conway & S. Gathercole, (Eds.), *Cognitive models of memory*. Hove, UK: Psychology Press.

Friston, K.J. (1997). Imaging cognitive anatomy. *Trends in Cognitive Sciences, 1*, 21–27.

Frith, C.D., Friston, K.J., Liddle, P.F., & Frackowiak, R.S.J. (1991). Willed action and the prefrontal cortex in man: A study with PET. *Proceedings of the Royal Society of London B Biol Sci, 244*, 241–246.

Gabrieli, J.D.E., Brewer, J.B., Desmond, J.E., & Glover, G.H. (1997). Separate neural bases of two fundamental memory processes in the human medial temporal lobe. *Science, 276*, 264–266.

Grady, C.L., McIntosh, A.R., Horwitz, B., Maisog, J.M., Ungerleider, L.G., Mentis, M.J., Pietrini, P., Schapiro, M.B., & Haxby, J. (1995). Age-related reductions in human recognition memory due to impaired encoding. *Science, 269*, 218–221.

Grasby, P.M., Frith, C.D., Friston, K.J., Bench, C., Frackowiak, R.S.J., & Dolan, R.J. (1993). Functional mapping of brain areas implicated in auditory-verbal memory function. *Brain, 116*, 1–20.

Grasby, P.M., Frith, C.D., Friston, K.J., Simpson, J., Fletcher, P.C., Frackowiak, R.S.J., & Dolan, R.J. (1994). A graded task approach to the functional mapping of brain areas implicated in auditory-verbal memory. *Brain, 117*, 1271–1282.

Gray, J.A. (1982). The neuropsychology of anxiety. Oxford: Oxford University Press.

Henke, K., Buck, A., Weber, B., & Wieser, H.G. (1997). Human hippocampus establishes associations in memory. *Hippocampus, 7*, 249–256.

Honey, R.C, Watt, A., & Good, M. (1998). Hippocampal lesions disrupt an associative-mismatch process. *Journal of Neuroscience, 18*, 2226–2230.

Isaac, C.L., & Mayes, A.R. (in press, a). Rate of forgetting in amnesia 1: Recall and recognition of prose. *Journal of Experimental Psychology: Learning, Memory and Cognition.*

Isaac, C.L., & Mayes, A.R. (in press, b). Rate of forgetting in amnesia 11: Recall and recognition of word lists at different levels of organization. *Journal of Experimental Psychology: Learning, Memory and Cognition.*

Jacoby, L.L., Kelley, C.M., & Dywan, J. (1989). Memory attributions. In H.L. Roediger III & F.I.M. Craik (Eds.), *Varieties of memory and consciousness: Essays in honour of Endel Tulving* (pp. 391–422). Hillsdale, NJ: Laurence Erlbaum.

Josephs, O., Turner, R., & Friston, K. (1997). Event-related fMRI. *Human Brain Mapping, 5*, 243–248.

Kapur, S., Craik, F.I.M., Jones, C., Brown, G.M., Houle, S., & Tulving E. (1994). Neuroanatomical correlates of encoding in episodic memory: Levels of processing effect. *Proceedings of the National Academy of Sciences USA, 91*, 2008–2011.

Kapur, S., Tulving, E., Cabeza, R., McIntosh, A.R., Houle, S., & Craik, F.I.M. (1996). The neural correlates of intentional learning of verbal materials: A PET study in humans. *Cognitive Brain Research, 4*, 243–249.

Kato, T., Erhard, P., Takayama, Y., Strupp, J., Le, T.H., Harada, M., Ogawa, S., & Ugurbil, K. (1997). Monitoring of cerebral multiphasic sustained responses (CMSR) in memory processing using fMRI. *Neuroimage, 5*, S593.

Kelley, W.M., Buckner, R.L., & Petersen, S.E. (1998a). Response from Kelley, Buckner and Petersen. *Trends in Cognitive Sciences, 2*, 421.

Kelley, W.M., Miezin, F.M., McDermott, K.B., Buckner, R.L., Raichle, M.E., Cohen, N.J., Ollinger, J.M., Akbudak, E., Conturo, T.E., Snyder, A.Z., & Petersen, S.E. (1998b). Hemispheric specialization in human dorsal frontal cortex and medial temporal lobe for verbal and nonverbal memory encoding. *Neuron, 20*, 927–936.

Kirchhoff, B., Stern, C.E., Kwong, K.K., & Gonzalez, R.G. (1998). A 3 Tesla functional MRI study of picture encoding. *Society for Neuroscience, 24*, 266.4.

Klingberg, T., Roland, P., & Kawashima, R. (1994). The human entorhinal cortex participates in associative memory. *Neuroreport, 6*, 57–60.

Knight, R.T. (1996). Contribution of human hippocampal region to novelty detection. *Nature, 383*, 256–259.

Kohler, S., Moscovitch, M., Winocur, G., Houle, S., & Macintosh, A.R. (1998). Networks of domain-specific and general regions involved in episodic memory for spatial location and object identity. *Neuropsychologia, 36*, 129–142.

Kopelman, M.D., Stevens, T.G., Foli, S., & Grasby, P. (1998). PET activation of the medial temporal lobe in learning. *Brain, 121*, 875–887.

Laurent-Demir, C., & Jaffard, R. (1997). Temporally extended retrograde amnesia for spatial information resulting from afterdischarges induced by electrical stimulation of the dorsal hippocampus in mice. *Psychobiology*, *25*, 133–140.

Lepage, M., Habib, R., & Tulving, E. (1998). Hippocampal PET activations of memory encoding and retrieval: The HIPER model. *Hippocampus*, *8*, 313–322.

Maguire, E.A., Burgess, N., Donnett, J.G., Frackowiak, R.S.J., Frith, C.D., & O'Keefe, J. (1998b). Knowing where and getting there: A human navigation network. *Science*, *280*, 921–924.

Maguire, E.A., Frith, C.D., Burgess, N., Donnett, J.G., & O'Keefe, J. (1998a). Knowing where things are: Parahippocampal involvement in encoding object locations in virtual large-scale space. *Journal of Cognitive Neuroscience*, *10*, 61–76.

Martin, A. (1999). Automatic activation of the medial temporal lobe during encoding: Lateralized influences of meaning and novelty. *Hippocampus*, *9*, 62–70.

Martin, A., Lalonde, F.M., Wiggs, C.L., Weisberg, J., Ungerleider, L.G., & Haxby, J.V. (1995). Repeated presentation of objects reduces activity in ventral occipital cortex: A MRI study of repetition priming. *Society for Neuroscience Abstracts*, *21*, 1497.

Martin, A., Wiggs, C.L., & Weisberg, J. (1997). Modulation of human medial temporal lobe activity by form, meaning, and experience. *Hippocampus*, *7*, 587–593.

Mayes, A.R. (1988). *Human organic memory disorders*. Cambridge: Cambridge University Press.

Mayes, A.R., & Downes, J.J. (1997). What do theories of the functional deficit(s) underlying amnesia have to explain? *Memory*, *5*, 3–36.

Mayes, A.R., Downes, J.J., Shoqeirat, M., Hall, C., & Sagar, H.J. (1993). Encoding ability is preserved in amnesia: Evidence from a direct test of encoding. *Neuropsychologia*, *31*, 745–759.

Mayes, A.R., Gooding, P., Gregory, L.J., Hunkin, N.M., Nunn, J.A., Van Eijk, R., Williams, S.C.R., Brammer, M., & Bullmore, E. (in press). The left hippocampus is activated by encoding verbal associations. *Behavioural Neurology*.

Meunier, M., Bachevalier, J., & Mishkin, M. (1997). Effects of orbital frontal and anterior cingulate lesions on object and spatial memory in rhesus monkeys. *Neuropsychologia*, *35*, 999–1015.

Mishkin, M., Vargha-Khadem, F., & Gadian, D.G. (1998). Amnesia and the organization of the hippocampal system. *Hippocampus*, *8*, 212–216.

Montaldi, D., Mayes, A.R., Barnes, A., Pirie, H., Hadley, D.M., Patterson, J., & Wyper, D.J. (1998a). Associative encoding activates the medial temporal lobes. *Human Brain Mapping*, *6*, 85–104.

Montaldi, D., Mayes, A.R., Pirie, H., Barnes, A., Hadley, D.M., Patterson, J., & Wyper, D.J. (1998b). Dissociating novelty detection and associative encoding in the processing of complex scenes. *Neuroimage*, *7*, S816.

Moscovitch, M., & Nadel, L. (1997). Memory consolidation and the hippocampal complex. *Current Opinions in Neurobiology*, *7*, 217–227.

Moser, M-B., & Moser, E.I. (1998). Functional differentiation in the hippocampus. *Hippocampus*, *8*, 608–618.

Murray, E.A. (in press). Memory for objects in nonhuman primates. In M. Gazzaniga (Ed.), *The cognitive neurosciences* (2nd Edn.) Cambridge, MA: MIT Press.

Nolde, S.F., Johnson, M.K., & Raye, C.L. (1998). The role of prefrontal cortex during tests of episodic memory. *Trends in Cognitive Sciences*, *2*, 399–406.

Nyberg, L., Cabeza, R., & Tulving, E. (1996). PET studies of encoding and retrieval: The HERA model. *Psychonomic Bulletin and Review*, *3*, 135–148.

Nyberg, L., Cabeza, R., & Tulving, E. (1998). Asymmetric frontal activation during episodic memory: What kind of specificity? *Trends in Cognitive Sciences*, *2*, 419–420.

Parker, A., Wilding, E., & Akerman, C. (1998). The von Restorff effect in visual object recognition memory in humans and monkeys: The role of frontal/perirhinal interaction. *Journal of Cognitive Neuroscience*, *10*, 691–703.

Parkinson, J.K., Murray, E., & Mishkin, M. (1988). A selective mnemonic role for the hippocampus in monkeys: Memory for the location of objects. *Journal of Neuroscience, 8,* 4159–4167.

Petersen, S.E., Fox, P.T., Posner, M.I., Mintun, M., & Raichle, M.E. (1988). Positron emission tomographic studies of cortical anatomy of single-word processing. *Nature, 331,* 585–589.

Petersson, K.M., Elfgren, C., & Ingvar, M. (1997). A dynamic role of the medial temporal lobe during retrieval of declarative memory in man. *Neuroimage, 6,* 1–11.

Petersson, K.M., Elfgren, C., & Ingvar, M. (1998). Practice related changes in the human brain during free recall of abstract designs. *Neuroimage, 7,* S831.

Phelps, E.A., LaBar, K.S., Anderson, A.K., O'Connor, K.J., Fulbright, R.K., & Spencer, D.D. (1998). Specifying the contributions of the human amygdala to emotional memory: A case study. *Neurocase, 4,* 527–540.

Raichle, M.E., Fiez, J.A., Videen, T.O., MacLeod, A.M.K., Pardo, J.V., Fox, P.T., & Petersen, S.E. (1994). Practice-related changes in human brain functional anatomy during nonmotor learning. *Cerebral Cortex, 4,* 8–26.

Reed, J.M., & Squire, L.R. (1997). Impaired recognition memory in patients with lesions limited to the hippocampal formation. *Behavioral Neuroscience, 111,* 667–675.

Roland, P.E., & Gulyas, B. (1995). Visual memory, visual imagery and visual recognition of large field patterns by the human brain: Functional anatomy by positron emission tomography. *Cerebral Cortex, 1,* 79–93.

Rolls, E.T. (1996). A theory of hippocampal function in memory. *Hippocampus, 6,* 601–620.

Rugg, M.D., Mark, R.E., Walla, P., Schloerscheidt, A.M., Birch, C.S., & Allan, K. (1998). Dissociation of neural correlates of implicit and explicit memory. *Nature, 392,* 595–601.

Schacter, D.L., Alpert, N.M., Savage, C.R., Rauch, S.L., & Albert, M.S. (1996). Conscious recollection and the human hippocampal formation: Evidence from positron emission tomography. *Proceedings of the National Academy of Sciences, USA, 93,* 321–325.

Schacter, D.L., & Buckner, R.L. (1998a). Priming and the brain. *Neuron, 20,* 185–195.

Schacter, D.L., & Buckner, R.L. (1998b). On the relations among priming, conscious recollection, and intentional retrieval: Evidence from neuroimaging research. *Neurobiology of Learning and Memory, 70,* 284–303.

Schacter, D.L., Buckner, R.L., Koutstaal, W., Dale, A.M., & Rosen, B.R. (1997). Late onset of anterior prefrontal activity during true and false recognition: An event-related fMRI study. *Neuroimage, 6,* 259–269.

Schacter, D.L., & Graf, P. (1986). Preserved learning in amnesic patients: Perspectives from research on direct priming. *Journal of Clinical and Experimental Neuropsychology, 6,* 727–743.

Schacter, D.L., Reiman, E., Uecker, A., Polster, M.R., Yun, L.S., & Cooper, L.A. (1995). Brain regions associated with retrieval of structurally coherent visual information. *Nature, 376,* 587–590.

Schacter, D.L., & Wagner, A.D. (1999). Medial temporal lobe activations in fMRI and PET studies of encoding and retrieval. *Hippocampus, 9,* 7–24.

Shallice, T., Fletcher, P., Frith, C.D., Grasby, P., Frackowiak, R.S.J., & Dolan, R.J. (1994). Brain regions associated with acquisition and retrieval of verbal episodic memory. *Nature, 368,* 633–635.

Shimamura, A.P. (1993). Neuropsychological analyses of implicit memory: History, methodology and theoretical interpretations. In P. Graf & M.E.J. Masson (Eds.), *Implicit memory: New directions in cognition, development, and neuropsychology.* Hillsdale, NJ: Lawrence Erlbaum Associates.

Squire, L.R., & Alvarez, P. (1995). Retrograde amnesia and memory consolidation: A neurobiological perspective. *Current Opinion in Neurobiology, 5,* 169–177.

Squire, L.R., Ojemann, J.G., Miezen, F.M., Petersen, S.E., Videen, T.O., & Raichle, M.E. (1992). Activation of the hippocampus in normal humans: A functional anatomical study of memory. *Proceedings of the National Academy of Science, USA, 89,* 1837–1841.

Stern, C.E., Corkin, S., Gonzalez, R.G., Guimaraes, A.R., Baker, J.R., Jennings, P.J., Carr, C.A.,

Sugiura, R.M, Vedantham, V., & Rosen, B.R. (1996). The hippocampal formation participates in novel picture encoding: Evidence from functional magnetic resonance imaging. *Proceedings of the National Academy of Sciences, USA, 93*, 8660–8665.

Sullivan, E.V., Marsh, L., Mathalon, D.H., Lim, K.O., & Pfefferbaum, A. (1995). Anterior hippocampal volume deficits in nonamnesic, aging chronic alcoholics. *Alcohol in Clinical & Experimental Research, 19*, 110–122.

Tulving, E., Kapur, S., Craik, F.I.M., Markowitsch, H.J., & Houle, S. (1994a). Hemispheric encoding/retrieval asymmetry in episodic memory: Positron emission tomography findings. *Proceedings of the National Academy of Sciences, USA, 91*, 2016–2020.

Tulving, E. & Markowitsch, H.J. (1997). Memory beyond the hippocampus. *Current Opinion in Neurobiology, 7*, 209–216.

Tulving, E., Markowitsch, H.J., Craik, F.I.M., Habib, R., & Houle, S. (1996). Novelty and familiarity activations in PET studies of encoding and retrieval. *Cerebral Cortex, 6*, 71–79.

Tulving, E., Markowitsch, H.J., Kapur, S., Habib, R., & Houle, S. (1994b). Novelty encoding networks in the human brain: Positron emission tomography data. *NeuroReport, 5*, 2525–2528.

Vargha-Khadem, F., Gadian, D.G., Watkins, K.E., Connelly, A., Van Paesschen, W., & Mishkin, M. (1997). Differential effects of early hippocampal pathology on episodic and semantic memory. *Science, 277*, 376–380.

Wagner, A.D., Poldrack, R.A., Eldridge, L.L., Desmond, J.E., Glover, G.H., & Gabrieli, J.D.E. (1998a). Material-specific lateralization of prefrontal activation during episodic encoding and retrieval. *NeuroReport, 19*, 3911–3717.

Wagner, A.D., Schacter, D.L., Rotte, M., Koutstaal, W., Maril, A., Dale, A.M., & Buckner, R.L. (1998b). Building memories: Remembering and forgetting of verbal experiences as predicted by brain activity. *Science, 281*, 1188–1190.

Wiggs, C.L., Weisberg, J., & Martin, A. (1999). Neural correlates of semantic and episodic retrieval. *Neuropsychologia, 37*, 103–118.

Wiggs, C.L. & Martin, A. (1998). Properties and mechanisms of perceptual priming. *Current Opinion in Neurobiology, 8*, 227–233.

MEMORY, 1999, 7 (5/6), 661–678

Direct Comparison of Episodic Encoding and Retrieval of Words: An Event-related fMRI Study

Kathleen B. McDermott, Jeffrey G. Ojemann, Steven E. Petersen,
John M. Ollinger, Abraham Z. Snyder, Erbil Akbudak,
Thomas E. Conturo, and Marcus E. Raichle

Washington University School of Medicine, USA

Functional magnetic resonance imaging (fMRI) was used to compare directly episodic encoding and retrieval. During encoding, subjects studied visually presented words and reported via keypress whether each word represented a pleasant or unpleasant concept (intentional, deep encoding). During the retrieval phase, subjects indicated (via keypress) whether visually presented words had previously been studied. No reliable differences were found during the recognition phase for words that had been previously studied and those that had not been studied. Areas preferentially active during encoding (relative to retrieval) included left superior frontal cortex, medial frontal cortex, left superior temporal cortex, posterior cingulate, left parahippocampal gyrus, and left inferior frontal gyrus. Regions more active in retrieval than encoding included bilateral inferior parietal cortex, bilateral precuneus, right frontal polar cortex, right dorsolateral prefrontal cortex, and right inferior frontal/insular cortex.

INTRODUCTION

Episodic memory refers to the type of long-term memory that allows a person to recollect personally experienced events (Tulving, 1983). It encompasses both the initial acquisition of information (encoding) and the subsequent remembering of the previous experiences (retrieval). The recent advent of neuroimaging techniques, e.g. positron emission tomography (PET) and functional magnetic resonance imaging (fMRI), has offered a new window through which to view episodic memory; we can now observe the living, awake brain as it encodes and later retrieves experiences. In the last decade, there has been a flurry of neuroimaging research designed to identify the neural substrates of episodic

Requests for reprints should be sent to Kathleen McDermott, Division of Radiological Sciences, Box 8225, 4525 Scott Ave., St Louis, MO 63110, USA. Email: kmcd@npg.wustl.edu

We thank Todd Braver, Randy Buckner, and Roddy Roediger for helpful comments on a previous version of this paper.

encoding and retrieval. Although the eventual goal is to understand the unique contributions of the individual structures contributing to encoding and retrieval, identification of the differences in activation patterns for the two processes is an important first step. It is this latter goal that is the primary focus of the present experiment.

Relatively little is known about the similarities and differences of the neural substrates underlying encoding and retrieval. The focus has generally been on two structures: hippocampus (and surrounding medial temporal regions) and frontal cortex. On the basis of lesion studies, we might expect the hippocampus and surrounding structures in the medial temporal lobe to contribute to encoding more than to retrieval; damage to these structures often renders one amnesic and unable to form lasting representations of newly encountered information. However, demonstrations of intact implicit memory in medial temporal amnesic patients (e.g. Warrington & Weiskrantz, 1968) could be taken as implicating medial temporal structures in conscious recollection (i.e. retrieval). Due to difficulties in attributing lesion-induced memory deficits to being encoding-or retrieval-based, as just demonstrated, the contribution of medial temporal structures to encoding and/or retrieval is unknown. Effects of frontal lobe damage have been reported to lead to memory disorders (Stuss et al., 1994), but this claim is controversial (Shimamura, Janowsky, & Squire, 1990). Lesion studies do not project a clear picture with respect to the role of frontal cortex in episodic memory.

On the basis of behavioural theories of memory (e.g. the encoding specificity principle, Tulving, 1983; transfer appropriate processing, Morris, Bransford, & Franks, 1977), we might expect the neural mechanisms in encoding and retrieval processes to overlap considerably (Roediger, Buckner, & McDermott, 1999). That is, retrieval will benefit to the extent that the cognitive operations performed reinstate those performed during encoding. Therefore, we might expect retrieval to involve a reactivation of processing areas used during encoding.

A complicating factor is that no single task captures the essence of encoding, and no single task captures the essence of retrieval. For example, both encoding and retrieval can be verbal or nonverbal, intentional or incidental. Further, encoding can be "deep" (meaning-based, Craik & Lockhart, 1972) or "shallow" (based on surface features); similarly, retrieval can be performed at a recollective level ("remembering" in Tulving's 1985 terminology) or a more heuristic level ("knowing"). Retrieval can be cued or noncued. Because all these variables interact behaviourally with encoding and retrieval they could be expected to differ somewhat in their neural substrates. In addition, encoding often involves a form of semantic retrieval, and episodic retrieval involves an element of encoding. Thus, no single study can definitively answer the question of how encoding and retrieval relate neurally.

Difficulties notwithstanding, the identification of structures differentially involved in encoding and retrieval has interested researchers and has both theoretical and clinical implications. However, direct, within-subject comparisons of the two tasks have been rarely reported (Fletcher et al., 1995b; Nyberg et al., 1996; Petrides et al., 1993; Shallice et al., 1994).

The present study was designed to compare encoding and retrieval of visually presented words. It builds on the existing studies in that it employs fMRI, which offers more observations per subject, and usually better spatial and temporal resolution than PET. In addition, fMRI permits the recognition test to closely approximate those typically given behaviourally. That is, old and new items can be randomly intermixed without sacrificing the ability to compare the two item types directly because selective averaging of trials is possible with fMRI (Dale & Buckner, 1997; Josephs, Turner, & Friston, 1997; Zarahn, Aguirre, & D'Esposito, 1997; for a review see Rosen, Buckner, & Dale, 1998). Following the scan, one can parse out certain types of trials (e.g. studied words) and compare them to others (e.g. nonstudied words). Designs that permit such analyses are typically called *event-related* designs. This type of design offers a significant methodological advance in that it minimises strategic differences that often plague blocked designs (in which a set, or block, of previously studied items occurs, followed by a block of nonstudied items).

In the present experiment, subjects studied (under intentional learning conditions) 64 words in four 295-second epochs (16 words per epoch, or "run"). Trials were spaced 16.5 seconds apart to allow the haemodynamic response from a given trial to peak and return to baseline before the subsequent trial (Buckner et al., 1996b). These encoding runs were compared to four retrieval runs (yes/no recognition memory), which were procedurally identical, with the exception of task instructions.

METHOD

Subjects

Eight subjects (three males, five females, mean age 22.3, ranging from 21 to 25 years) were recruited from the Washington University community in return for payment. All were right-handed, native speakers of English, had normal or corrected-to-normal vision, and reported no history of significant neurological problems. Subjects provided informed consent in accordance with the guidelines set by the Washington University Human Studies Committee.

Procedure and Materials

Scans were conducted on a Siemens 1.5 Tesla Vision System (Erlangen, Germany) with a standard circularly polarised head coil. A Power Macintosh computer (Apple, Cupertino, CA) and Psyscope software (Cohen et al., 1993) were used for display of visual stimuli. Subjects responded by pushing one of two keys on a fibre-optic light-sensitive keypress connected to a Psyscope Button Box (Carnegie Mellon University, Pittsburgh, PA). An LCD projector

(Sharp, model XGE850) projected stimuli onto a screen positioned at the head of the bore. Subjects viewed the screen via a mirror positioned on the head coil. A pillow was used to minimise head movement, and headphones dampened scanner noise and allowed for communication with subjects.

Structural images were acquired using the MPRAGE sequence with 2mm isotropic voxels (Mugler & Brookeman, 1990). Functional images were collected with an asymmetric spin-echo-planar sequence sensitive to blood oxygenation level-dependent (BOLD) contrast (TR = 2.364, 3.75 × 3.75mm in-plane resolution). In each functional run, 125 sets of 16 contiguous, 8mm-thick axial images were acquired parallel to the anterior–posterior commissure plane; this procedure offered whole-brain coverage at a high signal-to-noise ratio (Conturo et al., 1996). Each run lasted approximately five minutes (2.364 seconds per whole-brain acquisition, with 125 such acquisitions per run). There were approximately three minutes between runs, during which time subjects were allowed to rest.

Both encoding and retrieval runs were event-related. Trials occurred every 16.5 seconds to allow the haemodynamic response to rise and return to baseline before the next trial commenced. Trials began on (or near) the onset of the TR (or repetition time, the time required for one whole-brain scan), which allowed seven complete whole-brain acquisitions to occur for each (16.5-second) trial. In all runs, words were presented for one second, followed by a blank screen for three seconds and then a fixation point (a plus sign) for 12.5 seconds (see Fig. 1). Subjects were instructed to respond either while the word was on the screen or during the immediately following blank screen. Subjects were told that during the fixation phase they should look at the fixation point while remaining still. In the encoding runs, subjects were instructed to press one of two keys with their right hand to indicate whether the concept represented by the word was more "pleasant" or "unpleasant". They were also told to remember the words as well as possible for a later memory test. During the retrieval runs, subjects pressed one of two keys to indicate whether or not they had studied the word previously. Thus, there were visual, binary decision, and keypress components to both types of runs.

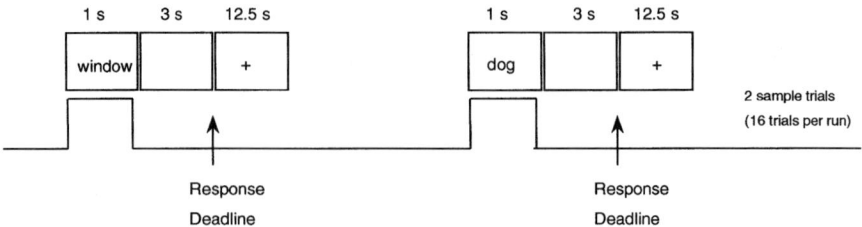

FIG. 1.   Schematic depiction of two trials. Trials occurred every 16.5 seconds, and each run included 16 trials.

As demonstrated in Fig. 2, half of the subjects participated in four encoding runs (or sets of 16 trials) followed by six retrieval runs, and the other half received the reverse order (six retrieval, then four encoding runs).[1] Because encoding runs sometimes followed retrieval runs, there were two types of encoding task: those scanned and those unscanned but later tested during retrieval runs (see Fig. 2). Similarly, there were two types of retrieval task: those scanned and unscanned. This manipulation was implemented primarily to control for order effects manifested in signal drift in the scanner; further, they helped control for other order effects (e.g. subject fatigue). Although the specific procedure is complex, the essence is that all subjects participated in three study–test cycles, and we varied which of the study and test episodes were scanned.

As depicted in the top row of Fig. 2, subjects in the encoding-first condition performed four encoding runs (64 words, 16 words/run, half high-frequency and half low-frequency of occurrence in the English language).[2] Subjects were instructed to try to remember the words for a later memory test; they also had to determine whether each word referred to a concept that was more "pleasant" or "unpleasant" and to indicate their decision with a keypress. Thus, intentional

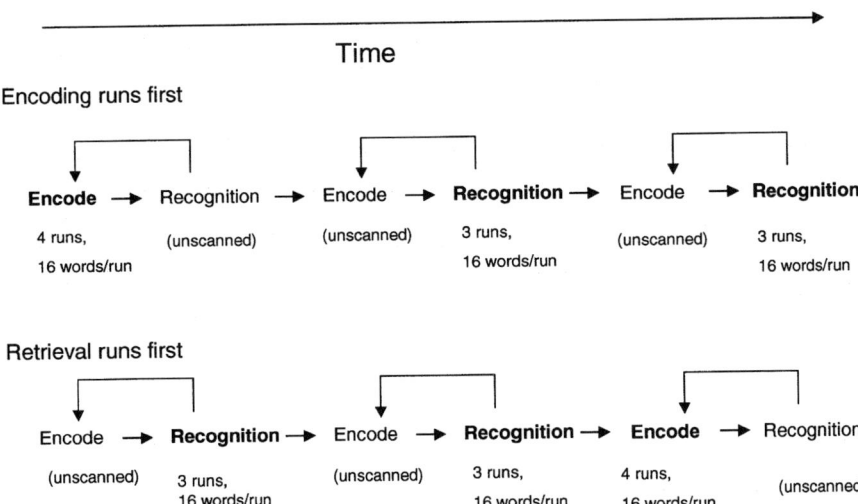

FIG. 2. Schematic depiction of the procedure for subjects receiving the encoding scans first, followed by retrieval scans (top row) and those scanned on the retrieval task first, followed by encoding scans (bottom row). Tasks in bold were those scanned; those in roman were not scanned.

---

[1]To equate power in the two conditions, we analysed only four retrieval runs per subject for the purposes of this paper.

[2]High frequency was defined as greater than 50 occurrences per million words; low frequency was defined as fewer than 10 occurrences per million words (Kučera & Francis, 1967).

semantic encoding was examined. A short recognition test followed the encoding scans (30 words, half old, not scanned); the purpose of the test was to ensure the words had been encoded effectively. Subjects then studied another set of words (24 words in an unscanned encoding task). Half of the encoded words were high-frequency and half low-frequency. Further, half were assigned to a deep level of processing and half to a shallow level. The deep condition required subjects to mentally determine (on a scale of 1 to 7) how pleasant the concept was, and the shallow task required them to count the number of vowels in the word. The encoding task was followed by three runs of memory tests. Subjects were required to determine whether the visually presented word had been previously studied or not, and to indicate their judgement via keypress. (Half of the tested words had been studied previously.) This final cycle repeated (unscanned encoding phase, three scanned recognition runs) with a different set of words.

For the "retrieval runs first" condition, which is depicted in the bottom row of Fig. 2, subjects studied 24 words (unscanned). Again, half were high-frequency and half low-frequency; further, half occurred under deep encoding and half shallow. Subjects were then tested on those words, via a recognition memory test, which was scanned. The test required subjects to determine whether visually presented words had been studied in the preceding session and to register the response via keypress (see Fig. 1). Again, half of the tested words had been studied in the preceding encoding session. This study (unscanned)–test (scanned) cycle then repeated, as shown in Fig. 2. Finally, these subjects participated in the four encoding scans, followed by an unscanned memory test to ensure instructions had been followed.

In summary, as depicted in Fig. 2, subjects either participated in the encoding first condition (n = 4; scanned encoding, then unscanned recognition; unscanned encoding, then scanned recognition; unscanned encoding, then scanned recognition) or in the retrieval first condition (n = 4, unscanned encoding, then scanned recognition; unscanned encoding, then scanned recognition; scanned encoding, then unscanned recognition).

Data Analysis

Data for each subject were subjected to the standard processing stream used at Washington University, which includes movement-correction within and across runs using an automated procedure (Snyder, 1996), whole brain normalisation to a common mode of 1000 to allow for comparisons across subjects, and temporal interpolation to correct for offsets in the acquisition times of individual slices (see Ojemann et al., 1997 for an overview).

The data were analysed using an in-house implementation of the general linear model. We began by identifying regions active in separate condition types (e.g. encoding relative to fixation). Specifically, we cross-correlated the timecourse of the BOLD response to each condition at each voxel (with lagged gamma function with a delay of 2.83 seconds and a width of 2 seconds, Dale & Buckner, 1997). The resulting magnitudes were then used to compute t-statistics to determine those reliably different from .00 (Friston, Jezzard, & Turner, 1994; Worsley & Friston, 1995).

In addition, comparisons between conditions were computed by assigning appropriate weights to each condition. This approach allowed for direct comparisons to determine regions differentially active in one condition relative to another (i.e. encoding to retrieval; high to low-frequency words; and, within retrieval, previously studied words to previously nonstudied words). The contrast of primary interest was the comparison of encoding and retrieval.

The resulting statistical images were warped into standardised atlas space (Talairach & Tournoux, 1988) and averaged across subjects. The resulting composite images were then corrected for multiple comparisons (Ollinger, 1997) such that $P < .05$ where P refers to the probability of a single erroneous activation in the image volume; in addition, single-voxel regions were rejected. The correction method uses a region-size dependent threshold to guarantee that the experiment-wide Type I error is $< .05$; this method provides weak Type I control at the voxel level but strong control at the cluster level. An automated peak-search algorithm (Mintun, Fox, & Raichle, 1989) identified the location (in atlas coordinates) of peak activations on the basis of level of statistical significance and cluster size.

RESULTS AND DISCUSSION

Behavioural Results

Due to equipment failure (in the fibre-optic light source), we obtained behavioural data for only four of our subjects; we therefore report only proportions of hits and correct rejections (and their median RTs) here. For the unscanned recognition tests following the encoding runs, the hit rate was 1.0 (761ms) and the correct rejection rate .98 (875ms). For the retrieval runs, the hit rate was .86 (1029ms) and the correct rejection rate .83 (1234ms). From these data we can conclude that subjects effectively encoded and retrieved in all phases of the experiment.

Imaging Results

When compared directly, both encoding and retrieval revealed several distinct regions more active than the other (Plate 7; Tables 1 and 2). We consider first regions more active in encoding than retrieval (Plate 7, Panel A; Table 1). Three of these regions have been reported previously as being associated with encoding processes: posterior cingulate (Shallice et al., 1995); left parahippocampal gyrus (Dolan & Fletcher, 1997; Kelley et al., 1998); and left inferior

TABLE 1
Regions More Active in Encoding than Retrieval

Location		Coordinates			Significance Level	
		x	*y*	*z*	*z-score*	*BA*
Frontal	Superior	−15	33	52	4.02	8
		−5	55	22	4.09	9/10
		5	53	28	3.81	9
		−17	45	46	4.61	8
	Medial	−3	49	28	4.73	9
		−1	55	14	3.84	10
	Inferior	−41	25	−6	3.64	47
		−51	23	10	3.41	45
Temporal	Superior	−43	−57	20	3.96	39
	Middle	−47	−61	14	3.94	39
	Parahippocampal gyrus	−19	−47	−4	3.76	19
Posterior Cingulate		−7	−53	6	4.03	30
		1	−61	14	3.6	30/23

Coordinates from the Talairach & Tournoux (1988) atlas; positive values refer to regions to the right of (x), anterior to (y), and superior to (z) the anterior commissure. The significance level for inclusion in the table was set to *P*<.001 (or *z* = 3.3). BA refers to approximate Brodmann area corresponding to atlas coordinates.

frontal cortex (in or near BA 45/47; Demb et al., 1995; Kapur et al., 1994; Nyberg, Cabeza, & Tulving, 1996). Three other regions found to be preferentially active in encoding have not been widely observed in other encoding studies: left superior frontal cortex (BA 8), medial frontal cortex, and left superior temporal cortex. Curiously, these three regions share another common feature: they seem to be de-activated in retrieval (see Fig. 3). We interpret these results cautiously, however, because the negative curves for retrieval do not follow the usual pattern for most negative curves. That is, typical curves for the BOLD signal (both positive and negative) have sharp onsets or offsets (as in the case for deactivations; Ojemann et al., 1998). That is, more typical negative curves would show sudden drops (much like a mirror reversal of the positive curves). Instead, the onset of these negative curves occurs more gradually.

Several regions were revealed as differentially active in retrieval relative to encoding (Plate 7, Panel B; Table 2). Timecourses for these regions can be seen in Fig. 4. The most robustly active regions were bilateral precuneus and bilateral inferior parietal cortex. In addition, right frontal polar cortex (specifically, anterior middle frontal gyrus, BA 10), right dorsolateral frontal cortex (BA 9/ 46), and right insular cortex (BA 45/47) were also more active in recognition memory than in encoding.

Encoding > Retrieval

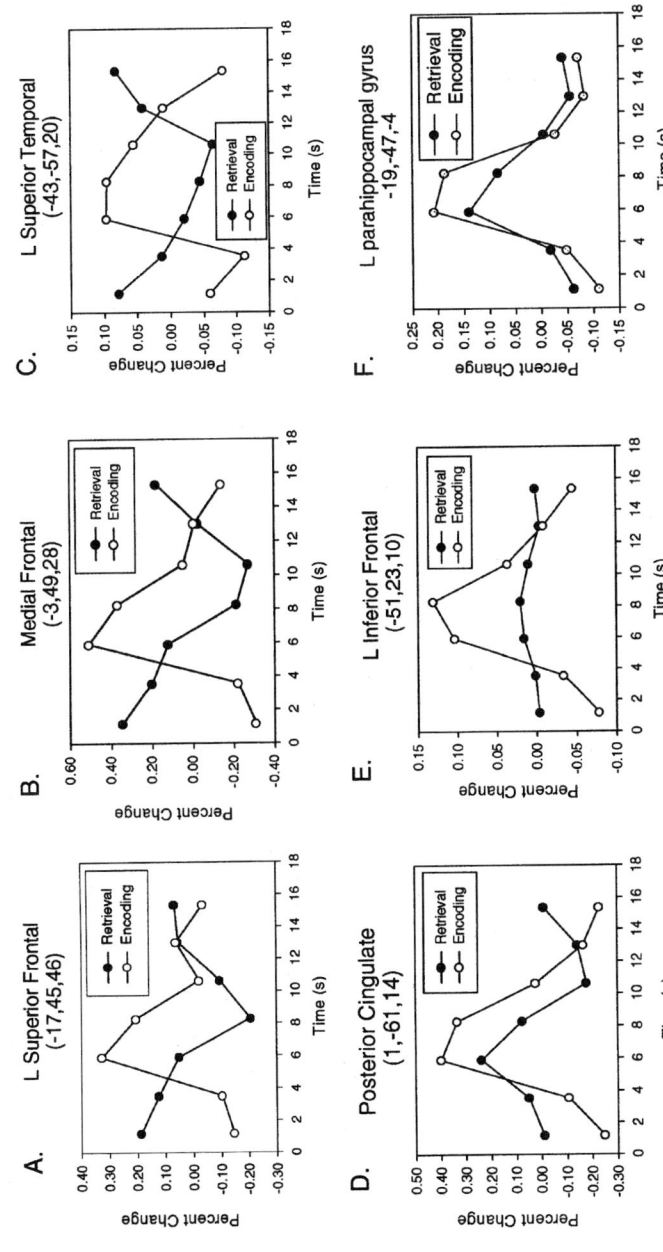

FIG. 3. Timecourses from selected peaks identified as more active in encoding than retrieval (see Plate 7, Panel A). Timecourses were obtained by defining a 15 × 15mm square region around the peak point on a 3mm axial slice and averaging the timecourse data for only the voxels that reached significance within that region. Note that peaks are plotted as percent change in signal, but because the images have been normalised to a common value, positive-going curves tend to start below .00, whereas negative-going curves tend to start above .00. Because each whole-brain scan took 2.36 seconds, positive-going curves tend to start below .00, whereas negative-going curves tend to start above .00. Because each whole-brain scan took 2.36 seconds, timepoints shown are the average timepoint for each of the seven scans within each trial (e.g. the first scan spanned from 0 to 2.36 seconds and is therefore plotted at 1.18 second). Note that the scale differs across graphs to highlight the response signal for each region. Alphabetic labels refer to the labels assigned in Plate 7.

669

TABLE 2
Regions More Active in Retrieval than Encoding

Location		Coordinates			Significance Level	
		x	y	z	z-score	BA
Frontal	Middle	41	31	30	4.38	9/46
		37	51	22	3.98	10
		−41	49	4	3.72	10/46
	Inferior/insular	31	21	2	3.4	45/47
Parietal	Superior	−19	−73	38	4.09	19
		31	−61	46	4.31	7
	Inferior	−33	−55	40	5.72	40
		37	−55	38	5.58	40
		41	−47	56	4.42	40
		53	−33	42	4.12	40
		−45	−49	40	4	40
	Medial/precuneus	−17	−67	48	3.52	7
		−7	−73	38	6.33	7/19
		9	−73	38	6.04	7/19
		13	−67	30	5.39	7/31
		−15	−69	28	4.95	31
		15	−61	24	4.37	31
		5	−69	28	3.98	31
Posterior Cingulate		−3	−29	24	3.97	23

Coordinates from the Talairach & Tournoux (1988) atlas; positive values refer to regions to the right of (x), anterior to (y), and superior to (z) the anterior commissure. The significance level for inclusion in the table was set to $P<.001$ (or $z = 3.3$). BA refers to approximate Brodmann area corresponding to atlas coordinates.

The activations in precuneus and inferior parietal cortex are especially interesting; although they have been reported in the retrieval literature (Andreasen et al., 1995; Buckner et al., 1996a; Fletcher, Frith, & Rugg, 1997; Fletcher et al., 1995b; Shallice et al., 1994; see Cabeza & Nyberg, 1997 for a review), they have not been explored to any extent. Receiving much more attention has been right frontal polar cortex (BA 10, see Plate 7, Panel B; Andreasen et al., 1995; Buckner et al., 1996a, 1998a,b; Nyberg et al., 1995; Rugg et al., 1996; Schacter et al., 1997; Squire et al., 1992) and, to a lesser extent, a more superior region in right dorsolateral prefrontal cortex (BA 9/46), also seen in the present data in Plate 7, Panel B (Buckner et al., 1998a; Wagner et al., 1999).

An interesting finding with respect to the right frontal polar activations in retrieval tasks has been the observation that the onset of the activation is late compared to signals in other cortical regions (Buckner et al., 1998b; Schacter et

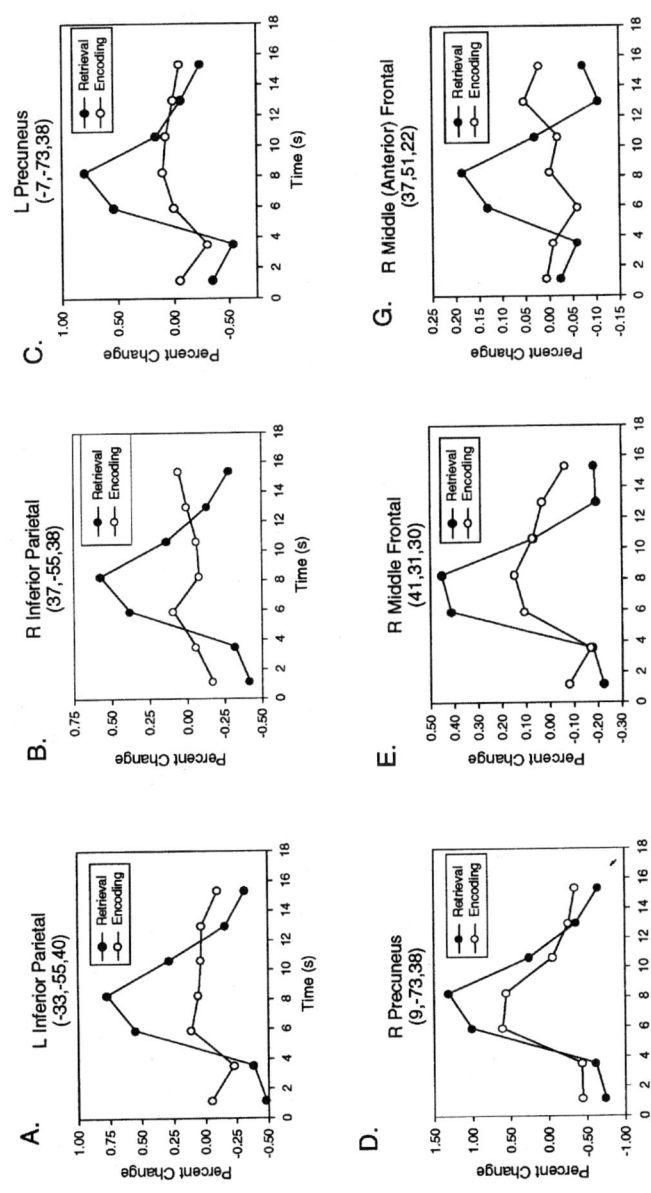

FIG. 4. Timecourses from selected peaks identified as more active in retrieval than encoding (see Plate 7, Panel B). Timecourses were obtained by defining a 15 × 15mm square region around the peak point on a 3mm axial slice and averaging the timecourse data for only the voxels that reached significance within that region. Note that peaks are plotted as percent change in signal, but because the images have been normalised to a common value, positive-going curves tend to start below .00, whereas negative-going curves tend to start above .00. Because each whole-brain scan took 2.36 seconds, timepoints shown are the average timepoint for each of the seven scans within each trial (e.g. the first scan spanned from 0 to 2.36 seconds and is therefore plotted at 1.18 second). Note that the scale differs across graphs to highlight the response signal for each region. Alphabetic labels refer to the labels assigned in Plate 7.

al., 1997). The late onset, however, was not observed in the present study (as shown in the curve in Fig. 4); in addition, we examined statistical activation images with gamma functions lagged at longer delays (3.83 and 5.83 seconds) and did not observe responses in this region. The reason for the discrepancy between our study and the two similar studies, which also employed event-related fMRI to examine verbal recognition memory, is unclear. Nevertheless, our frontal polar timecourse appears similar in nature to those in other regions.

Although substantial differences between encoding and retrieval were observed, a number of striking similarities were also observed (see Plate 8). When compared to the low-level baseline (i.e. fixating on a cross-hair), encoding and retrieval shared many activations in common (Plate 8). These similarities occurred in part by design so that differences between encoding and retrieval could be attributed to high-level cognitive processes and not motor or perceptual differences in the tasks. In this respect, many of the similarities speak to the reliability of the data. On another level, however, some similarities may be attributable to similarities in higher-level processing (e.g. posterior inferior frontal gyrus, insular responses, thalamus contralateral to the motor response). In sum, a visual comparison between encoding (relative to fixation) and retrieval (relative to fixation) demonstrates similar activation patterns.

A direct comparison of high-and low-frequency words (collapsing across the encoding/retrieval factor) revealed no reliable differences in activations. Similarly, a direct comparison of types of words on the retrieval test (i.e. "old" or previously studied words and "new" or nonstudied words) yielded no reliable activations. Schacter et al. (1997) and Buckner et al. (1998b) have conducted very similar comparisons and also did not observe differences as a function of hits and correct rejections (although see Friston et al., 1998). It now appears as though previously reported differences between old and new items, which were observed in blocked designs, may have been a product of the design (Buckner et al., 1998b). In blocked designs, many trials of the same type (e.g. old words) typically occur in immediate succession; thus, clusters of old words would be compared to clusters of new words. However, this type of design can lead to strategic differences on the part of the subject, which could account for differences in activation patterns for old and new words. That is, if subjects detect (consciously or not) that there is a pattern in the test sequence, their strategies for making the old/new judgement could change (Wagner et al., 1998). With event-related designs, strategic differences are minimised because the sequencing of words (with respect to prior study status) can occur in a random order, so subjects cannot predict or detect patterns in the testing sequence. The current data add to two previous reports using event-related fMRI that demonstrate equivalent activations for old and new items. This null effect, however, is likely not to be the true state of events; rather, subtle phenomenological differences such as these may not yet be detectable with current methodology. Another possibility is that when subjects attempt to recollect whether an item occurred previously, they think back to the list and retrieve some studied items (but not the item in question). Thus, they produce a correct rejection, but it is not the case that the retrieval attempt was wholly unsuccessful: some list words were accurately retrieved. This scenario could also explain the lack of old/new differences in recognition memory.

GENERAL DISCUSSION

The data reported here highlight both similarities and differences between intentional encoding and subsequent retrieval of visually presented words. The similarities are evident if one inspects the encoding activations relative to fixation and the retrieval activations relative to fixation. Differences between encoding and retrieval emerged when a direct comparison was performed. Areas more active in encoding than retrieval included left parahippocampal gyrus, posterior cingulate, left inferior frontal cortex, left superior frontal cortex, medial frontal cortex, and left superior temporal cortex. Regions more active in retrieval than encoding included bilateral precuneus, bilateral inferior parietal cortex, right frontal polar, right dorsolateral, and right insular cortex.

Curiously, right frontal polar cortex has received the most attention as a"retrieval" area, and there has been a controversy about its function in retrieval (Buckner et al., 1998a,b; Kapur et al., 1995; Nyberg et al., 1995; Rugg et al., 1996; Schacter et al., 1997). In addition, activations in this region during retrieval tasks have played a large role in the development of a widely known heuristic regarding the role of frontal cortex in episodic memory encoding and retrieval, which has been labelled Hemispheric Encoding/Retrieval Asymmetry (HERA) (Tulving et al., 1994; Nyberg, Cabeza, & Tulving, 1996). The claim is that left frontal areas are differentially involved in encoding, whereas right frontal areas are differentially involved in retrieval. Initially, HERA was intended to describe verbal episodic memory (Tulving et al., 1994), but it was later extended to episodic memory in general (whether verbal or nonverbal, Nyberg, Cabeza, & Tulving, 1996). To the extent that our data speak to this claim, there is some support for HERA. Verbal encoding activated left inferior and superior frontal gyri more than did retrieval; verbal retrieval activated right dorsolateral prefrontal regions (BA 9/46) and an anterior region of middle frontal gyrus (BA 10, R > L) in our study. However, our data suggest that frontal cortex may not be the most profitable area on which to focus when describing differences between encoding and retrieval (at least in the verbal domain). Intentional encoding and recognition memory also differ robustly in distinct regions of parietal cortex (i.e. bilateral precuneus and lateral inferior parietal regions).

Activations very similar to our parietal activations are often found in studies of working memory and have been attributed to verbal working memory (Jonides et al., 1997) and more specifically to phonological processing (Jonides et al., 1998). Fiez et al. (1996) surveyed the working memory literature and found the mean activation site across studies to be –33, –47, 37 and 36, –48, 41, coordinates that fall very close to the foci in the current experiment (i.e. –33, –55, 40 and 37, –55, 38 for left and right inferior parietal regions, respectively). It is not obvious, however, why phonological processing in retrieval should exceed that in encoding. Perhaps gist-or dual process-based theories of recognition memory (e.g. Reyna & Brainerd, 1995) might predict this pattern. That is, some theories of recognition memory hold that the task can, in some instances, be performed on a quick, automatic basis (e.g. whether the word "seems familiar"). These low-level familiarity judgements could be, in part, based on phonology. However, lateral inferior parietal activations have been reported in free recall (Andreasen et al., 1995), which would seem to rule out any gist-based accounts for the present activations because free recall is not thought to have a gist-like component, and instead to be almost wholly recollective. Admittedly, though, once words are successfully retrieved in free recall, they are most certainly processed phonologically. Therefore, although the source of the activation in retrieval is not obvious, the similarity in the region often attributed to phonological processing and our own activations in recognition memory is striking.

The more medial activations in precuneus are also interesting. A similar region (but about 15mm anterior to the activations in the present study) has been implicated in imaginal processing (Fletcher et al., 1995a). It would be a stretch to argue that imaginal processing should be greater in recognition memory than encoding. Nevertheless, there is some similarity in activated regions.

We should note that the activations in precuneus and inferior parietal cortex are distinct from other regions in the same general area, which have been found to be de-activated in retrieval tasks (e.g. Buckner et al., 1996a, 1998a). That is, in addition to the region of medial parietal cortex that is activated in retrieval, there is also a region de-activated; this de-activated region is slightly anterior to the activated region. In addition, the lateral inferior parietal activations occur near a more-lateral region that is de-activated.

One interesting null result is that the posterior and dorsal extent of the left inferior frontal gyrus (BA 6/44) was activated to an equivalent extent in encoding and retrieval. (This region is superior to the inferior frontal region observed to be preferentially active in encoding in the present study.) This equivalence is noteworthy because Kelley et al. (1998) found this region to be more active in intentional encoding of verbal materials, which led to a high level of performance on a recognition memory test, than incidental encoding of the same materials, which led to a low level of later recognition. Thus, one interpretation of their finding would be that this region of dorsal inferior frontal cortex is specifically involved in verbal episodic memory encoding (e.g. that it is the process of encoding, or maybe the intention to encode that activates this region). Further evidence for this claim can be found in Wagner et al. (1998b), who showed level-of-processing effects (Craik & Lockhart, 1972) in this same region, and, further, showed that greater activation in this region was predictive of later retrieval success. The current study suggests that it is neither encoding *per se* nor intent to encode that leads to activation here, but rather that active verbal processing in general elicits activation of dorsal inferior frontal cortex (see McDermott et al., in press).

In conclusion, our direct comparison of verbal episodic encoding and retrieval revealed many similarities and some differences between the two processes. Other similar comparisons, using different types of study and test materials, will be necessary to reveal the extent to which our results generalise across domains (e.g. verbal/nonverbal). Consistencies across studies will lead us to a better understanding of brain mechanisms underlying episodic encoding and retrieval. Our results highlight the importance of parietal cortex in episodic recognition of verbal materials; further comparisons will be necessary to establish the extent to which this observation generalises across different types of encoding and retrieval tasks.

REFERENCES

Andreasen, N.C., O'Leary, D.S., Arndt, S., Cizadlo, T., Hurtig, R., Rezai, K., Watkins, G.L., Ponto, L.L.B., & Hichwa, R.D. (1995). Short-term and long-term verbal memory: A positron emission tomography study. *Proceedings of the National Academy of Science, USA, 92*, 5111–5115.

Buckner, R.L., Bandettini, P.A., O'Craven, K.M., Savoy, R.L., Petersen, S.E., Raichle, M.E., & Rosen, B.R. (1996b). Detection of cortical activation during averaged single trials of a cognitive task using functional magnetic resonance imaging. *Proceedings of the National Academy of Sciences, USA, 93*, 1478–1483.

Buckner, R.L., Koutstaal, W., Schacter, D.L., Dale, A.M., Rotte, M., & Rosen, B.R. (1998b). Functional-anatomic study of episodic retrieval. II. Selective averaging of event-related fMRI trials to test the retrieval success hypothesis. *Neuroimage, 7*, 163–175.

Buckner, R.L., Koutstaal, W., Schacter, D.L., Wagner, A.D., & Rosen, B.R. (1998a). Functional anatomic study of episodic retrieval using fMRI: I. Retrieval effort versus retrieval success. *Neuroimage, 7*, 151–162.

Buckner, R.L., Raichle, M.E., Miezin, F.M., & Petersen, S.E. (1996a). Functional anatomic studies of memory retrieval for auditory words and visual pictures. *Journal of Neuroscience, 16*, 6219–6235.

Cabeza, R., & Nyberg, L. (1997). Imaging cognition: An empirical review of PET studies with normal subjects. *Journal of Cognitive Neuroscience, 9*, 1–26.

Cohen, J.D., MacWhinney, B., Flatt, M., & Provost, J. (1993). PsyScope: A new graphic interactive environment for designing psychology experiments. *Behavioral Research Methods, Instruments, and Computers, 25*, 257–271.

Conturo, T.E., McKinstry, R.C., Akbudak, E., Snyder, A.Z., Yang, T.Z., & Raichle, M.E. (1996). Sensitivity optimization and experimental design in functional magnetic resonance imaging. *Society for Neuroscience Abstracts, 22*, 7.

Craik, F.I.M. & Lockhart, R.S. (1972). Levels of processing: A framework for memory research. *Journal of Verbal Learning and Verbal Behavior, 4*, 671–684.

Dale, A.M. & Buckner, R.L. (1997). Selective averaging of rapidly presented individual trials using fMRI. *Human Brain Mapping, 5*, 329–340.

Demb, J.B., Desmond, J.E., Wagner, A.D., Vaidya, C.J., Glover, G.H., & Gabrieli, J.D.E. (1995). Semantic encoding and retrieval in the left inferior prefrontal cortex: A functional MRI study of task difficulty and process specificity. *Journal of Neuroscience, 15*, 5870–5878.

Dolan, R.J. & Fletcher, P.C. (1997). Dissociating prefrontal and hippocampal function in episodic memory encoding. *Nature, 388,* 582–585.

Fiez, J., Raichle, M.E., Miezin, F.M., & Petersen, S.E. (1996). PET studies of auditory and phonological processing: Effects of stimulus characteristics and task demands. *Journal of Cognitive Neuroscience, 7,* 808–822.

Fletcher, P.C., Frith, C.D., Baker, S.C., Shallice, T., Frackowiak, R.S., & Dolan, R.J. (1995a). The mind's eye—precuneus activation in memory-related imagery. *Neuroimage, 2,* 195–200.

Fletcher, P.C., Frith, C.D., Grasby, P.M., Shallice, T., Frackowiak, R.S.J., & Dolan, R.J. (1995b). Brain systems for encoding and retrieving auditory-verbal memory: An *in vivo* study in humans. *Brain, 118,* 401–416.

Fletcher, P.C., Frith, C.D., & Rugg, M.D. (1997). Functional neuroanatomy of episodic memory. *Trends in Neurosciences, 20,* 213–218.

Friston, K.J., Fletcher, P., Josephs, O., Holmes, A., Rugg, M.D., & Turner, R. (1998). Event-related fMRI: Characterizing differential responses. *Neuroimage, 7,* 30–40.

Friston, K.J., Jezzard, P., & Turner, R. (1994). Analysis of functional MRI time-series. *Human Brain Mapping, 1,* 153–171.

Janowsky, J.S., Shimamura, A.P., & Squire, L.R. (1989). Source memory impairments in patients with frontal lobe lesions. *Neuropsychologia, 27,* 1043–1056.

Jonides, J., Schumacher, E.H., Smith, E.E., Lauber, E.J., Awh, E., Minoshima, S., & Koeppe, R.A. (1997). Verbal working memory load affects regional brain activation as measured by PET. *Journal of Cognitive Neuroscience, 9,* 462–475.

Jonides, J., Schumacher, E.J., Smith, E.E., Koeppe, R.A., Wah, R., Reuter-Lorenz, P.A., Marschuetz, C., & Willis, C.R. (1998). The role of parietal cortex in verbal working memory. *The Journal of Neuroscience, 18,* 5026–5034.

Josephs, O., Turner, R., & Friston K. (1997). Event-related fMRI. *Human Brain Mapping, 5,* 243–248.

Kapur, S., Craik, F.I.M., Jones, C., Brown, G.M., Houle, S., & Tulving, E. (1995). Functional role of the prefrontal cortex in retrieval of memories: A Pet study. *Neuroreport, 6,* 1880–1884.

Kapur, S., Craik, F.I.M., Tulving, E., Wilson, A.A., Houle, S., Brown, G.M. (1994). Neuro-anatomical correlates of encoding in episodic memory: Levels of processing effect. *Proceedings of the National Academy of Sciences, USA, 91,* 2008–2011.

Kelley, W.M., Miezen, F.M., McDermott, K.B., Buckner, R.L., Raichle, M.E., Cohen, N.J., Ollinger, J.M. Akbudak, E., Conturo, T.E., Snyder, A.Z., & Petersen, S.E. (1998). Hemispheric asymmetry for verbal and nonverbal memory encoding in human dorsal frontal cortex. *Neuron, 20,* 927–936.

Kučera, H. & Francis, W.N. (1967). *Computational analysis of present-day American English.* Providence, RI: Brown University Press.

McDermott, K.B., Buckner, R.L., Petersen, S.E., Kelley, W.M., & Sanders, A.L. (in press). Set-specific and code-specific activation in frontal cortex: An fMRI study of encoding and retrieval of faces and words. *Journal of Cognitive Neuroscience.*

Mintun, M.A., Fox, P.T., & Raichle, M.E. (1989). A highly accurate method of localizing regions of neuronal activity in the human brain with positron emission tomography. *Journal of Cerebral Blood Flow and Metabolism, 9,* 96–103.

Morris, C.D., Bransford, J.D., & Franks, J.J. (1977). Levels of processing versus transfer appropriate processing. *Journal of Verbal Learning and Verbal Behavior, 16,* 519–533.

Mugler, J.P. & Brookeman, J.R. (1990). Three-dimensional magnetization-prepared rapid gradient-echo imaging (3d MP-RAGE). *Magnetic Resonance Medicine, 15,* 152–157.

Nyberg, L., Cabeza, R., & Tulving. E. (1996). PET studies of encoding and retrieval: The HERA model. *Psychonomic Bulletin & Review, 3,* 135–148.

Nyberg, L., McIntosh, A.R., Cabeza, R., Habib, R., Houle, S., & Tulving. E. (1996). General and specific brain regions involved in encoding and retrieval of events: What, where, and when. *Proceedings of the National Academy of Sciences, USA, 93,* 11280–11285.

Nyberg, L., Tulving, E., Habib, R., Nilsson, L.G., Kapur, S., Houle, S., Cabeza, R., & McIntosh, A.R. (1995). Functional brain maps of retrieval mode and recovery of episodic information. *Neuroreport*, *7*, 249–252.

Ojemann, J.G., Akbudak, E., Snyder, A.Z., McKinstry, R.C., Raichle, M.E., & Conturo, T.E. (1997). Anatomic localization and quantitative analysis of gradient refocused echo-planar fMRI susceptibility artifacts. *Neuroimage*, *6*, 156–167.

Ojemann, J.G., Buckner, R.L., Akbudak, E., Snyder, A.A., Ollinger, J.M., McKinstry, R.C., Rosen, B.R., Petersen, S.E., Raichle, M.E., & Conturo, T.E. (1998). Functional MRI studies of word-stem completion: Reliability across laboratories and comparison to blood flow imaging with PET. *Human Brain Mapping*, *6*, 203–215.

Ollinger, J.M. (1997). Correcting for multiple comparisons in fMRI activation studies with region-size dependent thresholds. *Proceedings of the International Society for Magnetic Resonance in Medicine Abstracts*, 1672.

Petrides, M., Alivisatos, B., Evans, A.C., & Meyer, E. (1993). Dissociation of human mid-dorsolateral from posterior dorsolateral frontal cortex in memory processing. *Proceedings of the National Academy of Sciences, USA*, *90*, 873–877.

Reyna, V.F. & Brainerd, C.J. (1995). Fuzzy-trace theory: An interim synthesis. *Learning and Individual Differences*, *7*, 1–75.

Roediger, H.L., Buckner, R.L., & McDermott, K.B. (1999). Components of processing. In J.K. Foster and M. Jelicic (Eds.), *Memory: Systems, process, or function?* (pp. 31–65). Oxford: Oxford University Press.

Rosen, B.R., Buckner, R.L., & Dale, A.M. (1998). Event related fMRI: Past, present, and future. *Proceedings of the National Academy of Sciences, USA*, *95*, 773–780.

Rugg, M.D., Fletcher, P.C., Frith, C.D., Frackowiak, R.S.J., & Dolan, R.J. (1996). Differential activation of the prefrontal cortex in successful and unsuccessful memory retrieval. *Brain*, *119*, 2073–2083.

Schacter, D.L., Buckner, R.L., Koutstaal, W., Dale, A.M., & Rosen, B.R. (1997). Late onset of anterior prefrontal activity during true and false recognition: An event-related fMRI study. *Neuroimage*, *6*, 259–269.

Shallice, T., Fletcher, P., Frith, C.D., Grasby, P., Frackowiak, R.S.J., & Dolan, R.J. (1994). Brain regions associated with acquisition and retrieval of verbal episodic memory. *Nature*, *368*, 633–635.

Shimamura, A.P., Janowsky, J.S., & Squire, L.R. (1990). Memory for the temporal order of events in patients with frontal lobe lesions and amnesic patients. *Neuropsychologia*, *28*, 803–813.

Snyder, A.Z. (1996). Difference image vs. ratio image error function forms in PET–PET realignment. In D. Bailey & T. Jones (Eds.), *Quantification of brain function using PET* (pp.131–137). San Diego: Academic Press.

Squire, L.R., Ojemann, J.G., Miezin, F.M., Petersen, S.E., Videen, T.O., & Raichle, M.E. (1992). Activation of the hippocampus in normal humans: A functional anatomical study of memory. *Proceedings of the National Academy of Sciences, USA*, *89*, 1837–1841.

Stuss, D.T., Alexander, M.P., Palumbo, C.L., Buckle, L., Sayer, L., & Pogue, J. (1994). Organizational strategies of patients with unilateral or bilateral frontal lobe injury in word list learning tasks. *Neuropsychology*, *8*, 355–373.

Talairach, J., & Tournoux, P. (1988). *Co-planar stereotaxic atlas of the human brain*. New York: Thieme.

Tulving, E. (1983). *Elements of episodic memory*. New York: Oxford University Press.

Tulving, E. (1985). Memory and consciousness. *Canadian Psychologist*, *26*, 1–12.

Tulving, E., Kapur, S., Craik, F.I.M., Markowitsch, H.J., & Houle, S. (1994). Hemispheric encoding/retrieval asymmetry in episodic memory: Positron emission tomography findings. *Proceedings of the National Academy of Sciences, USA*, *91*, 2016–2020.

Wagner, A.D., Desmond, J.E., Glover, G.H., & Gabrieli, J.D.E. (1998a). Prefrontal cortex and recognition memory: fMRI evidence for context-dependent retrieval processes. *Brain, 121*, 1985–2002.

Wagner, A.D., Schacter, D.L., Rotte, M., Koutstaal, W., Maril, A., Dale, A., Rosen, B., & Buckner, R.L. (1998b). Building memories: Remembering and forgetting of verbal experiences as predicted by brain activity. *Science, 281*, 1188–1191.

Warrington, E.K., & Weiskrantz, L. (1968). New method of testing long-term retention with special reference to amnesic patients. *Nature, 217*, 972–974.

Worsley, K.J., & Friston, K.J. (1995). Analysis of fMRI time-series revisited—again. *Neuroimage, 2*, 173–182.

Zarahn, E., Aguirre, G., & D'Esposito, M. (1997). A trial-based experimental design for fMRI. *Neuroimage, 6*, 122–138.

MEMORY, 1999, 7 (5/6), 679–702

A Positron Emission Tomography (PET) Study of Autobiographical Memory Retrieval

Martin A. Conway and David J. Turk

University of Bristol, UK

Shannon L. Miller, Jessica Logan, Robert D. Nebes,
Carolyn Cidis Meltzer and James T. Becker

University of Pittsburgh School of Medicine, USA

Memory for the experiences of one's life, autobiographical memory (AM), is one of the most human types of memory, yet comparatively little is known of its neurobiology. A positron emission tomography (PET) study of AM retrieval revealed that the left frontal cortex was significantly active during retrieval (compared to memory control tasks), together with activation in the inferior temporal and occipital lobes in the left hemisphere. We propose that this left frontal lobe activation reflects the operation of control processes that modulate the construction of AMs in posterior neocortical networks.

INTRODUCTION

The neuroanatomy of autobiographical memory (AM) is gradually being revealed in several converging lines of research. For instance, studies of retrograde amnesia in patients with brain damage demonstrate that networks in anterior and posterior cortical regions play important roles in autobiographical remembering (see Conway, in press, for a review). Similarly, a recent PET study of emotional AMs found large regions of frontal and temporal lobes in the right hemisphere to be active during memory retrieval (Fink et al., 1996). And, using EEG, Conway, Pleydell-Pearce, and Whitecross (1999) found that activation

Requests for reprints should be sent to Martin A. Conway, Centre for Learning and Memory, Department of Experimental Psychology, University of Bristol, 8 Woodland Road, Bristol BS8 1TN, UK. Email: M.A.Conway@bristol.ac.uk

This research was supported in part by funds from The Centre for Functional Brain Imaging (MH-49815), and the National Institute on Aging (AG13699). J.T.B. holds a Research Scientist Development Award (MH01 107). J.L. was a Summer Undergraduate Fellow in the Centre for the Neural Basis of Cognition (N.S.F. DBI-9605167) at the University of Pittsburgh and Carnegie-Mellon University.

flowed from the left frontal lobe to right temporal and occipital regions (with some weaker left hemisphere activation) as participants recalled a memory to a cue word and then held the memory in mind for a specified time. In this paper we report the first PET study to use the cue word method to elicit AMs. However, before turning to the study in detail we first review our model of AM which will be used to frame and interpret the findings.

CONSTRUCTING AUTOBIOGRAPHICAL MEMORIES IN A SELF-MEMORY SYSTEM

Autobiographical memories are transitory mental representations often effort-fully constructed and effortfully maintained in consciousness (Conway, 1992, 1996a; Conway & Fthenaki, in press; Conway & Pleydell-Pearce, 1999b; Hodges, 1995; Hodges & McCarthy, 1993; Kohler et al., 1998; Moscovitch, 1992, 1995). They contain knowledge at different levels of specificity in which more abstract knowledge about one's past provides a context for detailed event-specific knowledge (ESK). The nature of ESK is that it is near-sensory experience whereas other knowledge of *lifetime periods* (e.g. When I was at school, When I lived with "X", living in city "Y", working for company "Z", etc.) and *general events* (e.g. holiday in "A", shopping at "B", eating out at "C", etc.) is more conceptual and abstract than ESK. Figure 1 illustrates how these various types of knowledge might be organised in long-term memory. Note that lifetime period and general event knowledge are considered to have quite extensive local organisation whereas this is not the case for ESK—a point we shall briefly return to later (see Barsalou, 1988, Conway, 1992, 1996a, in press, Conway & Bekerian, 1987a, Conway & Pleydell-Pearce, 1999, and Conway, Pleydell-Pearce, & Whitecross, 1999, for further discussion). The central notion expressed by Fig. 1 is that knowledge held at higher more abstract levels can be used to access knowledge at more specific levels. So, for example, knowledge of goals, others, locations, activities, etc., common to a lifetime period can be used to access or index associated knowledge held at the general event level. In turn, knowledge held at the general event level can be used to access near-sensory-experience ESK and when a stable pattern of activation over these knowledge structures is established then a specific AM is formed. Indeed, neurological injury often selectively impairs different aspects of AM knowledge, although a general principle is that sensory-perceptual ESK is more frequently and more completely lost than abstract/conceptual personal knowl-edge. Moreover, these two broad classes of knowledge appear to be represented separately, with ESK located in posterior neocortical networks and abstract/conceptual knowledge in anterior networks. Figure 1 indicates this by depicting ESK as a separate memory system consisting of an undifferentiated pool of sensory-perceptual records—Conway (1992, in press) refers to these as "phenomenological records" to convey the idea that this knowledge is, in

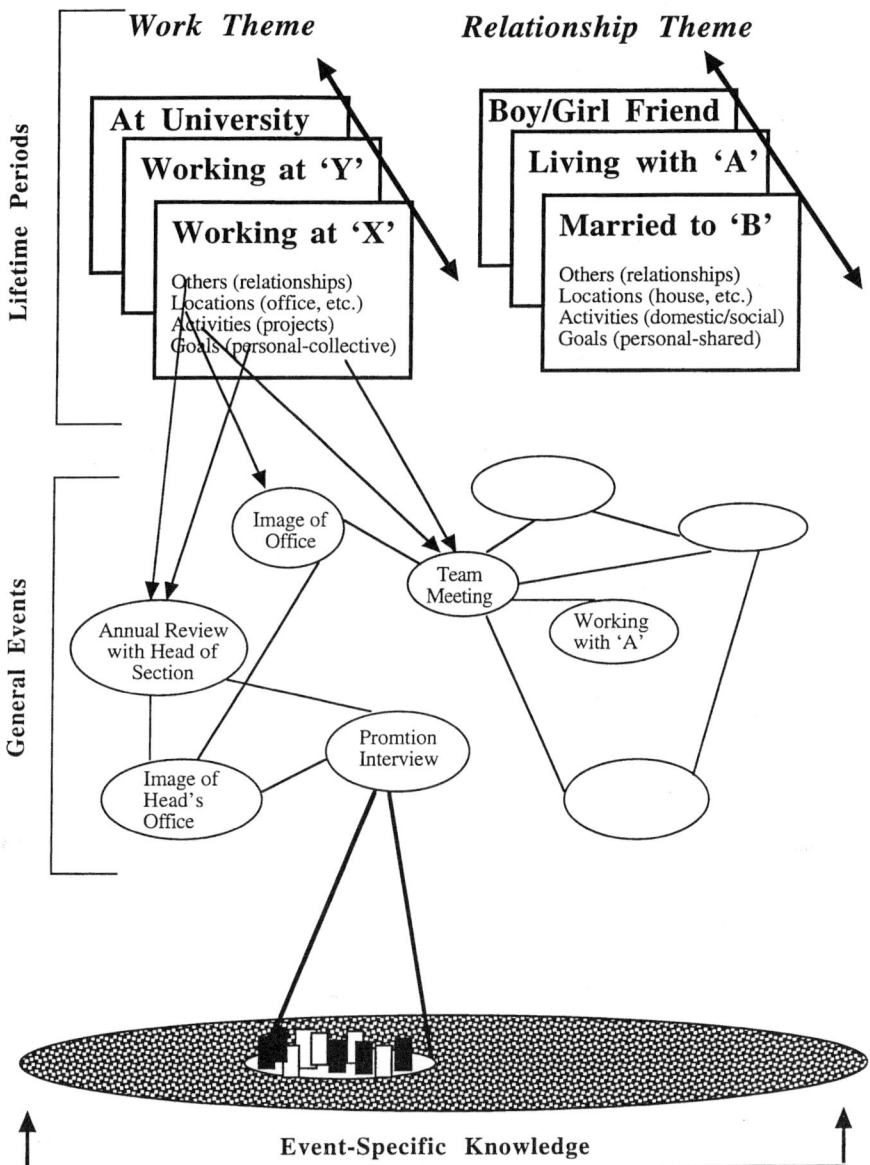

FIG. 1. Lifetime period, general event, and event-specific knowledge in the autobiographical knowledge base (after Conway 1996, Fig. 1).

681

part, a record of past conscious experience (see too Moscovitch, 1995, and also Fuster's, 1997, concept of a "netlet" which corresponds to notion of ESK developed in Conway, 1992, and 1996a).

The knowledge base depicted in Fig. 1 is accessed by a complex retrieval process (Burgess & Shallice, 1996; Conway & Bekerian, 1987a; Conway & Pleydell-Pearce, 1999) which operates when the system is in "retrieval mode" (Conway, in press; Moscovitch, 1995; Schacter, Norman, & Koustaal, 1998; Tulving, 1983). The process of *generative retrieval* is mediated by a search–evaluate–elaborate iterative cycle in which a cue is used to access knowledge, and accessed knowledge is then evaluated against some internal set of standards or criteria which specify abstract qualities of the memory, e.g. what it is to be about, as well as specific details such as a requirement for visual imagery. In generative retrieval a *retrieval template* is created by centrally located control processes and this modulates memory construction. When the outcome of the evaluation phase of retrieval does not lead to formation of an appropriate memory, i.e. the criteria of the retrieval template are not satisfied, then the accessed knowledge is elaborated upon and subsequently used as the new cue for the next search cycle (Burgess & Shallice, 1996; Conway, 1992, 1996b). For example, a person in an AM experiment in our laboratory was asked to say what came to mind while recalling a memory to the cue word *cinema*:

> When did I go to the cinema a lot? When I was a student. I lived in a student hall near Russell Square and we used to go to the art cinema there and I remember sitting in the dark in big red seats watching *The Spirit of the Beehive*.

This, typical, protocol, shows: (i) elaboration of the cue (When did I go to the cinema a lot?), (ii) access of a lifetime period (When I was a student), (iii) information common to the lifetime period, (iv) access of a general event (we used to go the art cinema), (v) access of sensory-perceptual details (sitting in the dark in big red seats) and other ESK (watching *The Spirit of the Beehive*).

Conway and Pleydell-Pearce (1999) propose that the process of generating retrieval templates and using them to modulate the search and evaluate cycles is a function of what they term the *working self*. The notion of a working self is derived from Markus and Ruvolo (1989) and refers to an individual's current set of active goals. These need not be conscious and are considered to be organised into complex goal hierarchies in the form of interlocking negative feedback loops, each of which seeks to reduce discrepancy between the aim of the goal and the state of the world, including internal states (see Carver & Scheier, 1982, 1990). In this way, what is remembered is controlled by the goals of the individual, but note that this only occurs at the point where knowledge is accessed in long-term memory: the model assumes that the search takes place automatically as activation is channelled through the indices of AM and control processes can only influence the search process by selecting particular cues.

Consequently, when activation is channelled from abstract to specific knowledge the mapping is one-to-many, e.g. one lifetime period to many general events, one general event to many records of ESK. So activation quickly dissipates and this is why a retrieval template is required: to supply the automatic search process with increasingly more elaborate and specific cues that focus and localise the activation leading to the formation of a stable pattern of activation in the knowledge base.

The generative retrieval process can, however, be bypassed if a sufficiently specific cue is encountered. The process of *direct retrieval* occurs when activation spreads from a single item or small set of ESK records to an associated general event and lifetime period. In this case a stable pattern of activation automatically forms, channelled by the organisation of knowledge in long-term memory which when emanating from ESK maps directly on to a single general event and single lifetime period. In direct retrieval AMs are formed outside the influence of the working self and once generated are experienced by the rememberer as spontaneously coming to mind. Berntsen (1996) found that such "spontaneous" remindings occurred with moderate frequency, once or twice a day, and Conway (1997) reviews a wide range of literary accounts of spontaneous recall, the most famous of which is, of course, Proust's (1913/81) spontaneous recovery of his childhood memories in response to smell and taste of a Madeleine cake dipped in warm tea. A striking demonstration of the power of specific cues in overcoming retrograde amnesia following brain injury can be found in Lucchelli, Muggia, and Spinnler (1995). On the other hand direct retrieval can have detrimental consequences and Markowitsch et al., (1997) report how cued recall of childhood traumatic memory led to dense retrograde amnesia. Traumatic memories may generally have the effect of triggering a stress response that increases glucosteroid release causing degenerative overstimulation if hippocampal and medial temporal lobe networks (Markowitsch, 1998; Sapolsky, 1996) and, indeed, hippocampal shrinkage has been found in soldiers with post-traumatic stress disorder (Gurvits et al., 1996) and survivors of childhood abuse (Bremner et al., 1995). More generally, the model we have outlined proposes that patterns of activation constantly arise and dissipate in response to internally generated and externally encountered cues. As constructing a full AM requires a direction of attention to the retrieval process and activated internal representations, then the potential for memory to capture attentional resources is high (Conway, in press). For this reason, and because recall of certain materials may be destabilising for the self, it is proposed that access to the AM knowledge base is, most of the time, inhibited and this inhibition is comparatively rarely overcome. If every cue activates AM knowledge to some extent then a spontaneous remembering rate of about twice a day (Berntsen, 1996) must be regarded as low.

In our model of AM there is, then, a hierarchically organised knowledge base, an iterative retrieval process, and the working self. Within this scheme specific

AMs can be constructed by the effortful process of generative retrieval in which a memory is intentionally established. This entails the creation of a retrieval template that corresponds to the goals of the working self and against which accessed knowledge is evaluated, elaborated, and then recycled in further attempts at knowledge access until an AM is judged to have been formed or the attempt is abandoned. On the other hand a cue may be of sufficient specificity to cause the spontaneous formation of a memory. Even in this case, however, it does not follow that such a construction will enter consciousness and capture attention. Spontaneously formed AMs must be evaluated too against the goals of the working self and this takes place outside conscious awareness. In both cases memories are constructed and evaluated in what we collectively refer to as the *Self-Memory System* (SMS) that is, the working self, the retrieval process, and its knowledge base.

NEUROANATOMY OF AUTOBIOGRAPHICAL MEMORY

A major hypothesis derived from our model of AM is that when memories are constructed activation will be present in both anterior and posterior regions and that, in generative retrieval, activation will progress over the retrieval interval from anterior to posterior sites. In a recent EEG study we monitored changes in slow cortical potentials (SCPs) as participants first recalled a specific AM to a cue word—e.g. restaurant, beach, train, etc.—then held the memory in mind for five seconds, and finally tried to remove the memory from mind for a further period of five seconds (Conway et al., 1999). We detected a complex pattern of SCPs that evolved and changed over time as memories were constructed, held in mind, and then inhibited: during the early phase of retrieval, after a cue had been read, anterior-temporal and frontal regions became active in the left hemisphere. Also present at this point was some weaker activation at right frontal sites, compared to same-side posterior regions. In our view the pattern of left hemisphere activity reflected the role of central control processes in generating a retrieval model within the SMS (see Heil, Rosler, & Hennighausen, 1997, Honda et al., 1996, for similar reports of left hemisphere activation during the retrieval of both verbal and nonverbal materials). The activation detected in right frontal regions (versus same-side posterior sites) may reflect, on the other hand, early attempts to access the autobiographical knowledge base and, possibly, evaluation of outputs is mediated by networks in both the frontal lobes. At the point of memory retrieval, especially for distinctive, important, vivid memories, there was a shift of activation to bilateral posterior regions and in particular to regions of the occipital lobes. According to our model this is the moment when a stable pattern of activation is formed in the autobiographical memory knowledge base and linked to the frontally generated retrieval model. Very rapidly after memory formation activation shifted to the right hemisphere and, while a memory was held in mind, activation was detectable through right frontal regions, temporal lobes (bilaterally but more extensive on the right than left), and in the occipital lobes (also bilateral). This right hemisphere pattern of activation represents the fusion of activation across several different systems and is perhaps held in place by a retrieval model local to right frontal networks. To be more specific, it may be that general event knowledge is held in regions of temporal cortex (see Moscovitch, 1995), and ESK in occipital sites. When the cue to forget the memory was presented there was a growth of positivity in centro-parietal and right hemisphere regions, and this may reflect an attempt to inhibit a memory retrieval model as a way of "removing a memory from mind". This flow of activation, over the course of the retrieval period, from left frontal networks to right frontal, temporal, and occipital lobes, is exactly what our cognitive model of AM predicts and, as we shall see, the initial left frontal activation is especially interesting.

Currently the only other specifically AM neuroimaging (PET) study has been reported by Fink et al. (1996). In Fink et al. participants read sentences that named events from either another person's biography (Impersonal) or events from their own life (Personal). In both cases participants were to imagine what happened in the named event. Very extensive right hemisphere activation unique to the Personal condition was detected, and this activation was particularly marked in the right prefrontal cortex and right temporal lobe, especially the right temporopolar cortex, and right hippocampal formation. These findings fit well with the SCP data reported earlier but they also differ in that no left frontal activation was detected. It seems to us that reason for this is that the stimuli used in the Fink et al. study considerably minimised generation of a retrieval model. This is because the sentences named (highly emotional) events from the participants' own autobiographical memory, and this is known to speed AM construction and reduce the number of search and verify iterations needed in evolving an effective retrieval model (Conway & Bekerian, 1987a). Direct access to AM knowledge effectively bypasses the search phase of generative retrieval and leads to a single verification phase producing a retrieval model in which the influence of the goals of the working self are reduced, although it seems unlikely that these would be completely absent. This line of reasoning suggests that networks in the left frontal lobe may play an important role in generative retrieval but have very little influence in direct retrieval. Other recent work also supports this point (Craik et al., 1998; Maguire & Mummery, 1999; see too Nolde, Johnson, & D'Esposito, 1998) and, later, we consider it in some detail.

It seems possible, then, that networks mediating the working self might be located in left frontal regions, as it is this region that becomes active early in generative retrieval as a memory template is constructed. Later in retrieval activation switches to the right frontal cortex and, once a memory is formed and held in mind, activation rises in the temporal lobes bilaterally and regions of the occipital lobes (Conway et al., 1999; Fink et al., 1996). Of particular importance in this sequence of memory formation are networks at the temporofrontal junction (Kroll, Markowitsch, Knight, & von Cramon, 1997), basal forebrain and ventral regions of the frontal lobes (Damasio, 1994; Eslinger & Damasio, 1985; Moscovitch & Melo, 1997), connections between temporal and occipital cortices (Conway, 1996a,b; Rubin & Greenberg, 1998), and the MTL memory system (Moscovitch, 1995; Squire, 1992). During the course of retrieval, activation flows from anterior networks in the frontal lobes to posterior networks in temporal and occipital networks to which it becomes localised when a specific memory is held in conscious awareness.

NEUROIMAGING AUTOBIOGRAPHICAL MEMORY CONSTRUCTION: TWO HYPOTHESES

We describe a positron emission tomography (PET) study of AM retrieval that sought to test two different hypotheses. The first hypothesis relates to our cognitive model of AM retrieval and proposes that there will be widespread activation of neocortex during the construction of AMs. Note that as retrieval is cued by non-personal word cues that name common objects, actions, and locations, we expect to induce generative retrieval and, therefore, activation of left frontal networks. Because the temporal resolution of PET is not sufficiently detailed we will not be able to examine this activation as it unfolds over time. Nevertheless, it is expected that widespread activation in addition to left frontal activity will be detected. The second hypothesis is derived from McClelland, McNaughton, and O'Reilly (1995) who argued that the hippocampal formation is critical to the consolidation of memories, but once memories are consolidated they become represented in neocortical areas and their retrieval then becomes independent of hippocampal networks. If this is correct then hippocampal activation should be present in the retrieval of recent memories (McClelland et al., 1995, consider 12–24 months as recent) but not in the retrieval of remote memories. We examine this hypothesis by manipulating the age of recalled memories and note that, even apart from the McClelland et al., conjecture, whether different brain regions mediate the recall of recent and remote memories is a question of interest in its own right and one that has not been addressed previously.

A PET STUDY OF AUTOBIOGRAPHICAL MEMORY RETRIEVAL

The basic experimental task is one commonly used in the study of autobiographical memory: the cue word retrieval task (see Conway, 1990; 1996b). In this procedure a participant is presented with a series of cue words and required to recall a specific AM to each word. They respond as soon as an AM occurs to them, usually by pressing a button or describing their memory aloud. As our aim is to study generative rather than direct retrieval, the cue word task is highly appropriate as it requires a great deal of generative retrieval. However, a feature of the task is that memories retrieved to different cues take different amounts of time and, moreover, it is known that there are in any case large individual differences in speed of AM retrieval (see Conway, 1996b). neither of these would normally be a problem but within the context of a PET study in which the activation is sampled in 90-second blocks it means that there is a potential for some participants to recall very few memories whereas others may recall a great deal more. In order to reduce the effects of this potential imbalance we used a deadline procedure in which participants were timed out if they had not retrieved a specific AM within five seconds. As AM retrieval times in the cue word procedure typically have a mean of about five seconds, the consequence of the deadline was that on at least some occasions retrieval stopped before a memory was fully formed. This was not considered a major problem as the purpose of the experiment was to investigate the retrieval process, which would have been common to all trials, only more extensive on some rather than others. Nevertheless, the sum of activation over all trials (15 at five seconds each) should reflect the full retrieval process up to and including formation of specific AMs.

A further issue here relates to the nature of the various control tasks to be used as baselines in the analyses of the PET data. For our second hypothesis concerning the role of the hippocampal formation in the retrieval of recent and remote memories there is no problem, and the pattern of activation for recent AMs can be subtracted from that for remote and vice versa. In this way their unique patterns of activation can be established. The issue is more difficult in establishing the patterns of brain activation for AM on its own. As the cue word retrieval task requires participants to read a word, it seemed reasonable that we should include a task in which individual words were simply read. Subtracted out from the AM conditions this would leave activation unique to AM. This, however, would still not reveal activation unique to AM recall compared to recall of any other type of knowledge. For instance, in by far the majority of memory PET studies participants learn and recall word lists (Nyberg, Cabeza, & Tulving, 1996), but is this comparable to recalling events from one's life? We think not, as at a very minimum it entails recall of very highly specific information that typically would be lost over a period of hours and days. AMs in contrast, although also often containing specific knowledge, are durable and informationally more complex. Despite this it was decided to use cued recall of word paired-associates as one of the control conditions in order to remove from the AM patterns of activation any activity due to short-and medium-term memory systems. This also provides a way of comparing traditional word-list recall with AM recall and established whether or not the two actually do differ.[1] In addition to these control conditions we included a rest condition in which participants looked at a display of white noise while being scanned. This too is a commonly used control condition, although we noted that it is very unlikely that the participant is doing nothing while studying the dynamically changing white noise patterns. Instead, they very often daydream and this in itself may give rise to activations that inadvertently remove in the subtractive analysis areas of interest from the experimental task. Our view is that careful use of all three control conditions will allow us to identify patterns of activation unique to AM.

Method

Participants.   There were six participants (three males, three females); all were healthy (no history of neurological or psychiatric disorders), young (age = 34.3 years, s.d. = 8.66, range = 25–43), right-handed, and native English speaking. Informed consent was obtained prior to the start of the study. Each female volunteer had a negative serum pregnancy test on the day of the PET scan. This research had been approved by the Radiation Dosimetry Review Committee and the Institutional Review Board of the University of Pittsburgh Medical Centre.

PET Procedures.   Each participant was scanned 10 times measuring regional cerebral blood flow (relCBF) using O^{15}-water with standard laboratory procedures (Becker, Mintun, & Diehl, 1994). Participants were placed in the supine position on a Siemens HR + PET scanning table. The scanner collects 63 parallel planes over a 15.2cm axial field of view. An intravenous catheter was placed in the left antecubital vein for radiopharmaceutical injection. The head was positioned within the head holder and a softened thermoplastic mask fitted over the face, moulded to the patient's facial contours (with cutouts for the eyes, ears, and mouth) and fastened to the head holder. The PET scanner table was moved so that the highest imaging plane was at the vertex of the head, with the result that the entire brain volume was scanned. Transmission scanning was done in all PET studies prior to radiopharmaceutical injection using three rotating rod sources of 68Ge/68Ga.

---

[1]There are several other control tasks that could be used in a comparison with the AM conditions. For instance, participants might be asked to recall stories that they had learned previously, pictures, even fabricated AMs or the AMs of others. At this point and in this initial study, which transfers the AM cue word procedure to PET for the first time, we are more concerned to use standard tasks that have been used before in PET. Nonetheless, it might be noted that future studies employing more complex control tasks may tell us more about AM than is revealed by the present contrast with the recall of paired associates. Of course, such studies will have to draw on an understanding of the neuroanatomical basis of their complex control tasks if the resulting patterns of activation are to be of use.

Measurements of relCBF were made after an intravenous bolus injection of 10–11 mCi of H^2O^{15} water in 5–7ml of saline. The start of each scan was triggered when the total counts measured exceeded twice the background count, approximately 30 seconds after each injection. The data acquired in the 60-second sampling frame were used as the qualitative map of cerebral blood flow (Fox & Mintun, 1989). Data were acquired and reconstructed in full three-dimensional mode (Townsend et al., 1991). Each participant also had a magnetic resonance image (MRI) scan of the head. The PET and MRI data were co-registered, and used to aid in the alignment of the PET images. The PET images from each subject were centred (left–right), vertically aligned to correct for movement in the transverse and coronal planes, and co-registered to one another to correct for slight head movement during the scan (Miroshima, Berger, Lee, & Mintun, 1992; Woods, Cherry, Mazziotta, 1992). The rest of the PET scans collected were mathematically registered to the first scan by PET-to-PET alignment (Woods et al., 1992). These processes centred the images and oriented them in the same coordinate system for later processing. The statistical analysis of the data was carried out using the Statistical Parametric Mapping program (SPM95; Friston, Frith, Liddle, & Frackowiak, 1991) in PRO MATLAB (Mathworks Inc, Sherborn, Mass., USA). The scans were spatially normalised using linear transformation, which removed individual variability and transformed each brain into the Talairach and Tournoux atlas reference space (Talairach & Tournoux, 1988). We used the linear transformation to avoid loss of information at the top and bottom-most images. The scans were then smoothed with a three-dimensional Gaussian filter with a 16mm full-width half maximum (inplane) to suppress noise and minimise effects of normalisation errors by increasing the sensitivity of the signal. Differences in global activity within and between subjects were removed by analysis of covariance (ANCOVA) on a voxel-by-voxel basis with global counts as covariate and regional activity across participants for participant being studied in all conditions. Comparisons of the means across selected conditions were made on a voxel-by-voxel basis using the t-statistic. The resulting values constituted a statistical parametric map (SPM; Friston et al., 1991).

Activation Task Procedures. Test materials were presented on a video monitor above the participant's head in the PET scanner. In all conditions, each stimulus was on-screen for 200ms, with 4800ms between presentations and there was a total of 15 trials during each scan. There were two blocks of five scans; scan order was different between blocks. All words and letter strings appeared in uppercase print. For the Visual Baseline Rest Condition, subjects saw a rectangular-shaped box containing pixels of random intensity (Becker et al., 1994). For the Paired-Associate Recall Task (PA), the subjects were taught a set of 15 verbal paired associates prior to being placed in the scanner. The word–word pairs (e.g. "FLOWER"–"CLOCK") were presented for two seconds, and after the entire list of pairs had been presented, subjects were given a test list. During the test phase the subjects saw the first word of each pair (e.g. ''FLOWER''–?) and were asked to speak the second word. After five seconds, the word–word pair was presented again, regardless of whether the subject had correctly recalled the response word. The entire list of pairs was presented repeatedly until the participant either recalled all 15 pairs correctly in a single test trial, or made only one error in each of three consecutive trials. During the PET scans, the cued recall of PAs condition consisted of showing the first word of a pair (e.g. ''FLOWER''–?) to which the second associated word was recalled and then spoken aloud. The response words were not presented during the scan phases.

For the autobiographical memory tasks, the participants were trained prior to scanning that they were to recall an event from their past in response to a cue word. They were instructed to recall a specific episode, and to be able to report as much detail about the episode as possible. Further, they were told that they should respond to the cue word with a word of their own that would allow them to later remember the event that had come to mind. For the ''recent'' task (AM-recent), the subjects were instructed to recall events that had occurred during the 12 months prior to the scan. For the ''remote'' condition (AM-remote), the participants were asked to recall events that had occurred when they were aged 15 years or younger. During the PET scans themselves, therefore, participants responded with a single word upon retrieving a specific memory. The experimenter recorded each response word, and then debriefed the participant immediately after the scan was finished (i.e. while still in the scanner, and before the next injection). All of the verbal responses were recorded for later transcription and scoring.

Materials. All the words used in this experiment were selected in an unsystematic way from a larger pool of words previously used in AM experiments in the first author's laboratory. This pool contains words that name common objects, actions, and locations (common emotion words were excluded) selected so as to be likely to correspond to common experiences and, therefore, common AMs. Frequency, imagability etc., were not controlled, but the words used had been successfully used in other AM retrieval experiments.

Results

The analyses of relCBF reported in this section focus on autobiographical memory retrieval compared to the control tasks, and second on differences in the recall of recent and remote memories.

Patterns of Activation in Autobiographical Recall. By examining relCBF during AM retrieval relative to that measured during PA recall, it was possible to compare and contrast the neuroanatomical bases of these two types of episodic remembering. Because both of these recall tasks are thought to involve the same cognitive processes (Howe & Courage, 1996), i.e. those involved in episodic memory retrieval, then there should be few, if any, differences in the brain structures activated by these sets of tasks. Accordingly, we subtracted the patterns of activation arising in the PA condition from those present during retrieval of AMs. (Note that recent and remove AMs were grouped together for this contrast and this was because when analysed separately the findings were the same as when analysed together.) The upper panel of Fig. 2 shows that relative to the PA condition, there was an extensive network of brain regions specifically responsible for the retrieval of AMs. A large volume of left frontal lobe was significantly more active in both AM conditions than in the cued recall of PAs with a region of activity extending through the left convexity from Brodmann Area (BA) 6 to BA44/45; significant peak foci were observed in BA45, BA45/47 in the inferior regions, and BA9 and 6 in the middle and superior regions (see Table 1 for Talaraich & Tournoux coordinates). A second large significant region of relCBF was present at the posterior to middle temporal gyrus in the left anterior occipital lobe and left posterior parietal lobe at BA39. In addition to this a region of inferior left temporal lobe, BA20, with coordinates –40/–4/–28 had Z scores of $P < .003$, which although above our cut-off (see Table 1), nevertheless strongly suggested that networks in this region might also play a unique role in AM retrieval. Other reliable regions of activation were also detected in left occipital lobe with foci in BA18. In order to better visualise the extent of the unique left frontal involvement in AM retrieval, Plate 9 shows SPM-generated foci overlaid onto the co-registered summed MRI derived from all participants' data. It can be seen from Plate 9 that the area of activation extends throughout the medial-posterior left frontal cortex encompassing orbital, ventral-lateral, and dorsal-lateral networks. Note too the pattern of activation in the anterior left occipital lobe which is at the occipital–parietal juncture. The comparisons between AM and the visual noise and word reading tasks gave rise to highly similar findings with the same left hemisphere regions activated to the same extent but with a few new smaller areas of activation now present in the AM data. For example, AM minus the pattern of activations for word reading produced the same unique pattern of left hemisphere activation plus some small isolated areas of right frontal (central) activity and some left parietal spots of activation. In general, the visual noise and word reading conditions were associated with bilateral posterior temporal and parietal activation with some occipital activation (see Fig. 3 ahead) but this did not seem to greatly overlap with the pattern of activation of central control processes that direct, evaluate, and elaborate iterative searches of the AM knowledge base during memory retrieval. Furthermore, the data show, strikingly, that these processes are characteristic of AM recall but are not present in the recall of other types of episodically encoded information.

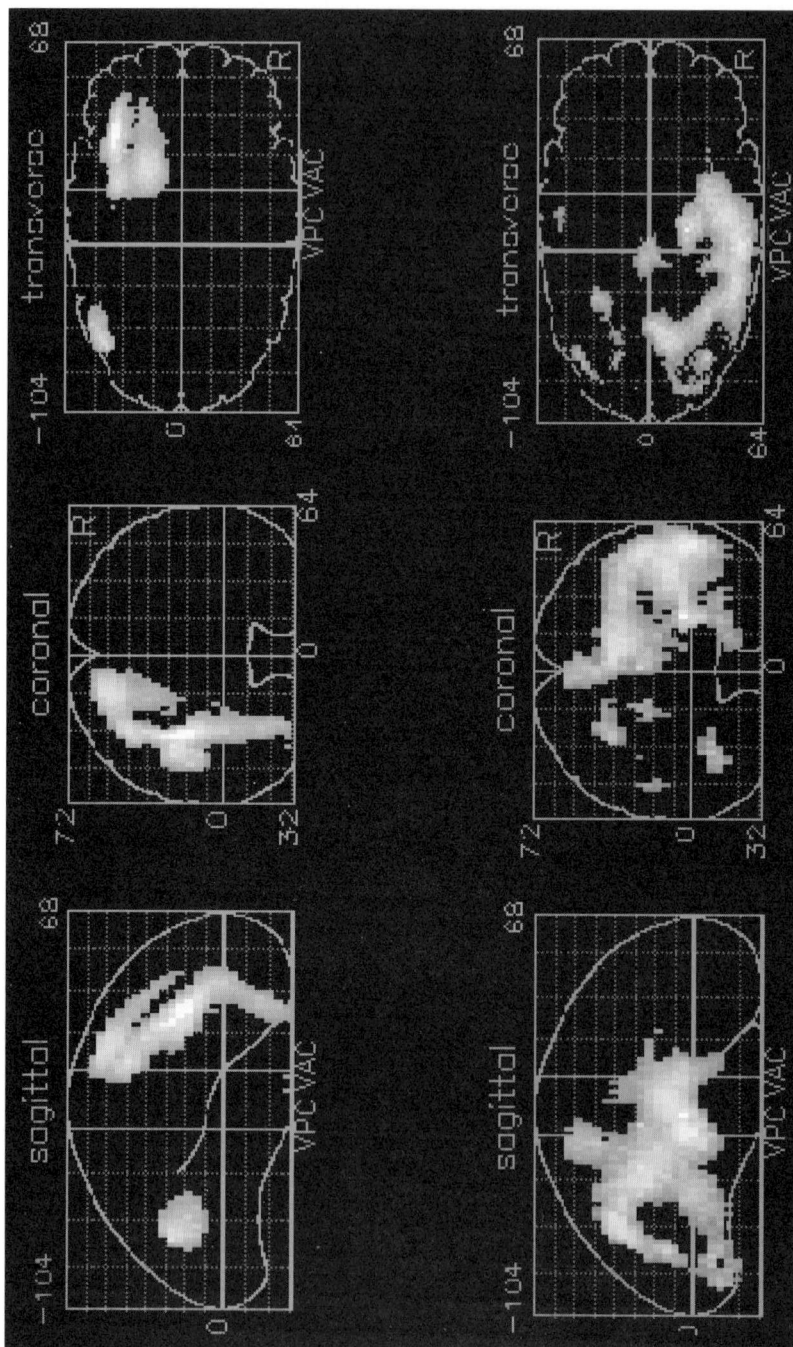

FIG. 2. Graphical representations of voxels with a significantly different relCBF ($P<.001$) in standard SPM "glass" images. Each view displays all voxels with statistically significant differences in blood flow. Views are the coronal, sagittal, and axial planes. The top panel displays the results of the contrast AM–PA; that is, those voxels whose relCBF was significantly greater in the two AM conditions compared with that seen in the PA condition. The lower panel displays the results of the opposite contrast (i.e. PA–AM).

TABLE 1

Increases in Brain Activity Associated with Recall of Autobiographical Memories (AMs) and Paired Associates (PAs)

Contrast	Region	Side	Coordinates			
			X	Y	Z	Z statistic
Recent plus Remote AMs minus cued recall of PAs						
	BA39	L	−40	−74	24	4.81
		L	−48	−64	16	4.29
	BA45	L	−36	24	20	5.38
	BA45/47	L	−34	36	0	4.32
	BA47	L	−32	30	−16	3.96
	BA6	L	−18	6	56	4.74
		L	−34	2	44	4.72
		L	−14	14	52	4.41
	BA9	L	−34	12	36	4.66
		L	−20	30	36	3.74
		L	−22	36	28	3.43
Cued recall of PAs minus recent plus remote AMs						
	Putamen	R	22	−18	4	4.23
		R	28	−12	4	3.58
	BA21	R	52	−26	0	4.16
		R	48	−50	0	3.42
	BA22	R	48	−48	20	3.84
		R	48	−32	16	3.69
		R	34	−34	16	3.25
	BA40	R	48	−40	24	3.98
	BA39/40	R	34	−54	32	3.58
		R	42	−48	32	3.55
	Insula	R	40	−10	12	3.95
		R	36	−34	16	3.34
	BA42	R	50	−16	8	3.88
		R	42	−26	8	3.50
	Precuneus	R	12	−68	32	3.89
		R	20	−64	36	3.48

Coordinates in standard stereotactic space identify statistically significant foci within areas of activation. For all comparisons $P<.001$ and BA = Brodmann Area.

Turning now to the reverse contrast of the cued recall of PAs condition minus the summed AM conditions we find, in marked contrast to the left-sided pattern of activation during AM retrieval, significantly greater relCBF in the *right* cortical hemisphere (see lower panel of Fig. 2 and Table 1 for Talaraich & Tournoux coordinates) particularly in temporal, parietal, and occipital lobes. There was bilateral activation of the posterior/medial temporal lobes, BA11/21, with a peak focus on the right side. Increases in relCBF in the parietal lobes were largely posterior on the right side and towards the midline with a peak focus in BA40. There were also bilateral increases in relCBF in the occipital lobes with right side foci in precuneus, and again with right side foci, activation of the insula and BA42. This pattern of activation changed somewhat when the two other control conditions were subtracted from it. For example when visual noise was subtracted, only bilateral activation in the medial temporal lobes remained significant and when word reading was subtracted bilateral temporal and parietal activation was observed.

Finally, and in order to bring these findings together in a single comparison, an eigenimage analysis was conducted. A number of factors were extracted in this analysis, however, two factors accounted for the majority of the variance in the relCBF data. The first factor accounted for 60% of the variance and was essentially a left frontal/right posterior factor; this is shown in Fig. 3. The autobiographical memory conditions loaded only on the left frontal end of the factor whereas the other control conditions loaded only on the right posterior end. Figure 3 also shows some midline and posterior activation for the AM conditions, although this is not of the intensity or extent of that observed in the other control conditions. We return to this later finding subsequently and here simply note that the eigenimage analysis confirms what the individual contrasts revealed, namely that AM retrieval uniquely and extensively engages left frontal networks, whereas the other conditions are associated with activation bilaterally in temporal, parietal, and occipital, lobes.

Patterns of Activation in the Recall of Recent and Remote Autobiographical Memories.   It has often been suggested that there are important differences in the way recent and remote AMs are represented in long-term memory, and current theories of the function of the hippocampus in memory storage and retrieval make different predictions about the relCBF in this brain region during the different task conditions. On the one hand (Squire, 1992), it is argued that hippocampal system networks are only involved in the retrieval of recently acquired information and are not invoked for more remote knowledge that has been "consolidated" in neocortical networks (McClellan et al., 1995), so can be retrieved via neocortical pathways that do not rely on the limbic system. In contrast, a more recent theory (Nadel & Moscovitch, 1997) argues that hippocampal networks are always involved in memory retrieval regardless of the age or state of consolidation of the retained information. By the first view then

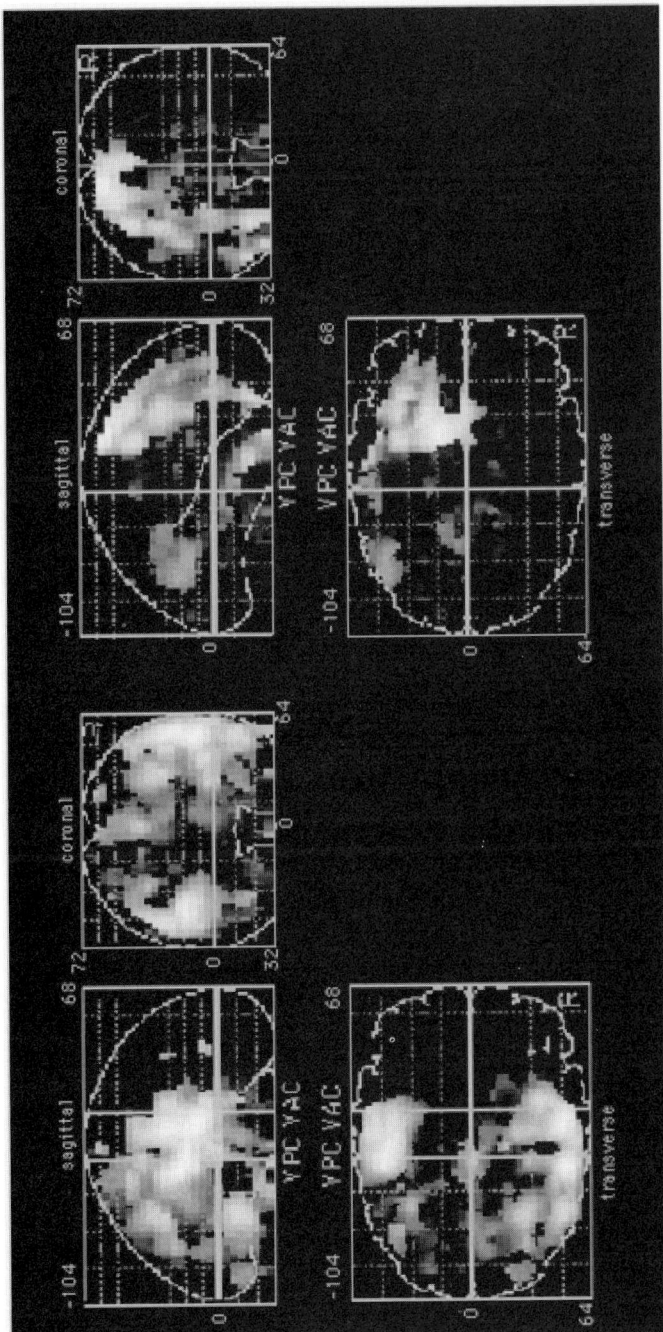

FIG. 3. Graphical representations of voxels with a significantly different relCBF ($P<.001$) in standard SPM "glass" images at either end of the single factor accounting for 60% of the total variance over all conditions.

we would expect to detect increases in hippocampal relCBF in the retrieval of recent but not remote memories, whereas according to the second view no such differences will be detected and hippocampal networks should be equally active in both conditions.

In fact, the contrasts between recent and remote, and remote and recent, AMs produced few differences and of these only those arising from the subtraction of remote from recent proved reliable. Unique to the retrieval of recent AMs (memories of events occurring in the last 12 months) were increases in relCBF in small regions of the occipital/parietal lobes in BA19 and brain stem; no differences in hippocampal relCBF were observed. A region-of-interest analysis found that the hippocampal system was reliably active during all the task conditions used in this study with an average relCBF 8% over baseline. Lack of differential activation of the hippocampal system in the recall of AMs of different ages and an overall task-independent activation of this system suggests that the system, which is critical to the encoding of new knowledge, may be constantly active in all on-going experience during which it mediates the encoding of that experience. If this is the case then it will prove extremely difficult to establish a differential role for the hippocampal formation in the retrieval of recent compared to remote memories. Current neuroimaging techniques do not have the sensitivity to detect subtle changes in processing of the type that may be involved and it may be that other types of data will be required to test this hypothesis (cf. Nadel & Moscovitch, 1997). All we can conclude is that the present study does not provide any confirmatory support for the view that the hippocampus is active in the recall of recent memories but not in the recall of remote memories: in the present experiment the hippocampal formation was active in all conditions.

Discussion

We found extensive and intense activation in the left frontal lobe during the recall of both recent and remote AMs. This pattern of activation was not observed in the recall of paired associates nor was it observed in other tasks such as word reading and studying patterns of visual noise. Left frontal activation is, then, a distinguishing feature of AM recall and this finding stands in striking contrast to many, but not all, previous neuroimaging studies of memory retrieval. Thus, the typical pattern in word recognition and cued recall is that of right hemisphere activation in regions of the temporal lobe and frontal lobe, especially prefrontal areas (cf. Nyberg et al., 1996). Similarly in the Fink et al. (1996) PET study of the cued recall of details of highly emotional memories mainly right side frontal and temporal activation was detected. However, more recent experiments, some of which are in progress (Markowitsch, personal communication), have detected extensive left hemisphere activation in self-referring memory tasks. For instance, Craik et al. (1998), in a PET study in which participants encoded materials in either a self-referring way or in other ways that did not increase self-reference, found bilateral frontal activation during the encoding of high self-referent materials. Bilateral activation of the medial frontal lobe, middle frontal gyrus, in BA10 on the left side and BA9 on the right, with additional right inferior frontal gyrus activation, all occurred during self-referent encoding. Craik et al. (1998) concluded that a general schematic representation of the self (the working self), primarily in left frontal regions, influences encoding. The data from Craik et al. fit well with other recent findings such as those of Maguire and Mummery (1998) who also observed primarily left frontoparietal activations when self-referring items were processed.

Related to this is a proposal of Gabrieli and colleagues (e.g. Gabrieli, Poldrack, & Desmond, 1998) that the left prefrontal cortex acts as a domain-specific semantic working memory. In their review of the imaging data they identify BAs 9 and 10, 24/32 (cingulate gyrus), and 43 (left caudate nucleus) as critical sites. As far as AM is concerned these could be areas where abstract/conceptual knowledge, perhaps that of lifetime periods, is used to contextualise and frame the construction of more detailed memories. This (complex) process could be influenced by working self structures stored in the same or adjacent regions. Indeed, Nolde et al. (1998) found both left and right prefrontal cortical activation during retrieval. However, the left prefrontal region was more active during the recall of memory details, leading Nolde et al. (1998) to conclude that the left prefrontal cortex (BAs 46, 44, 10, & 9) was important in complex problem-solving types of remembering, whereas the right prefrontal cortex (BAs 45, 44, 10, 9, & 8) mediated simpler memory tasks such as recognition. Other work by this group (Nolde, Johnson, & Raye, 1998) has further established that the left prefrontal cortex is frequently differentially active in complex or difficult retrieval tasks, and an area that is often activated is BA10, although in some experiments the activation is bilateral. Taken together these studies all point to a major role for frontal networks, especially on the left side, in complex self-referring memory tasks such as the construction of AMs.

Thus, the differences between the present findings and those of Fink et al. can be explained in several ways, all of which may be correct. In the Fink et al. study participants imagine ''what happens next'' when provided with a sentence from a description of a memory of emotional event which they had provided earlier. This not only bypasses generative retrieval, because of the specificity of the cue, but it may also make the retrieval task much simpler and, following Nolde et al., we might therefore expect to observe right frontal activation. Had Fink et al. cued their participants to recall emotional memories with emotion words, e.g. Sad, Frightened, Happy, etc. (see Conway & Bekerian, 1987b), they might have additionally observed the extensive pattern of left frontal activation we have reported here. A further difference between Fink et al. and the present findings is that we did not detect extensive right hemisphere activation. Our suggestion is that this may be because we did not sample AMs of highly emotional experiences, AMs that in the Fink et al. study would, we assume, have been mostly of negative experiences. The AMs recalled by our participants (which they described after the scans in response to the words they had provided naming the AMs during the scans) were of comparatively mundane everyday events, which although distinctive did not generally contain mentions of intense—and often did not feature any—emotions. Finally, there is a discrepancy between the present study and the findings of Conway et al. (1999) who observed a flow of activation during retrieval from left frontal areas to right hemisphere posterior (temporal/occipital) regions. In the Conway et al. study, however, the right posterior activation only became present shortly after a memory had been formed and while it was held in mind. In the present study the pace of presentation of cues may have limited or prevented memories being held in mind and perhaps it is for this reason that only left hemisphere occipital activation was detected rather than bilateral, but greater on the right than left, temporal/occipital activation. Despite this, the striking left frontal activation found in the AM conditions of the present study parallels that activation observed by Conway et al. (1999) who, we note, also used a cue word AM retrieval procedure similar to the one used here.

Also of interest was the failure to find any substantial differences in the patterns of activation for recent compared to remote memories. This, as we noted earlier, does not provide support for the view that certain brain areas, i.e. the hippocampal formation, are only active in the recall of recent not-yet-consolidated memories. Also it does not fit well with the suggestion that older AMs, especially those from childhood, have by some process of rehearsal become represented semantically. This null finding is, then, somewhat unexpected, although with the relatively small sample of AMs used in the present study it is suggestive rather than definitive. Nevertheless, if no differences were observed in a wider sample of AMs of different ages then current theories about the representation of recent and remote memories would require modification. A further null finding that departs from previous studies was the failure to detect activation in the right frontal lobe during the cued recall of paired associates. A difference in our study that may account for this is that, unusually for this type of study, our participants learned the PAs until they could recall them either without error or with only a minor omission. The reason for this was to create stable memory representation that might, at least partly, be similar to well learned AMs. This over-learning may have facilitated direct access to these items in memory and made redundant any monitoring of active representations prior to output. Possibly it is this monitoring of accessed information in long-term memory that is undertaken by right frontal networks in the cued recall of words (e.g. Rugg et al., 1996).

Overall, then, we have found that different types of episodic remembering (AM versus cued recall of recently learned words) engage different brain systems. This is surprising, as it shows that not all types of episodic memory share the same processing sequences, as previously assumed. The effortful construction of AMs is heavily reliant on the operation of control process sited in networks in the left frontal lobes: regions of temporal and occipital lobes, also on the left side, may be sites at which autobiographical knowledge is stored. Cued recall of recently learned words, by contrast, does not entail processing in frontal networks and instead is associated with relatively stronger activation of right temporal lobe and of the occipital lobes (bilaterally) and, to a lesser extent, parietal lobes. This pattern in cued recall may reflect direct access to and re-experience of a very recent episode. In contrast to these striking differences hippocampal activation was found to be common to all the tasks we used and did not vary with age of memory. This favours the view that networks in this system are active in all forms of remembering. In conclusion, AM retrieval is distinguished by activation of sites in the left cortical hemisphere and, in our view, this reflects an involvement of aspects of self in remembering, aspects that act to control what is remembered and how.

REFERENCES

Barsalou, L.W. (1988). The content and organization of autobiographical memories. In U. Neisser & E. Winograd (Eds.), *Remembering reconsidered: Ecological and traditional approaches to the study of memory* (pp.193–243). Cambridge: Cambridge University Press.

Becker, J.T., Mintun, M.A., Diehl, D.J., et al. (1994). Functional neuroanatomy of verbal free recall: A replication study. *Human Brain Mapping, 1*, 284–292.

Berntsen, D. (1996). Involuntary autobiographical memories. *Applied Cognitive Psychology, 10*(5), 435–454.

Bremner, J.D., Krystal, J.H., Southwick, S.M., & Charney, D.S. (1995). Functional neuroanatomical correlates of the effects of stress on memory. *Journal of Traumatic Stress, 8*, 527–553.

Burgess, P.W., & Shallice, T. (1996). Confabulation and the control of recollection. *Memory, 4*(4), 359–411.

Carver, C.S. & Scheier, M.F. (1982). Control theory: A useful conceptual framework for personality-social, clinical, and health psychology. *Psychological Bulletin, 92*, 111–135.

Carver, C.S. & Scheier, M.F. (1990). Origins and functions of positive and negative affect: A control-process view. *Psychological Review, 97*, 19–35.

Conway, M.A. (1990). *Autobiographical memory: An introduction.* Buckingham, UK: Open University Press.

Conway, M.A. (1992). A structural model of autobiographical memory. In M.A. Conway, D.C. Rubin, H. Spinnler & W.A. Wagenaar (Eds.), *Theoretical perspectives on autobiographical memory* (pp. 167–194). Dordrecht, The Netherlands: Kluwer Academic Publishers.

Conway, M.A. (1996a). Autobiographical memories and autobiographical knowledge. In D.C. Rubin (Ed.), *Remembering our past: Studies in autobiographical memory* (pp. 67–93). Cambridge: Cambridge University Press.

Conway, M.A. (1996b). Failures of autobiographical remembering. In D. Herrmann, M. Johnson, C. McEvoy, C. Hertzog, & P. Hertel (Eds.), *Basic and applied memory: Theory in context* (pp. 295–315). Hillsdale, NJ: Erlbaum.

Conway, M.A. (1997). Past and present: Recovered memories and false memories. In M.A. Conway (Ed.), *False and recovered memories* (pp. 150–191). Oxford: Oxford University Press.

Conway, M.A., & Fthenaki, I. (in press). Disruption and loss of autobiographical memory. In L. Cermak (Ed.), *Handbook of neuropsychology: Memory.* Amsterdam: Elsevier.

Conway, M.A. (in press). Phenomenological records and the self-memory system. In T. McCormack & C. Hoerl (Eds.), *Time and memory: Issues in philosophy and psychology.* Oxford: Oxford University Press.

Conway, M.A., & Bekerian, D.A. (1987a). Organization in autobiographical memory. *Memory & Cognition, 15*(2), 119–132.

Conway, M.A., & Bekerian, D.A. (1987b). Situational knowledge and emotions. *Cognition and Emotion, 1*(2), 145–191.

Conway, M.A., Pleydell-Pearce, C.W., & Whitecross, S.E. (1999). *The neuroanatomy of autobiographical memory: A slow cortical potentials (SCPs) study of autobiographical memory retrieval.* Manuscript submitted for publication.

Conway, M.A., & Pleydell-Pearce, C.W. (1999). *On the construction of autobiographical memories: A motivational/cognitive/neuroscience model.* Manuscript submitted for publication.

Craik, F.I.M., Moroz, T.M., Moscovitch, M., Stuss, D.T., Winocur, G., Tulving, E., & Kapur, S. (1998). In search of self: A PET investigation of self-referential information. *Psychological Science, 10*(1), 26–34.

Damasio, A.R. (1994). *Descartes' error.* London: Papermac.

Eslinger, P.J., & Damasio, A.R. (1985). Severe disturbance of higher cognition after bilateral frontal lobe ablation: Patient EVR. *Neurology, 35,* 1731–1741.

Fink, G.R., Markowitsch, H.J., Reinkemeier, M., Bruckbauer, T., Kessler, J., & Heiss, W. (1996). Cerebral representation of one's own past: Neural networks involved in autobiographical memory. *Journal of Neuroscience, 18*(13), 4275–4282.

Fox, P.T., & Mintun, M.A. (1989). Noninvasive functional brain mapping by change-distribution analysis of averaged PET images of H2150 tissue activity. *Journal of Nuclear Medicine, 30,* 141–149.

Friston, K.F., Frith, C.D., Liddle, P.F., & Frackowiak, R.S.J. (1991). Comparing functional (PET) images: The assessment of significant change. *Journal of Cerebral Blood Flow Metab., 10,* 458–466.

Fuster, J.M. (1997). Network memory. *Trends in Neuroscience, 20*(10), 451–459.

Gabrieli, J.D.E., Poldrack, R.A., & Desmond, J.E. (1998). The role of the left prefrontal cortex in language and memory. *Proceedings of the National Academy of Sciences, 95,* 906–913.

Gurvits, T.V., Shenton, M.E., Hokama, H., Ohta, H., Lasko, N.B., Gilbertson, M.W., Orr, S.P., Kikinis, R., Jolesz, F.A., McCarley, R.W., & Pitman, R.K. (1996). A magnetic resonance imaging study of hippocampal volume in chronic, combat related, post-traumatic stress disorder. *Biological Psychiatry, 40,* 1091–1099.

Heil, M., Rosler, F., & Hennighausen, E. (1997). Topography of brain electrical activity dissociates the retrieval of spatial versus verbal information from episodic long-term memory in humans. *Neuroscience Letters, 222,* 45–48.

Hodges, J. (1995). Retrograde amnesia. In A.D. Baddeley, B.A. Wilson, & F.N. Watts (Eds.), *Handbook of memory disorders* (pp.81–108). Chichester, UK: John Wiley & Sons.

Hodges, J.R., & McCarthy, R.A. (1993). Autobiographical amnesia resulting from bilateral paramedian thalamic infarction. *Brain, 116,* 921–940.

Honda, M., Barrett, G. Yoshimura, N., Ikeda, A., Nagamine, T., & Shibasaki, H. (1996). Event-related potentials during paired associate memory paradigm. *Electroencephalography and Clinical Neurophysiology, 100,* 407–421.

Howe, M.L., & Courage M.L. (1996). The emergence and early development of autobiographical memory. *Psychological Review, 104,* 499–523.

Kohler, S., McIntosh, A.R., Moscovitch, M., & Winocur, G. (1998). Functional interactions between the medial temporal lobes and posterior neocortex related to episodic memory retrieval. *Cerebral Cortex, 8,* 451–461.

Kroll, N.E.A., Markowitsch, H.J., Knight, R.T., & von Cramon, D.Y. (1997). Retrieval of old memories: The temporofrontal hypothesis. *Brain, 120*, 1377–1399.

Lucchelli, F., Muggia, S., & Spinnler, H. (1995). The 'Petites Madeleines' phenomenon in two amnesic patients. Sudden recovery of forgotten memories. *Brain, 113*, 1673–1794.

Maguire, E.A., & Mummery, C.J. (1999). Differential modulation of a common memory retrieval network revealed by PET. *Hippocampus, 9*, 54–61.

Markowitsch, H.J. (1998). Cognitive neuroscience of memory. *Neurocase, 4*, 429–435.

Markowitsch, H.J., Thiel, A., Kessler, J., von Stockhausen, H.-M., & Heiss, W.-D. (1997). Ecphorising semi-conscious episodic information via the right temporopolar cortex: a PET study. *Neurocase, 3*, 445–449.

Markus, H., & Ruvolo, A. (1989). Possible selves: Personalized representations of goals. In L.A. Pervin (Ed.), *Goal concepts in personality and social psychology* (pp.211–242). Hillsdale, NJ: Lawrence Erlbaum Associates.

McClelland, J.L., McNaughton, B.L., O'Reilly, R.C. (1995). Why there are complementary learning systems in the hippocampus and neocortex: Insights from the successes and failures of connectionist models of learning and memory. *Psychological Review, 102*(3), 419–457.

Miroshima, S., Berger, K.L., Lee, K.S., & Mintun, M.A. (1992). An automated method for rotational correction and centering of three-dimensional functional brain images. *Journal of Nuclear Medicine, 33*, 1579–1585.

Moscovitch, M. (1992). Memory and working-with-memory: A component process model based on modules and central systems. *Journal of Cognitive Neuroscience, 4*, 257–267.

Moscovitch, M. (1995). Recovered consciousness: A hypothesis concerning modularity and episodic memory. *Journal of Clinical and Experimental Neuropsychology, 17*, 276–290.

Moscovitch, M., & Mello, B. (1997). Strategic retrieval and the frontal lobes: Evidence from confabulation and amnesia. *Neuropsychologia, 35*(7), 1017–1034.

Nadel, L., & Moscovitch, M. (1997). Consolidation, amnesia, and the hippocampal complex. *Current Opinion in Neurobiology, 7*, 217–227.

Nolde, S.F., Johnson, M.K., & D'Esposito, M. (1998). Left prefrontal activation during episodic remembering: An event-related fMRI study. *NeuroReport, 9*, 509–514.

Nolde, S.F., Johnson, M.K., & Raye, C.L. (1998). The role of prefrontal cortex during tests of episodic memory. *Trends in Cognitive Sciences, 2*, 399–406.

Nyberg, L., Cabeza, R., & Tulving, E. (1996). PET studies of encoding and retrieval: The HERA model. *Psychonomic Bulletin and Review, 3*, 135–148.

Proust, M. (1913/1981). *Rememberance of things past* [C.K. Scott-Moncrieff, T. Kilmartin, & A. Mayor, Trans]. New York: Random House.

Rugg, M.D., Fletcher, P.C., Frith, C.D., Frackowiak, R.S.J., & Dolan, R.J. (1996). Differential activation of the prefrontal cortex in successful and unsuccessful memory retrieval. *Brain, 119*, 2073–2083.

Rubin, D.C., & Greenberg, D.L. (1998). Visual-memory-deficit amnesia: A distinct amnesic presentation and etiology. *Proceedings of the National Academy of Sciences, 95*, 1–4.

Sapolsky, R.M. (1996). Stress, glucocorticoids, and damage to the nervous system: The current state of confusion. *Stress, 1*, 1–19.

Schacter, D.L., Norman, K.A., & Koutstaal, W. (1998). The cognitive neuroscience of constructive memory. *Annual Review of Psychology, 49*, 289–318.

Squire, L.R. (1992). Memory and the hippocampus: A synthesis from findings with rats, monkeys, and humans. *Psychological Review, 99*, 195–231.

Talairach, J., & Tournoux, P. (1988). *Co-planar stereotactic atlas of the human brain: 3-dimensional proportional system: An approach to cerebral imaging.* New York: Thieme Medical Publishers.

Townsend, D.W., Geissbuhler, A., Defrise, M., et al. (1991). Fully three-dimensional reconstruction for a PET camera with retractable septa. *IEEE Transactions on Medical Imaging, 10*(4), 505–512.

Tulving, E. (1983). *Elements of episodic memory.* Oxford: Clarendon Press.

Woods, R.P., Cherry, S.R., & Mazziotta, J.C. (1992). Rapid automated algorithm for aligning and reslicing PET images. *Journal of Computer Assisted Tomography, 16*(4), 620–633.

MEMORY, 1999, 7 (5/6), 703–713

Right Prefrontal Cortex Responds to Item Familiarity During a Memory Encoding Task

P.C. Fletcher

Institute of Neurology, London, UK

R.J. Dolan

Institute of Neurology, and Royal Free Hospital Medical School, London, UK

In a previous word-pair encoding study (Dolan & Fletcher, 1997), we examined the effect of introducing novelty, either in studied words or in their mutual associations. A left medial temporal lobe (MTL) sensitivity to novel words and left prefrontal cortex (PFC) to novel associations was observed. In this further report on the data, we explored the extent to which the right PFC, more generally implicated in retrieval operations (Fletcher, Frith, & Rugg, 1997), was sensitive to these manipulations. Specifically, we characterised changes associated with increasing familiarity of study material. We demonstrate that the response in right ventrolateral PFC is preferentially sensitive to a condition in which all material was familiar (that is, in which all material had been presented prior to scanning). A more dorsal region in right PFC was found to be relatively more active in association with a condition in which one item in the pair was familiar but was paired with a novel associate. Our results suggest that sensitivity to stimulus familiarity is expressed in right PFC, even within the context of an encoding task. The data also provide further evidence for functional heterogeneity within right PFC, with a more ventral region responding to familiarity of complete word pairs and a more dorsal region responding to familiar single words occurring in the context of new associative relationships.

INTRODUCTION

Activation of right PFC during memory retrieval is widely observed across a number of functional neuroimaging studies employing a range of psychological paradigms and test modalities (Fletcher et al., 1997; Tulving et al., 1994a). The functional significance of these observations has remained unexplained. One suggestion is that the predominance of right PFC activation during retrieval

Requests for reprints should be sent to Paul Fletcher, C. und O. Vogt Institut Für Hirnforschung, Heinrich-Hein Universitat, Universitatsstrasse 1, D 40225, Dusseldorf, Germany. Email: fletcher@hirn.uni-duesseldorf.de

PCF and RJD are supported by the Wellcome Trust.

experiments reflects the adoption of a "retrieval mode", necessary for the initiation and maintenance of retrieval processes (Kapur et al., 1995; Nyberg et al., 1995). However, it has also been argued that right prefrontal activation is sensitive to the degree of retrieval success (Rugg et al., 1996) although it seems that retrieval occurring intentionally is associated with greater levels of right PFC activation than retrieval that is incidental to task demands (Rugg et al., 1997). It seems, therefore, that existing evidence supports the position that right PFC involvement in memory retrieval reflects both the processes involved in attempting to recall study material and those that may be contingent on the actual successful retrieval of material. Other work has suggested that right PFC shows a non-linear response to difficulty of paired associate retrieval as measured by the "semantic relatedness' of pair members (Fletcher et al., 1996). This latter response was interpreted as a reflection of post-retrieval error-checking with the non-linearity of response reflecting at least two different types of possible error which each varied differently as a function of semantic relatedness. Other work has suggested that the region is also sensitive to processes necessary for retrieval of information regarding feature rather than location information (Nyberg et al., 1996; Owen et al., 1996).

The picture is further complicated by evidence that there is heterogeneity within right PFC with respect to sub-processes occurring in episodic memory retrieval (Fletcher et al., 1998). Tasks necessitating "monitoring" processes (Burgess & Shallice, 1996) have been associated with activation of dorsal right PFC whereas simpler, externally specified retrieval processes, not necessitating monitoring, are associated with activation of more ventral PFC.

Clearly, our understanding of the significance of right PFC activation in association with memory retrieval is incomplete with respect to the processes subserved and to the functional heterogeneity within PFC. The current experiment was designed to explore brain systems associated with the encoding of word paired associates and has already been reported as such (Dolan & Fletcher, 1997). However, the basic study design, which characterised the effects of novelty, may also produce interesting effects with respect to growing familiarity of study material and the possibility of this engendering retrieval, whether incidental or intentional, even though such retrieval would be occurring in the face of an encoding task. In this treatment of the data, we examine effects associated with this familiarity. During positron emission tomography (PET) scanning, subjects were presented with lists of word pairs, each pair consisting of a category and an exemplar. These pairs were, in the context of the experiment, novel or familiar with respect to both the words themselves and the semantic linkages between them. We showed that left dorsolateral prefrontal cortex (DLPFC) was sensitive to a manipulation of the association between category and exemplar, that is, maximal activation in this region was seen in scans involving a change in category–exemplar pairings. By contrast the medial temporal cortex, including the hippocampus and parahippocampal region, showed a response that was maximal when the entire word pair was novel. This analysis of the data has been reported and discussed elsewhere (Dolan & Fletcher, 1997). The present analysis of the data thus involves a reversal of our previous analyses. In simple terms, instead of characterising brain changes occurring in association with novel compared to familiar stimuli, we now explored changes occurring in association with familiar compared to novel stimuli. This extension of our original analysis was motivated by post hoc reports from all subjects that they frequently, and spontaneously, recalled previous presentations of familiar items in response to cueing even though the experimental task did not explicitly require this. This observation is of particular interest in the light of the aforementioned confusion regarding the role of right PFC in episodic memory retrieval and the array of functional neuroimaging studies that have shown this region to be involved in many different retrieval situations (Buckner et al., 1996; Fletcher et al., 1996, 1998; Kapur et al., 1995; Nyberg et al., 1996; Rugg et al., 1996; Shallice et al., 1994; Tulving et al., 1994a,b; Wheeler, Stuss, & Tulving, 1997). Most previous studies have examined retrieval-related brain systems in the context of tasks that have explicitly required subjects to recall previously presented material (Fletcher et al., 1997). In the current study, any retrieval was incidental to the task demands and, thus, provides a different setting in which to explore retrieval-related brain responses.

METHOD

PET Scanning

Six healthy male right-handed volunteers were studied using a SIEMENS/CPS ECAT EXACT HR+ (MODEL 962) PET scanner in 3-D mode with a 15cm axial field of view. Relative rCBF was measured from the distribution of radioactivity after slow bolus i.v. injection of $H_2^{15}O$ (9mCi per scan, each lasting 90 seconds). Attenuation-corrected data were reconstructed into 63 image planes with a resulting resolution of 6mm at full-width-half-maximum. For each subject, structural magnetic resonance (MR) images were obtained with a 2 T Magnetom VISION (Siemens, Germany).

Psychological Tasks

Prior to each PET scan, subjects were presented verbally with a list of category–exemplar word pairs (e.g. DOG. . .BOXER). The list was presented twice, during a 90-second lead-in period, with a third presentation timed to coincide with the onset of PET scanning. Subjects were instructed to try to remember material for later testing. They were unaware of when scanning was actually occurring, in order to ensure, as far as possible, that they attended to each of the list presentations. During the third presentation (that is, during scanning), one of the following manipulations was made:

1. The same list was presented for the third time. That is, all material was familiar. We shall henceforth refer to this condition as the *Wholly Familiar* condition.

2. For each pair, either the category or the exemplar was changed. (Thus, for example, DOG...BOXER might become DOG...LABRADOR or SPORTSMAN...BOXER). In this case, material was partly familiar. Although the [New Category...Old exemplar and [Old Category...New Exemplar] conditions were actually scanned separately, we have collapsed them for the purposes of the current analysis and would point out, with respect to the prefrontal regions discussed, that there was no difference in levels of activity between them. We shall refer to this condition as the *Partially Familiar* condition.

3. An entirely new list of word pairs was presented. We shall refer to this as the *Wholly Novel* condition.

The order of the presentation of experimental conditions was counterbalanced both within and across subjects.

Data Analysis

Statistical parametric mapping (SPM96) software was used for image realignment, transformation into standard stereotactic space, smoothing, and statistical analysis (Friston et al., 1995). All measurements per condition were averaged across subjects. State-dependent differences in global flow were co-varied out using ANCOVA. Main effects and interactions were assessed with contrasts of the adjusted task means using t-statistic subsequently transformed into normally distributed Z statistic. The resulting set of Z values constituted a statistical parametric map [$SPM_{(z)}$] which was then thresholded at $P < .001$. The following comparisons were made. Scans in which presented material was wholly familiar and those in which material was partly familiar were compared separately with those in which material was completely novel. A further comparison was made directly between the wholly and partially familiar conditions.

RESULTS

Behavioural Results

The effectiveness of encoding was assessed using a cued retrieval task after a five-minute interval. These data showed recall was 95% for the wholly novel condition, 78% for the partially familiar condition, and 93% for the wholly familiar condition. It should be noted that the significantly lower level of recall with respect to the partially familiar condition reflects proactive interference and has been discussed elsewhere (Dolan & Fletcher, 1997).

Neuroimaging Results

Unless otherwise stated, the statistical parametric maps were thresholded at $P < .001$, uncorrected for multiple comparisons.

Wholly Familiar vs *Wholly Novel.*   Wholly familiar stimuli were associated with relatively greater activation in bilateral anterior PFC, in dorsal and ventral regions of the right middle frontal gyrus and in medial and lateral parietal cortex (see Table 1 and Plate 3).

Partially Familiar vs *Wholly Novel.*   Partially familiar stimuli were associated with relatively greater activation in bilateral anterior PFC, in a dorsal region of the right middle frontal gyrus and in medial and lateral parietal cortex (see Table 2 and Plate 4).

TABLE 1

Regions Showing Significantly Greater Activity in Association with the Presentation of Wholly Familiar Compared to Wholly Novel Material

Region	Coordinates*	Z Score
R. Middle frontal gyrus (BA 10)	40, 56, −4	4.5
L. Middle frontal gyrus (BA 10)	−32, 58, 0	4.1
R. Inferior frontal gyrus (BA 44/45)	48, 12, 12	3.3
R. Middle frontal gyrus (BA 9/46)	44, 24, 30	3.3
Medial parietal cortex (BA 7)	−2, −74, 52	3.3

*Talairach and Tournoux, 1988.

TABLE 2

Regions Showing Significantly Greater Activity in Association with the Presentation of *Partially Familiar* Compared to *Wholly Novel* Material

Region	Coordinates*	Z Score
R. Middle frontal gyrus (BA 10)	30, 58, −2	4.1
L. Middle frontal gyrus (BA 10)	−32, 58, 0	5.5
R. Middle frontal gyrus (BA 9/46)	44, 20, 26	4.0
	42, 8, 36	3.2
L. Middle frontal gyrus (BA 9)	−46, 20, 40	4.9
Medial parietal cortex (BA 7)	0, −70, 48	6.2
R. Lateral parietal cortex (BA 7)	28, −54, 50	4.2
L. Lateral parietal cortex (BA 7)	−36, −54, 48	4.2

*Talairach and Tournoux, 1988.

Wholly familiar vs *Partial Familiar.*   Compared to the partial familiar condition, the wholly familiar condition was associated with relatively greater levels of activity in bilateral anterior temporal regions and right medial parietal cortex.

Partially Familiar vs *Wholly Familiar.*   This comparison showed the partially familiar condition to be associated with greater activity in left dorsolateral prefrontal cortex, left medial and lateral parietal cortex.

In view of the particular interest in right PFC with respect to item familiarity, we repeated the last two contrasts at a reduced level of significance ($P < .05$, uncorrected), concentrating solely on the dorsal and ventral right PFC which had been shown to be activated in the two familiar conditions (*wholly familiar* and *partially familiar*) compared to the wholly novel condition. These comparisons showed a dissociation in the ventral and dorsal regions with greater levels of activity in ventral right PFC in the wholly compared to the partially familiar condition, and greater levels of activity in the dorsal right PFC in the reverse contrasts. These results are summarised in Plates 3 and 4.

DISCUSSION

Our data demonstrate that right PFC is sensitive to the degree of stimulus familiarity and that this sensitivity can be seen even in a task designed to engage encoding processes. Moreover, there was subtle evidence of a dissociation in the observed patterns of activity occurring in dorsal and ventral right PFC. The latter showed an apparently linear relationship with the degree of stimulus familiarity. Activity here was maximal when all pair members presented during the scan had already been presented twice during the lead-in period. The more dorsal region, on the other hand, was maximally sensitive to the condition in which subjects had become familiarised with only part of the stimuli (i.e. one item in each pair).

Before discussing these results in greater detail, it is important to raise a number of caveats. Primarily, the experiment was designed to look at the effects of stimulus novelty during memory encoding and the condition that has been considered as the ''activation'' task in the current treatment of the data was originally used as the ''baseline''. The current analysis is reported because of the interesting findings with respect to right PFC but we are suitably cautious about drawing firm conclusions over an issue that the experiment was not designed to address. In addition, the subtlety of the findings (most particularly with reference to the ventral–dorsal dissociation, which only survived a lenient statistical threshold for significance) is another reason for caution. Nevertheless, we believe that the results bear further discussion for a number of reasons. First, it is both interesting and potentially informative that the left and right prefrontal regions are responding to task demands with highly different qualitative patterns of response. Second, it is a reminder that task manipulations may produce effects associated with processes beyond those that the tasks are explicitly designed to engage, even though the task may be designated and considered as a fairly low-level baseline condition. Finally, the observation of different patterns of familiarity response in ventral and dorsal regions of right PFC is worth speculating upon.

Overall, the right PFC region showing a response to familiarity encompassed the ventral areas of the inferior frontal gyrus, bordering upon and, perhaps, extending into the insula, and a more dorsal region of the inferior frontal sulcus. In previous studies, activation of right PFC has been found in association with memory retrieval (Fletcher et al., 1997; Fletcher et al., 1998; Shallice et al., 1994; Squire et al., 1992; Tulving et al., 1994b). The finding has been framed in terms of the adoption of a retrieval mode or of processes subserving an active search of memory contents. However, our data suggest that right prefrontal activation can occur in association with the presentation of previously learned material even in the context of a task in which these processes are not explicitly operative. Rather, it is possible that incidental retrieval will also engage right prefrontally mediated processes. An important question here is whether subjects were actually retrieving material incidentally. Incidental retrieval can refer to retrieval that is incidental to task demands (i.e. not required to perform the allotted task) or retrieval that occurs incidentally without subjects engaging in an effortful memory search (that is, incidental as opposed to intentional retrieval). With respect to the first definition, we can be confident that the retrieval was incidental. However, with respect to the second and more interesting definition, the case is less clear cut. Although subjects reported that, in the *Wholly Familiar* condition, presentation of one item was often associated with effortless retrieval of its pair, it is nevertheless possible that the right PFC activation actually reflects a more effortful process. Moreover, recent findings have suggested that right PFC (in a dorsal region close to the one reported here) shows higher levels of activity in intentional compared to incidental retrieval (Rugg et al., 1997). Aside from post hoc subjects' reports, we have no clear way of addressing the question of to what extent subjects' retrieval was truly incidental. Nevertheless, the different patterns of activity observed in the dorsal and ventral foci of activation may offer some clues as will be discussed next.

One possibility, concerning the functional significance of our findings, is that the activations simply reflect the recognition, during scanning, of items that had been presented during the lead-in period. This would be consistent with a previous study of word recognition memory (Rugg et al., 1996) where word lists containing a higher density of previously presented items were associated with activation of right PFC when compared to lists consisting entirely of previously unseen items. However, it should also be noted that other experiments with similar designs have concluded that the right PFC activation reflects retrieval effort rather than the actual recognition of items (Kapur et al., 1995; Nyberg et al., 1995). A related but alternative possibility is that activation of right PFC reflects automatic item retrieval in response to verbal cueing. Thus, for example, when a word pair such as DOG...BOXER was presented for the third time (the third presentation occurring during scanning), the presentation of the category DOG results in automatic retrieval of the exemplar BOXER. Indeed subjects reported, at debriefing, that this was so in the *Wholly Familiar* condition, remarking that presentation of the categories resulted in the automatic retrieval of the appropriate exemplar, pre-empting its presentation by the experimenter. Thus, right PFC activity may reflect recognition or cued retrieval of paired associates. If it reflects cued retrieval then, as remarked earlier, it is not entirely clear whether this is incidental or intentional.

However, the observed functional heterogeneity within right PFC is interesting and possibly informative with respect to this uncertainty. The more ventral region showed a greater sensitivity to the *Wholly Familiar* condition, whereas the more dorsal region showed greater sensitivity to the *Partially Familiar* condition. This observation of a dissociation between more dorsal and ventral regions is in keeping with previous functional neuroimaging experiments of episodic memory retrieval (Fletcher et al., 1998) and with evidence from monkey experiments which have suggested that, in working memory tasks, dorsal and ventral regions of PFC subserve qualitatively different processes (Petrides, 1994, 1995). Moreover, it suggests that the two regions subserve qualitatively different processing.

Regarding the more ventral right PFC activation, it was preferentially sensitive to lists in which items were wholly familiar. Recall that this was the condition in which subjects reported incidental retrieval occurring in anticipation of the experimenter's presentation of the exemplar. By contrast, in the condition where material was only partly familiar, they reported that they tended to do this less as it was unhelpful to the experimental task—the task instructions being to encode the new category–exemplar pairings (although subjects were not made aware of when scanning was occurring, nor were they informed as to the nature of the experimental manipulations, the blocked presentations meant that they nevertheless realised the nature of changes and that these changes occurred during the third presentation of a list). This suggestion, that the more ventral activation reflects automatic retrieval of exemplars in response to category presentation, is in keeping with a previous study (Fletcher et al., 1998) showing that right ventral PFC is most active with cued paired associate retrieval. Our interpretation was that the activation in this region reflected retrieval specification (as determined by each successive category cue) across the course of the scan. The present finding is consistent with this interpretation in regard to the *Wholly Familiar* condition. On the other hand, the absence of ventral PFC activation in the *Partially Familiar* condition (at the pre-set threshold for statistical significance) is consistent with the subjective reports of participants that automatic retrieval of paired associates was unhelpful to the experimental task in this condition. However, it should be noted that right ventral PFC activity in this condition was intermediate between the *Wholly Familiar* and *Wholly Novel* conditions and, at a lower threshold for significance ($P < .01$, uncorrected) activation was seen here in association with the *Partially Familiar* condition. In this condition, the familiarity of the presented categories may have led to some spontaneous recovery of their previous associates but, as subjects found this unhelpful, there may have been an active suppression of this phenomenon. Alternatively, it might simply be the case that this region was responsive purely to the amount of familiar material within a scanning block. That is, it is possible that every time subjects recognised an item that had been previously presented, then activation occurred irrespective of whether or not presentation of that item provoked cued retrieval of its previously learned associate.

With respect to the pattern of activity seen in the more dorsal region of right PFC, these two possible interpretations are less plausible. Activity here was greater in both the *Wholly* and the *Partially Familiar* conditions when compared separately with the *Wholly Novel* condition. A direct comparison of the *Wholly* and the *Partially Familiar* conditions at a reduced threshold for significance ($P < .05$, uncorrected) showed a relatively greater activation of the dorsal region in response to the latter condition. This is a complex finding which cannot be attributed simply to stimulus familiarity, as activity was maximal in the condition where only half of the material was familiar. It also seems unlikely that the observed pattern of activity in this region reflects automatic cued retrieval, as the extent to which such retrieval was occurring was maximal in the *Wholly Familiar* condition. Rather, we suggest that activity here reflects a more active processing. More specifically, if the activation in this region reflected purely retrieval-related processing (whether recognition, incidental, or intentional cued retrieval, as discussed earlier) then it would be maximal in the *Wholly Familiar* condition. The *Partially Familiar* condition, in which it achieved peak activation, is one in which these forms of automatic retrieval would be unhelpful, and, perhaps, a hindrance. We suggest, therefore, that the dorsal right PFC activation might reflect processes that check/monitor (Burgess & Shallice, 1996) the products of this unnecessary and unhelpful retrieval. This, of course, is highly speculative but it is noteworthy that, in a recent study (Fletcher et al., 1998), we demonstrated greater activation of right dorsal PFC in a retrieval task that required monitoring of retrieval products. In the case of the *Partially Familiar* condition, such monitoring would, we suggest, be engaged to a greater extent than in the *Wholly Familiar* condition. In the *Partially Familiar* condition, word pairs each contained one new item and, therefore, a new associative relationship. Thus, in this condition, the previously learned association to each item would need to be suppressed or adjusted. In our previous reporting of these data (Dolan & Fletcher, 1997), we noted that this condition was most prominently associated with activation of left PFC and we interpreted this observation in terms of proactive interference or the active formation of new semantic associations to stimuli that had been previously presented with different associations. It seems plausible that this condition also engages right dorsal PFC to a lesser extent (which did not survive our previously more stringent statistical threshold), and that left and right prefrontal cortices act in conjunction, the latter involved in the retrieval and monitoring of previously learned associations and the former engaged in the formation of the new ones and, perhaps, suppression of the previously learned responses.

In summary, these data indicate that right PFC activation associated with explicit memory retrieval may occur in the absence of an experimental requirement to retrieve material. That is, certain processes, subserved by right prefrontal function may be engaged automatically and/or incidentally when familiar items are presented. Further, the precise regions of prefrontal cortex activated are anatomically distinct, and dependent on the nature of these processes and the extent to which they are appropriate to the context of the experiment. Although these findings must be treated with all due caution, arising as they do from a post hoc analysis of data, we suggest that they may nevertheless be informative with respect to the frequently reported activation of right PFC in association with memory retrieval.

REFERENCES

Buckner, R.L., Raichle, M.E., Miezin, F.M., & Petersen, S.E. (1996). Functional anatomic studies of memory retrieval for auditory words and visual pictures. *Journal of Neuroscience, 16*(19), 6219–6235.

Burgess, P.W., & Shallice, T. (1996). Confabulation and the control of recollection. *Memory, 4*(4), 359.

Dolan, R.J., & Fletcher, P.C. (1997). Dissociating prefrontal and hippocampal function in episodic memory encoding. *Nature, 388,* 582–585.

Fletcher, P.C., Frith, C.D., & Rugg, M.D. (1997). The functional neuroanatomy of episodic memory. *Trends in Neurosciences, 20*(5), 213–218.

Fletcher, P.C., Shallice, T., Frith, C.D., Frackowiak, R.S.J., & Dolan, R.J. (1996). Brain activity during memory retrieval: The influence of imagery and semantic cueing. *Brain, 119,* 1587–1596.

Fletcher, P.C., Shallice, T., Frith, C.D., Frackowiak, R.S.J., & Dolan, R.J. (1998). The functional roles of the prefrontal cortex in episodic memory: II Retrieval. *Brain, 121,* 1249–1256.

Friston, K.J., Holmes, A.P., Worsley, K.J., Poline, J.B., Frith, C.D., & Frackowiak, R.S.J. (1995). Statistical parametric maps in functional imaging; a general linear approach. *Human Brain Mapping, 2,* 189–210.

Kapur, S., Craik, F., Brown, G.M., Houle, S., & Tulving, E. (1995). Functional role of the prefrontal cortex in memory retrieval: A PET study. *NeuroReport, 6,* 1880–1894.

Nyberg, L., McIntosh, A.R., Cabeza, R., Habib, R., Houle, S., & Tulving, E. (1996). General and specific brain regions involved in encoding and retrieval of events: What, where and when. *Proceedings of the National Academy of Science*, USA, *93,* 11280–11285.

Nyberg, L., Tulving, E., Habib, R., Nilsson, L.G., Kapur, S., Cabeza, R., & McIntosh, A.R. (1995). Functional brain maps of retrieval mode and recovery of episodic information. *NeuroReport, 7,* 249–252.

Owen, A.M., Milner, B., Petrides, M., & Evans, A.C. (1996). Memory for object features versus memory for object location: A positron emission tomography study of encoding and retrieval processes. *Proceedings of the National Academy of Science*, USA, *93,* 9212–9217.

Petrides, M. (1994). Frontal lobes and working memory: Evidence from investigations of the effects of cortical excisions in non-human primates. In F. Boller & J. Grafman (Eds.), *Handbook of neuropsychology (Vol. 9)* (pp.59–82). Amsterdam: Elsevier Science.

Petrides, M. (1995). Impairments on non-spatial self-ordered working memory tasks after lesions to the mid-dorsal part of the lateral frontal cortex in the monkey. *Journal of Neuroscience, 15*(1), 359–375.

Rugg, M.D., Fletcher, P.C., Frith, C.D., Frackowiak, R.S.J., & Dolan, R.J. (1996). Differential activation of the prefrontal cortex in successful and unsuccessful memory retrieval. *Brain, 119*, 2073–2083.

Rugg, M.D., Fletcher, P.C., Frith, C.D., Frackowiak, R.S.J., & Dolan, R.J. (1997). Brain regions supporting intentional and incidental memory: A PET study. *NeuroReport, 8*(5), 1283–1287.

Shallice, T., Fletcher, P., Frith, C.D., Grasby, P., Frackowiak, R.S.J., & Dolan, R.J. (1994). Brain regions associated with acquisition and retrieval of verbal episodic memory. *Nature, 368*, 633–635.

Squire, L.R., Ojemann, J.G., Miezin, F.M., Petersen, S.E., Videen, T.O., & Raichle, M.E. (1992). Activation of the hippocampus in normal humans: A functional anatomical study of memory. *Proceedings of the National Academy of Science, USA, 89*, 1837–1841.

Talairach, J., & Tournoux, P. (1988). *Co-planar stereotaxic atlas of the human brain.* Stuttgart: George Theme Verlag.

Tulving, E., Kapur, S., Craik, F.I.M., Moscovitch, M., & Houle, S. (1994a). Hemispheric encoding/retrieval asymmetry in episodic memory: Positron emission tomography findings. *Proceedings of the National Academy of Science, USA, 91*, 2016–2020.

Tulving, E., Kapur, S., Markovitsch, H.J., Craik, F.I.M., Habib, R., & Houle, S. (1994b). Neuroanatomical correlates of retrieval in episodic memory: Auditory sentence recognition. *Proceedings of the National Academy of Science, USA, 91*, 2012–2015.

Wheeler, M.A., Stuss, D.T., & Tulving, E. (1997). Towards a theory of episodic memory: The frontal lobes and autonoetic consciousness. *Psychological Bulletin, 121*(3), 331–354.

MEMORY, 1999, 7 (5/6), 715–732

The Hippocampus and Delayed Recall: Bigger is not Necessarily Better?

Jonathan K. Foster, Andrew Meikle, and Gregory Goodson

University of Manchester, UK

Andrew R. Mayes

Royal Hallamshire Hospital, University of Sheffield, UK

Matthew Howard

University of Liverpool, UK

Sandra I. Sünram

University of Manchester, UK

Enis Cezayirli and Neil Roberts

University of Liverpool, UK

Healthy young female participants were tested on a measure of delayed verbal recall and then received volumetric Magnetic Resonance Imaging (MRI) scans. The analysis of the MRI scans focused on the volume of the hippocampus. Left hippocampal volume was negatively associated with the level of delayed verbal recall performance. This relationship was confirmed in further testing. This finding is consistent with a previous report of a similar relationship in healthy elderly individuals, but not in patients with Alzheimer's disease, in whom the opposite relationship was observed. An explanation of these findings in terms of impaired neural pruning of the hippocampus is advanced, whereby insufficient pruning of the hippocampus during childhood and adolescence (following adequate growth) may lead to reduced mnemonic efficiency.

Requests for reprints should be sent to Jonathan K. Foster, Department of Psychology, University of Manchester, Oxford Road, Manchester M13 9PL, UK. Email: foster@psy.man.ac.uk

We wish to acknowledge the contributions of research, clinical, and support staff at the Magnetic Resonance and Image Analysis Research Centre (MARIARC) at the University of Liverpool, UK, for their assistance in this work. We are grateful to Professor Robb of the MAYO Foundation, Minnesota, USA for provision of a collaborative agreement (through the Magnetic Resonance and Image Analysis Research Centre at the University of Liverpool) for the development of the ANALYZE software. We also thank Clare Isaac for permitting us to use her story test materials, and undergraduate students at the University of Manchester for participating in the study. We are grateful to Stefan Kohler and Lars Nyberg for their comments on an earlier draft of this paper. This work was supported by an MRC Programme grant (G9300193).

INTRODUCTION

There has been longstanding neuropsychological interest in the relationship between a structure's volume and its functional efficiency. In the nineteenth century, phrenologists such as Gall believed that the size of a specific brain structure determined the efficiency with which the structure performed its functions. In recent years, it has become possible to address this question in vivo using non-invasive brain imaging techniques such as Magnetic Resonance Imaging (MRI). These techniques have enabled researchers to investigate much more systematically than has been possible hitherto the relationship between the volume and other anatomical characteristics of specific brain regions and the particular psychological processes that those regions are thought to subserve. Regional brain volume is likely to be a function of the number of neurones and the complexity of these neurones' interconnections. It seems in turn reasonable to suppose that network efficiency (and, consequently, level of psychological performance) will, in part, be a function of the number of components in a neural network, and in part related to the complexity of the neurones' interconnections. This means that, when other factors are controlled, individuals with larger brain regions should perform the functions mediated by those regions better.

There is some support for this line of reasoning, based on findings drawn from a number of studies of memory disorders. In particular, volumes measured in this way for the hippocampus have been found to be directly proportional to neuronal number (Kuzniecky & Jackson, 1995). It is widely believed that damage to the hippocampus causes anterograde amnesia (Eichenbaum, Otto, & Cohen, 1994; Squire, 1992; see also Mayes, 1988). This notion is supported by the findings of recent functional brain imaging research which have implicated the hippocampus in mediating aspects of long-term memory (Gabrieli et al., 1997; Nyberg et al., 1996; Owen et al., 1996; Schacter et al., 1996; Stern et al., 1996; Tulving et al., 1996). The hippocampus seems to be involved with explicit memory, as is implied by the positive correlation between its volume and explicit memory performance, found in several studies of patient groups in whom this structure is likely to be damaged (Deweer et al., 1995; Foster et al., 1997; Lencz et al., 1992; Nestor et al., 1993; Sass et al., 1992). Furthermore, a recent meta-analysis has argued that hippocampal circuit lesions particularly disrupt recall (Aggleton & Shaw, 1996). Left- and right-sided lesions of medial temporal lobe structures are associated respectively with verbal and non-verbal memory, as many studies show that left-sided medial temporal lobe lesions impair explicit memory for verbal information whereas right-sided lesions impair explicit memory for hard-to-verbalise information such as spatial location (see Mayes, 1988).

The view that the hippocampus is concerned primarily with delayed free recall is quite well supported by work on temporal lobe epilepsy and other conditions (Baxendale, 1997; Lencz et al. (1992); Miller, Munoz, & Finmore 1993). There is further evidence from work on temporal lobe epilepsy that hippocampal lesions disrupt explicit memory only after a delay (Pigott & Milner, 1993). Work conducted in non-human species also indicates that the hippocampus is primarily involved with the mediation of delayed rather than immediate memory (Colombo & Gross, 1994). This notion is also consistent with the work of Isaac (1994), who previously found that amnesics with probable or certain damage to the hippocampus or hippocampal circuit of Papez (which projects from the hippocampus via the fornix to the thalamus and maxillary bodies) showed accelerated loss of free recall of stories and organised word lists at filled delays between 15–20 seconds and 10 minutes (see also Isaac & Mayes, in press a, b). However, patients' recognition performance was equally impaired at both delays. In conjunction with the work of Pigott and Milner (1993) and other studies, this suggests that one deficit, linked to hippocampal circuit damage, is related to accelerated loss of some forms of explicit memory. One theoretical explanation of this is that whereas recall requires retrieval of complex associations, recognition typically involves item retrieval, and the hippocampus only stores complex associations (Cohen et al., 1997).

In a recent study of Alzheimer's disease patients and age-matched controls, Foster and colleagues (1997) observed a positive association between hippocampal volume and delayed memory. Volumetric MRI procedures showed that delayed non-verbal recall scores, based on reproduction of figures from the WMS-R, correlated specifically with volume of the hippocampus on both the left and the right sides. A more specific correlation was observed for verbal recall, in that the volume of the left (but not right) hippocampus correlated with a delayed verbal recall measure derived from the California Verbal Learning Test. A follow-up study by Kohler et al. (1998) confirmed that delayed verbal recall correlated with hippocampal volume in a group of Alzheimer patients alone. However, in normal elderly controls, the relationship went in the opposite direction (i.e. there was a negative relationship between hippocampal volume and delayed memory performance). By contrast, Golomb et al. (1994) observed, in a large group of older participants, that hippocampal (but not superior temporal gyrus) volumes were associated positively with delayed memory performance. There was no association between hippocampal volume and either short-term memory or relatively immediately tested long-term memory in this study. Taken together, these studies suggest a relationship between hippocampal volume and delayed explicit memory, and particularly recall, although the nature of this relationship requires further research. This was the primary goal of the study reported here.

In temporal lobe epilepsy and Alzheimer's disease, it can be argued that the volume of the hippocampus varies partly because of natural variations in its premorbid volume, but mainly because its circuitry has been deranged by neuropathology to varying degrees. The same argument might be applied more weakly to "normal" ageing. This would suggest that in these three groups of participants, hippocampal volume relates to measures of delayed memory mainly because the volume measure closely reflects the degree to which the functioning of the hippocampal circuitry has been disrupted pathologically. In these brain-damaged people, however, if there is a part of the relationship between volume and delayed memory that may be determined by variations in the premorbid volume of the basically intact hippocampus, this is extremely difficult to identify. In order to isolate and examine this factor, in the study reported here we decided to determine whether a significant relationship also exists between hippocampal volume and delayed recall in young people with no evidence of brain damage. If such a relationship does exist, this would imply that the volume of the hippocampus is at least a partial determinant of individual differences in normal levels of delayed explicit memory.

A previous study that we conducted using MRI revealed considerable variation both in memory performance and in the size of brain structures (including the hippocampus) across healthy, young individuals (Mackay et al., 1998). In the previous study, we identified people with widely differing levels of face recognition performance and then referred them for brain scanning. Initially, 200 students were tested. From these individuals, those who scored worst and those who scored best on a delayed face recognition test were selected to undergo MRI scanning. These comprised a total of 29 participants. Although the volumes of the hippocampus varied considerably across individuals, there was little difference in the hippocampal volumes of good and poor face recognisers. The two groups were also compared with respect to the volumes of the hippocampus as a proportion of whole brain volume; i.e. they were normalised. This analysis also revealed no significant differences in proportional hippocampal volume between good and poor face recognisers.

Several factors emerged from the aforementioned study (see Mackay et al., 1998). First, it was possible to develop reliable MRI volumetric measurements of medial temporal lobe structures using the procedures we had adopted. Second, the volume of the left and right hippocampus was found to be highly variable even in healthy young participants. This has been found more generally with both human and non-human primate brains (Amaral, personal communication). Furthermore, the values we found for the hippocampal volume corresponded well with those reported by Bhatia et al. (1993) for a similar group of healthy young participants. With respect to the hippocampus, volumes varied from less than 2ml to 5ml across the 29 individuals who had been scanned. It seems probable that this individual variability has functional implications, and that significant neuropsychological relationships would be revealed using appropriate memory measures. Third, there was evidence that participants were consistent in their memory performance across test sessions, and that their memory performance was not measurably influenced by variations in alertness and motivation. Fourth, and most important from a neuropsychological perspective, the findings from this first study are consistent with the hypothesis that the hippocampus is minimally involved in subserving recognition memory (Aggleton & Shaw, 1996).

The findings of the first young control study prompted some modifications for the investigation reported here. First, we decided to focus on recall rather than recognition, because of recent evidence that recall but not recognition is mediated via the hippocampus. Second, we determined in the first study (Mackay et al., 1998) that coronal MRI slices need to be reformatted in a plane orthogonal to the long axis of the hippocampus, because comparison of these images with standard coronal slices showed that the reformatting procedure makes it easier to discriminate the boundaries of the hippocampus and amygdala at the anterior end of the hippocampus. Third, we also discovered in the Mackay et al. (1998) investigation that it is possible to measure the left and right hippocampus to a high degree of accuracy by re-orienting the coronal images according to the location of the hippocampus on one side of the brain only. As in the previous investigation, the present study used stereological techniques to measure hippocampal volume (see Mackay et al., 1998, for further details concerning this important measurement technique).

Our central objective in the present study was to determine whether the volume of the left hippocampus correlated with delayed story recall in healthy normal individuals. Although the rate at which verbal recall fades almost certainly depends on the operation of other structures as well as the hippocampus, based on previous findings in epilepsy, Alzheimer's disease, and normal ageing, we still expected to observe a significant relationship between left hippocampal volume and delayed recall. Furthermore, given the previous findings obtained with non-brain-damaged controls in the Kohler et al. (1998) paper, we concluded that, contrary to the clinical literature, the evidence is more convincing that controls show a negative relationship between hippocampal volume and delayed recall, and this is what we expected to find in the current study.

METHOD

In this section, the four phases of the experiment will be referred to as Phase One (i.e. neuropsychology test session one), Phase Two (i.e. volumetric MRI brain scanning), Phase Three (i.e. neuropsychology test session two) and Phase Four (i.e. neuropsychology test session three). These phases correspond to the sequence in which the study was conducted.

Participants

A total of 74 female undergraduates and one postgraduate student at the University of Manchester were tested during Phase One of the experiment. The participants were aged between 18 and 30 years of age, with a mean age of 19.8

years. All participants were tested in the same room. Prior to testing, participants were asked to read and sign a written consent form. This included full reference to the fact that, depending on their test performance, participants may subsequently be asked to attend for MR brain scanning. Psychometric testing then commenced.

A selection process of 18 participants (9 with relatively fast rates of forgetting and 9 with relatively slow rates of forgetting) took place based on individual performance in Phase One of testing. These 18 participants were then referred for MRI brain scanning. The goal of the scanning selection process was to focus on a sample of participants who showed a good range in performance on memory testing. We also attempted to match scanned participants in other abilities that could have confounded verbal memory performance (for example, verbal ability, intelligence, arousal, alertness, and motivation) in order to maximise "signal" versus "noise" in the memory test data. MRI scanning of these 18 participants took place approximately four months after the original testing session, in Phase Two of the experiment. Of the 18 participants referred for MRI, 17 were classified as right-handed, based on their performance on the Edinburgh Handedness Inventory (short form).

Subsequently, it proved possible to recall 8 of the original 18 individuals for follow-up testing approximately six months after the original test session, in Phase Three of the study. Finally, 10 of the original 18 participants were recalled for testing approximately 18 months after the original test session, in Phase Four of the study. The test sessions conducted in Phases Three and Four were undertaken in order to investigate the consistency of memory performance within individuals. We used different but equivalent materials to evaluate delayed recall in the three memory test sessions. (We consider this consistency testing an important methodological procedure, although it is undertaken in few other neuroimaging studies of which we are aware.

Apparatus and Materials

Recall memory was evaluated using three different vignettes (one story in each of Phases One, Three, and Four) taken from the battery of stories developed by Isaac (1994; see also Isaac & Mayes, in press a, b). These stories were designed to evaluate verbal episodic memory, and have been shown to be reliable in previous studies of amnesia. Each story was separated into 20 components, and for each component that was recalled verbatim, participants received one mark. The maximum possible score per vignette was therefore 20. In Phase Three, performance on the Isaac stories was also scored for gist as well as verbatim, in order to ensure reliability of performance on a complementary measure of memory performance.

Neuropsychology Procedure

The procedure was similar in Phases One, Three, and Four. There was a delay of approximately 6 months between Phases One and Three, and approximately 12 months between Phases Three and Four.

Participants were tested individually in the experimental testing cubicle. Each participant sat in the same position, faced by the experimenters on the opposite side of the table. Participants were first shown the consent form and asked to complete the form if they wished to continue with the experiment. They were also told that even after signing the consent form they could withdraw from the experiment at any stage without prejudice.

Participants were informed that they would be read aloud a short story at different times in the experiment, and that they would later be asked to remember this story as well as they could. Participants were also told that they would be asked to judge subjectively whether the events and characters described were "pleasant", "neutral", or "unpleasant" directly after they had heard each story (this procedure was conducted in order to ensure that the target stories were attended to and processed to an approximately equivalent degree across all participants; see Craik & Lockhart, 1972; Craik & Tulving, 1975). Each participant was informed of the duration of the test session and asked to raise any questions with the experimenters before the start of testing.

Each vignette was read by the experimenter in a steady, even tone, and took approximately 20 seconds to complete. After participants had heard each vignette, they were asked respond to the emotional judgement question about the story (i.e. "pleasant", "neutral", or "unpleasant"). Participants then took part in a series of additional verbal tests during the memory delay which were designed to provide distraction (i.e. to prevent verbal rehearsal of memory materials) but not interference. Delayed recall testing began 20 minutes after the experimenter had finished reading the story.

MR Image Acquisition and Processing Procedure

Participants were selected for MR scanning in Phase Two on the basis of their test performance in Phase One. Approximately six months after Phase One, 18 participants from Phase One of the experiment were imaged on a 1.5 T GE SIGNA Whole Body imaging System (General Electric, Milwaukee, USA) using a proprietary quadrature head coil. A total of 124 coronal T-1 weighted images 1.6mm thick were acquired throughout the brain using a 3D spoiled gradient echo sequence (3D-SPGR) with the following parameters (TE=9ms, TR=34msec, flip angle =30°, 1 NEX). The field of view (FOV) of the image is 20cm, made up of a 256 × 256 pixel matrix. The SPGR sequence used provides optimum contrast between tissues on the basis of the value of their T1 relaxation times. The shorter the T1 the higher the signal intensity, so that white matter appears brighter than grey matter, and CSF appears black. The images show no evidence of movement or chemical shift artifact, and partial voluming effects are minimal.

MR images were transferred to ANALYZE (MAYO Foundation, Minnesota, USA) software running on a SPARC 10 workstation (SUN Microsystems, CA, USA) for reformatting and image analysis. For optimal visualisation of the hippocampus, the volume dataset was resized to create isotropic voxels, and re-aligned orthogonal to the longitudinal axis of the hippocampus (Bartzokis et al, 1993; Kuzniecky & Jackson, 1995). Correction for asymmetric head position in the x, y, and z planes was carried out at this time. (Reformatting stages are further detailed and illustrated in Mackay et al., 1998.) Post transformation voxel size was $0.781 \times 0.781 \times 0.781$mm.

Hippocampal Anatomy and Definition

The hippocampus comprises the areas CA1, CA2, CA3, and CA4, dentate gyrus, subiculum, presubiculum, and parasubiculum. Even with the high-resolution 3D SPGR scan these individual areas are often indistinguishable. The entire hippocampus was measured throughout its complete rostro-caudal extent as follows: the posterior limit of the hippocampus was demarcated by the first slice upon which the lateral ventricles were separated into the body of the lateral ventricle and the temporal horns. In the medial aspect, the hippocampus is well delineated by the CSF space of the wings of the ambient cistern, and supero-laterally by the temporal horn of the lateral ventricle. The subiculum is separated from the entorhinal cortex, from where the cortical grey matter ribbon of the parahippocampal gyrus extends inferiorly. At anterior hippocampal slices, the subiculum ends where the uncal sulcus meets the ambient cistern. The anterior hippocampus is delineated from the amygdala by the alveus and the CSF of the uncal sulcus in the superior extent. The head of the anterior hippocampus is eventually replaced by the amygdaloid nuclei in the AP plane.

Further detail on the protocol for hippocampal morphometry used in this study is provided in Mackay et al., 1998.

Precise Volume Estimation

Hippocampal volumes were estimated using the Cavalieri method of modern design stereology. This technique enables rapid, unbiased estimation of the volume of a structure of arbitrary shape and size. The method requires that the structure is sectioned from end to end with a series of parallel planes a constant distance apart. Provided that the position of the first section is random within the sectioning interval, an unbiased estimate of volume is obtained by multiplying the total area of the transects through the structure on all the sections by the sectioning interval. Section areas are estimated by point counting. An array of test points is lain over the image, and points falling within the boundary of the structure are counted and multiplied by the area per point to provide an unbiased estimate of consecutive section areas. Volume is estimated in an unbiased fashion as the sum of the section areas multiplied by the section interval. The precision of a volume estimate obtained using the Cavalieri method may be measured by its coefficient of error (CE) or "relative standard error." Further detail concerning the accuracy and efficiency of this volumetric technique are provided in Mackay et al (1998), and Roberts et al., (1994). In the present study point counting was carried out via stereology menus within ANALYZE (MAYO Foundation, Minnesota, USA). An illustration of the application of the stereological point-counting technique to three sections through the hippocampus is illustrated in Plate 10.

Mackay et al. (1998) also provide detail on the use of stereology for the calculation of left and right cerebral hemisphere and total brain volumes. These volumes were used as the arithmetic denominator when calculating normalised hippocampal volumes. These normalised volumes were used in statistical analyses in addition to raw volumes to investigate the relationship between hippocampal morphology and memory performance.

Reliability

Hippocampal and hemisphere volume measurements were conducted by an experienced researcher (MH), for whom measures of high intra- and inter-rater reliability have been obtained (intraclass correlation coefficient for hippocampal volumes >0.7 and for cerebral hemisphere volumes >0.75). The intraclass correlation coefficient (ICC) expresses the proportion of total measurement variability attributable to true biological variability in volume (Fleiss, 1986). As the amount of random error in measurements decreases, their reliability increases and the ICC approaches 1.

RESULTS

We focus here on delayed recall performance (see Table 1), as this was the measure on which Kohler et al. had reported a negative association with hippocampal volume in the healthy elderly (Kohler et al., 1998). In addition, this was the measure which produced the most reliable levels of performance across the three memory test sessions in the present study. Nevertheless, we acknowledge that, although well motivated by the extant literature, by focusing on one memory measure (delayed recall) and one brain structure (hippocampus), we restrict the degree to which functional specificity can be inferred from the present findings. Therefore, the findings of the current study must be interpreted with some degree of caution. Note also that, given the previous findings observed by Kohler et al. (1998), we here computed one-tailed analyses. However, the reader should note that even using two-tailed tests, the main findings presented below still hold.

Left hippocampal volume was negatively correlated with delayed story recall in all three memory test sessions. This was the case whether raw left hippocampal volume was analysed or whether left hippocampal volume was

TABLE 1
Individuals' Memory Performance Across the Three Test Sessions

	Mean	Standard Deviation	Minimum	Maximum
Delayed Recall 1	8.2	2.4	4	13
Delayed Recall 2	5.1	1.1	4	7
Delayed Recall 3	7.1	2.5	4	11
LH	2.2	0.3	1.7	2.6
LH/LCH	0.5	0.1	0.4	0.6
LH/TBV	0.2	0.04	0.2	0.3

Descriptive statistics for the brain measures of central interest are also shown. Delayed Recall 1, Delayed Recall 2, and Delayed Recall 3 refer to memory performance during test sessions 1, 2, and 3, respectively. LH = raw left hippocampal volume; LH/LCH = left hippocampal volume normalised for volume of left cerebral hemisphere; LH/TBV = left hippocampal volume normalised for total brain volume.

normalised for (i) left hemisphere volume or (ii) total brain volume (normalisation was performed by dividing raw hippocampal volume by the volume of the corresponding cerebral hemisphere or by the volume of the whole brain). The consistency of these negative correlations suggests that these findings are stable. However, only some of these negative correlations were statistically significant; namely, the negative relationships between left hippocampal volume and delayed recall performance observed in Phase One (i.e. memory test session 1; see Table 1). This is perhaps not surprising, given that a relatively small number of participants received MR scanning, and the largest number of participants was tested in this first test session. In Phases Three and Four (i.e. memory test sessions 2 and 3), there were similar correlations between delayed recall performance and left hippocampal volume to those observed in Phase One, but these correlations did not reach statistical significance (see Table 1). There was some suggestion that the correlations observed for memory test sessions 2 and 3 were somewhat reduced in size compared with test session 1, and this may have related to changes in the level of variability in the behavioural data as testing progressed, and participants became more accustomed to the general format of the memory testing. However, note that this systematic decline in the level of correlations over testing was not observed for the correlations between delayed recall and left hippocampal raw volume (see Fig. 1 and Table 2).

The test session 1 correlations reached statistical significance when session 1 delayed recall was correlated with left hippocampal volume normalised for (i) left hemisphere and (ii) whole brain. There was also a statistical trend in the same direction when the raw left hippocampal volume was used in the correlational analyses.

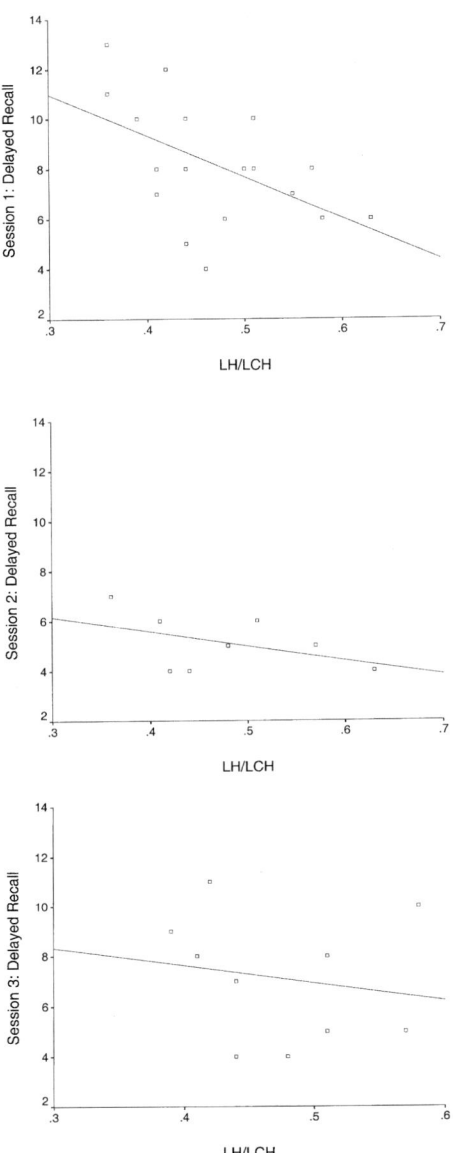

FIG. 1.   Scatterplots, including lines of best fit, showing the relationship between the volume of the left hippocampus normalised for the volume of the left cerebral hemisphere and (a) session 1 delayed recall, (b) session 2 delayed recall, and (c) session 3 delay recall performance. The volume of the left hippocampus normalised for the volume of the left cerebral hemisphere is shown throughout, as this parameter showed the largest overall correlation with delayed recall performance ($r = .5231$ in session 1). The equations describing the lines of best fit are as follows: (a) session 1 delayed recall $= -16.5 LH/LCH + 15.9$, (b) session 2 delayed recall $= -5 LH/LCH + 7.9$, (c) session 3 delayed recall $= -7.0 LH/LCH + 10.4$.

TABLE 2
Correlations Between Delayed Recall Performance and Hippocampal Volumes in Test Sessions 1, 2, and 3

	Session 1 (n = 18)	Session 2 (n = 8)	Session 3 (n = 10)
LH	−0.3496 (P=0.077)	−0.4562 (P=0.128)	−0.3937 (P=0.130)
LH/LCH	−0.5231 (P=0.013)	−0.4648 (P=0.123)	−0.1835 (P=0.306
LH/TBV	−0.5219 (P=0.13)	−0.4401 (P=0.138)	−0.2380 (P=0.254)

LH = raw left hippocampal volume; LH/LCH = left hippocampal volume normalised for volume of left cerebral hemisphere; LH/TBV = left hippocampal volume normalised for total brain volume. In session 1 (Phase One of the experiment), 18 participants were tested, in session 2 (Phase Three of the experiment) 8 participants were tested, and in session 3 (Phase Four of the experiment) 10 participants were tested. One-tailed Pearson's product moment correlation coefficients are cited in each case.

Right hippocampal volume was also negatively associated with delayed recall performance (one-tailed Pearson's correlation coefficient with delayed recall performance in test session 1: with raw right hippocampal volume $r=-.2990$, $P=.114$; with right hippocampal volume normalised for right hemisphere volume $r=-.3774$, $P=.061$; with right hippocampal volume normalised for total brain volume $r=-.3961$, $P=.052$). However, importantly, the significant relationship between delayed recall performance and left hippocampal volume was at the cusp of statistical significance when right hippocampal volume was partialled out of the analysis (one-tailed $r=-.1902$, $P=.232$; $r=-.4075$, $P=.052$; $r=-.3799$, $P=.066$ for raw left hippocampal volume, left hippocampal volume normalised for left cerebral volume, left hippocampal volume normalized for total brain volume, respectively). The converse was not the case; i.e. when left hippocampal volume was partialled out, the negative relationship between right hippocampal volume and delayed recall performance was reduced beyond chance levels (one-tailed $r=-.0089$, $P=.486$; $r=.1242$, $P=.317$; $r=.0919$, $P=.363$ for raw right hippocampal volume, right hippocampal volume normalized for right cerebral volume, right hippocampal volume normalised for total brain volume, respectively).

When independent t-tests were computed to compare the delayed recall performance of the relatively "fast" (n=9) and "slow" (n=9) forgetting groups, there were significant group differences (1-tailed) between the left hippocampal volume normalised for left cerebral volume ($t=1.901$, $P=.0375$), left hippocampal volume normalized for total brain volume ($t=1.823$, $P=.0435$), right hippocampal volume normalised for right cerebral volume ($t=2.065$, $P=.028$) and right hippocampal volume normalised for total brain volume ($t = 1.937$, $P = .0355$). The group of relatively "fast" forgetters (i.e. those participants with lower levels of delayed recall performance) had a larger hippocampus in each case.

Further statistical information concerning individuals' recall performance across the three test sessions is provided in Table 2.

DISCUSSION

This study reports the findings that in healthy young people hippocampal volume may be negatively associated with delayed memory performance. This finding runs directly counter to what one might expect on the basis of the amnesia, temporal lobe epilepsy, and Alzheimer literatures. Although both the left and right hippocampus were measured, the negative correlation observed between hippocampal volume and delayed recall was strongest for the left hippocampus. Despite the relatively small sample size, and the restricted number of anatomical and mnemonic indices that are reported here, these findings are important for theories concerning the neural mediation of episodic memory, as well as for the significance of the volume of the hippocampus in healthy young individuals. It is interesting that, overall, normalised hippocampal volumes showed the stronger relationships with memory, perhaps suggesting that it is the amount of cortically projected information processed by the hippocampus per unit volume that determines delayed recall performance. In addition, impaired delayed recall has been cited as an important feature of anterograde amnesia caused by medial temporal lobe damage. This represents an intriguing comparison with the current findings, although clearly the mechanisms that are operating in healthy young controls and in patients with amnesia must be different. Specifically, in the former group, larger hippocampal volume appears to be associated with worse delayed recall performance, whereas the opposite relationship seems to obtain in brain-damaged amnesic patients.

The findings reported here do however echo the previous observations of Kohler et al. (1998) in a population of healthy elderly controls, and therefore cannot easily be dismissed as being spurious. In the Kohler et al. study, there was a positive relationship between hippocampal volume and delayed verbal recall in patients with Alzheimer's disease, but an opposite relationship was observed in healthy age-matched control participants. In particular, in the 26 elderly controls who were reported in the Kohler et al. investigation, there was a negative correlation of $-.55$ between hippocampal volume and delayed recall performance on the CVLT (this correlation was significant at the $P < .01$ level of significance). These values compare with a strength of association of $-.5231$ (normalised left hippocampus) and $-.3774$ (normalised right hippocampus) in the 18 healthy young individuals who were tested in Phase One of the present investigation. The first of these values is clearly very close to the size of the negative correlation observed by Kohler et al. (note that Kohler et al. used a combined volume of the left and right hippocampus in their calculations).

By contrast, in the Kohler et al. study, in Alzheimer patients there was a positive correlation of 0.61 between hippocampal volume and delayed recall performance (this correlation was significant at the $P < .001$ level). As well as extending the findings of Kohler et al. to a younger population, the present study also permitted us to focus more on whether the left or right hippocampus is mediating the delayed recall association. The volume of both left and right hippocampus showed a negative correlation with delayed recall performance. However, we observed in Mackay et al. (1998) that anatomically the volumes of the left and right hippocampus are strongly associated within an individual. When the volume of the left hippocampus was partialled out in the present study, the relationship of the right hippocampus with delayed recall no longer reached statistical significance. However, the converse was not the case. Therefore, it was the left hippocampus that showed the strongest relationship with delayed recall performance. This is consistent with previous findings concerning the role of left- and right-sided medial temporal lobe structures in memory for verbal versus non-verbal materials (see Mayes, 1988).

Work that has previously been conducted into the relationship between the volume of the hippocampus and memory performance in controls has tended to produce a somewhat equivocal pattern of findings. Although, as far as we are aware, no previous studies have focused specifically on this issue in healthy young controls alone, Golomb et al. (1993, 1994) have studied this in the healthy elderly, and have suggested a positive association between hippocampal volume and delayed memory performance in this population. Similar findings were reported in follow-up studies conducted by Golomb and colleagues (Convit et al., 1997; de Leon et al., 1996, 1997). It is possible of course that observations of this kind can be contaminated by the presence of individuals with incipient Alzheimer's disease or other forms of pathological memory (such as Age Associated Memory Impairment) in the healthy control group. Another study by Raz et al. (1998) found no association between hippocampal volume and performance on various delayed memory tasks in a large sample of normal controls varying in age from 18–77 years. Although Raz et al. (1998) found no association between hippocampal volume and delayed memory performance in their total sample, these researchers noted that reduction in the volume of limbic structures did predict declines in explicit memory in participants over 60 years old. Raz et al. (1998) argued that only participant sub-groups in which there is evidence for poor memory performance may reveal a positive association between episodic memory and the volume of medial temporal lobe structures. As well as their own findings, this argument might explain the findings of the studies conducted by Golomb and colleagues. In addition, another study observed age-related decline in MRI volumes of temporal lobe grey matter but no significant volume reductions in the hippocampus, although age-related declines in verbal and nonverbal "working memory" were observed (Sullivan et al., 1995).

Taken together with the present findings, and the results obtained by Kohler et al. (1998), the data obtained by Golomb, Raz, Sullivan, and colleagues seem consistent with the proposition that there may be (at least) two different mechanisms operating in determining the relationship between hippocampal volume and delayed recall performance. In healthy young people, the primary factor in determining the relationship between the volume of the hippocampus and delayed memory performance may be the degree of neural pruning that has taken place during childhood and adolescence (following adequate hippocampal growth). This may occur through a mechanism such as programmed cell death, on which much interest has been focused recently in the research literature. Indeed, it is known that during development more neurones, axons, synapses, and receptors are generated than are subsequently retained in the brain during adulthood (Cowan et al., 1984). It may be that an inadequately pruned hippocampus mediates delayed memory less efficiently than a well pruned hippocampus. This could explain why there is a negative relationship between hippocampal volume and delayed memory performance in healthy young people. However, clearly one can not extrapolate this relationship indefinitely in a linear fashion: suboptimal memory performance would obviously be likely to occur in an individual with no hippocampus! Although the current study indicates a broadly linear relationship within the current data, clearly the specific parameters of this relationship will need to be worked out in future research.

By contrast, in pathological conditions such as Alzheimer's disease, the primary factor in determining the relationship between delayed recall performance and hippocampal volume may be the degree of circuit disruption that has taken place as a consequence of the disease in question, such that the lower volume threshold for efficient hippocampal functioning is exceeded. This effect—which is likely to be considerably greater in scale than any reduction in volume due to neural pruning in early life—might explain why there is a positive relationship between hippocampal volume and delayed memory performance in these individuals. The healthy elderly may represent a hybrid population, located somewhere between these two groups; therefore, the nature of the relationship that is observed in elderly "controls" may depend on the proportion of individuals falling into the "non-pathological" versus "pathological" categories. This could explain the mixed pattern of findings that have been reported in previous studies of the elderly.

This account is speculative but plausible. However, other possible explanations for the present data must also be considered. For example, it is possible that the modulatory effects of hormonal processes could be relevant here (McEwen & Sapolsky, 1995). These processes (which might be especially relevant in post-menarchal female participants) could render the volume of the hippocampus variable over time. Indeed, results from endocrinological studies in non-human animals suggest that experimentally induced changes in hippocampal size are not necessarily permanent (McEwen, 1997). However, this explanation may be less applicable here when one considers that a broadly comparable relationship between memory performance and hippocampal volume was observed in the present study when memory was tested on several occasions, separated by approximately 18 months in total. Therefore, although hippocampal volumes may be affected not only by early developmental processes but also by physiological effects occurring at later stages in life, hormonal considerations seem unlikely to provide a full explanation in the current context.

In summary, this report presents an intriguing finding concerning the relationship between hippocampal volume and delayed recall performance in healthy young individuals. These findings complement previous findings reported in studies of the elderly and brain-damaged individuals. In the future, additional replications and extensions of these findings, measuring a greater number of brain regions and their relative volumes, and testing additional aspects of memory in larger and more wide-ranging samples of participants, are clearly required. Such investigations will enable us to probe systematically the relationship between medial temporal lobe structures and memory functioning in the young, the elderly, and following different aetiologies of brain injury.

REFERENCES

Aggleton, J.P., & Shaw, C. (1996). Amnesia and recognition memory: A re-analysis of psychometric data. *Neuropsychologia, 34*, 51–62.

Bartzokis, G., Mintz, J., Marx, P., Osborn, D., Chiang, F., Phelan, C., & Marder, S. (1993). Reliability of in vivo volume measures of hippocampus and other brain structures using MRI. *Magnetic Resonance Imaging, 11*, 933–1006.

Baxendale, S. (1997). The role of the hippocampus in recognition memory. *Neuropsychologia, 35*, 591–598.

Bhatia, S., Bookheimer, S.Y., Gaillard, W.D., & Theodore, W.H. (1993). Measurement of whole temporal-lobe and hippocampus for MR volumetry—normative data. *Neurology, 43*, 2006–2010.

Cohen, N.J., Poldrack, R.A., & Eichenbaum, H.J.N. (1997). Memory for items and memory for relations in the procedural/declarative memory framework. *Memory, 5*, 131–178.

Colombo, M., & Gross, C. (1994). Responses of inferior temporal cortex and hippocampal neurones during delayed matching-to-sample in monkeys. *Behavioral Neuroscience, 108*, 443–455.

Convit, A. et al. (1997). Specific hippocampal volume reductions in individuals at risk for Alzheimer's disease. *Neurobiology of Aging, 18*, 131–138.

Cowan, W.M., Fawcett, J.W., O'Leary, D.D.M., & Stanfield, B.B. (1984). Regressive events in neurogenesis. *Science, 225*, 1258–1265.

Craik, F.I.M., & Lockhart, R.S. (1972). Levels of processing: A framework for memory research. *Journal of Verbal Learning and Verbal Behavior, 11*, 671–684.

Craik, F.I.M., & Tulving, E. (1975). Depth of processing and the retention of words in episodic memory. *Journal of Experimental Psychology: General, 104*, 268–294.

De Leon, M.J., Convit, A., George, A.E., Golomb, J., DeSanti, S., et al. (1996). In vivo structural studies of the hippocampus in normal aging and in incipient Alzheimer's disease. *Annals of the New York Academy of Sciences, 777*, 1–13.

De Leon, M.J., George, A.E., Golomb, J., Tarshish, C., Convit, A., et al. (1997). Frequency of hippocampal formation atrophy in normal aging and Alzheimer's disease. *Neurobiology of Aging, 18,* 1–11.

Deweer, B., Lehericy, S., Pillon, B., Baulac, M., Chiras, J., Marsault, C., Agid, Y., & Dubois, B. (1995). Memory disorders in probable Alzheimer's disease—the role of hippocampal atrophy as shown with MRI. *Journal of Neurology, Neurosurgery and Psychiatry, 58,* 590–597.

Eichenbaum, H., Otto, T., & Cohen, N.J. (1994). Two functional components of the hippocampal memory system. *Behavioral and Brain Sciences, 17,* 449–517.

Fleiss, J.L. (1986). *The design and analysis of clinical experiments.* New York: John Wiley & Sons.

Foster, J.K., Black, S.E., Buck, B.H., & Bronskill, M.J. (1997). Executive and associated functions in normal and pathological aging: A neuroimaging perspective. In P. Rabbitt (Ed.), *Methodology of frontal and executive functions.* Hove, UK: Lawrence Erlbaum.

Gabrieli, J.D.E., Brewer, J.B., Desmond, J.E., & Glover, G.H. et al. (1997). Separate neural bases of two fundamental memory processes in the human medial temporal lobe. *Science, 276,* 264–266.

Golomb, J., de Leon, M.J, Kluger, A., George, A.E., Tarshish, M.A., & Feris, S.H. (1993). Hippocampal atrophy in normal aging: An association with recent memory impairment. *Archives of Neurology, 50,* 967–973.

Golomb, J., Kluger, A., de Leon, M.J., Feris, S.H., Convit, A., Mittleman, M.S., Cohen, J., Rusinek, H., De Santi, S., & George, A.E. (1994). Hippocampal formation size in normal human aging: A correlate of delayed secondary memory performance. *Learning and Memory, 1,* 45–54.

Isaac, C.L. (1994). *Rate of forgetting in organic amnesia.* Unpublished PhD thesis, University of Manchester, UK.

Isaac, C.L., & Mayes, A.R. (in press, a). Rate of forgetting in amnesia I: Recall and recognition of prose. *Journal of Experimental Psychology: Learning, Memory & Cognition.*

Isaac, C.L., & Mayes, A.R. (in press, b). Rate of forgetting in amnesia II: Recall and recognition of word lists at different levels of organization. *Journal of Experimental Psychology: Learning, Memory & Cognition.*

Kohler, S., Black, S.E., Sinden, M., Szekely, C., Kidron, D., Parker, J.L., Foster, J.K., Moscovitch, M., Winocur, G., Szalai, J.P., & Bronskill, M.J. (1998). Memory impairments associated with hippocampal versus parahippocampal-gyrus atrophy: An MR volumetry study in Alzheimer's disease. *Neuropsychologia, 36,* 901–914.

Kuzniecky, R.I., & Jackson, G.D. (1995). *Magnetic resonance in epilepsy.* New York: Raven Press.

Lencz, T., McCarthy, G., Bronen, R.A., Scott, T.M., Inserni, J.A., Sass, K.J., Novelly, R.A., Kim, J.H., & Spencer, D.D. (1992). Quantitative magnetic resonance imaging in temporal lobe epilepsy: Relationship to neuropathology and neuropsychological function. *Annals of Neurology, 31,* 629–637.

Mackay, C.E., Roberts, N., Mayes, A.R., Downes, J.J., Foster, J.K., & Mann, D. (1998). An exploratory study of the relationship between face recognition memory and the volume of medial temporal lobe structures in healthy young males. *Behavioural Neurology, 11,* 3–20.

Mayes, A.R. (1988). *Human organic memory disorders.* Cambridge: Cambridge University Press.

McEwen, B.S. (1997). Possible mechanisms for atrophy of the human hippocampus. *Molecular Psychiatry, 2,* 255–262.

McEwen, B.S., & Sapolsky, R.M. (1995). Stress and cognitive function. *Current Opinion in Neurobiology, 5,* 205–216.

Miller, L.A., Munoz, D.G., & Finmore, M. (1993). Hippocampal sclerosis and human memory. *Archives of Neurology, 50,* 391–394.

Nestor, P.G., Shenton, M.E., McCarley, R.W., Haimson, R., Smith, S.R., O'Donnell, B., Kimble, M., Kikinis, R., & Ferec, A.J. (1993). Neuropsychological correlates of MRI temporal lobe abnormalities in schizophrenia. *American Journal of Psychiatry, 150,* 1849–1855.

Nieuwenhuys, R., Voogel, J., & Van Huijzen, C. (1988). *The human central nervous system: A synopsis and atlas* (3rd Ed., Revised). Berlin: Springer-Verlag.

Nyberg, L., McIntosh, A.R., Houle, S., Nilsson, L.G., & Tulving, E.J.N. (1996). Activation of medial temporal structures during episodic memory retrieval. *Nature, 380*, 715–717.

Owen, A.M., Milner, B., Petrides, M., & Evans, A.C. (1996). A specific role for the right parahippocampal gyrus in the retrieval of object location: A positron emission tomography study. *Journal of Cognitive Neuroscience, 8*, 588–602.

Pigott, S., & Milner, B. (1993). Memory for different aspects of complex visual scenes after unilateral temporal- or frontal-lobe resection. *Neuropsychologia, 31*, 1–15.

Raz, N., Gunning-Dixon, F.M., Head, D., Dupuis, J.H., &Acker, J.D. (1998). Neuroanatomical correlates of cognitive aging: Evidence from structural magnetic resonance imaging. *Neuropsychology, 12*, 95–114.

Roberts, N., Garden, A.S., Cruz-Orive, L.M., Whitehouse, G.H., & Edwards, R.H.T. (1994). Estimation of fetal volume by magnetic resonance imaging and stereology. *British Journal of Radiology, 67*, 1067–1077.

Sass, K.J., Sass, A., Westerveld, M., Lencz, T., Novelly, R.A., Kim, J.H., & Spencer, D.D. (1992). Specificity in the correlation of verbal memory and hippocampal neuron loss: Dissociation of memory, language and verbal intellectual ability. *Journal of Clinical and Experimental Neuropsychology, 14*, 662–672.

Schacter, D.L., Alpert, N.M., Savage, C.R., Rauch, S.L., & Albert, M.S. (1996). Conscious recollection and the human hippocampal formation: Evidence from positron emission tomography. *Proceedings of the National Academy of Sciences, 93*, 321–325.

Squire, L.R. (1992). Memory and the hippocampus: A synthesis from findings with rats, monkeys and humans. *Psychological Review, 99*, 195–231.

Stern, C.E., Corkin, S., Gonzalez, R.G., Guimares, A.R., Baker, J.R., et al. (1996). The hippocampal formation participates in novel picture encoding: evidence from functional magnetic resonance imaging. *Proceedings of the National Academy of Sciences, 93*, 8860–8665.

Sullivan, E.V., Marsh, L., Mathalon, D.H., Lim, K.O., & Pfefferbaum, A. (1995). Age-related decline in MRI volumes of temporal lobe gray matter but not hippocampus. *Neurobiology of Aging 16*, 591–606.

Tulving, E., Markowitsch, H.J., Craik, F.I.M., Habib, R., & Houle, S. (1996). Novelty and familiarity activations in PET studies of memory encoding and retrieval. *Cerebral Cortex, 6*, 71–79.

MEMORY, 1999, 7 (5/6), 733–740

Memory, Imaging, and the Mind-Brain: In Conclusion

Jonathan K. Foster

University of Manchester, UK

Over the past decade, neuroimaging technologies have enabled researchers to examine the spatial and temporal mechanisms of cognitive functioning and, in so doing, to probe on-line the relationship between mind and brain. Neuroimaging techniques are important, because if harnessed properly to address appropriate research issues, they enable one to tackle more precisely cognitive and neurobehavioural questions that have previously been amenable only through techniques such as lesion methods. The focus of this special issue has been the use of these rapidly emerging methodologies to examine questions about the cognitive architecture of memory and the implementation of different mnemonic processes by the brain. A number of important issues have been tackled, including the relationship between different neurological "hard" signs (as indexed through neuroimaging) and types of memory dysfunction, the relationship of different types of neuroimaging signs to each other, the role of the hippocampus in mediating memories from different autobiographical periods, the use of novel statistical protocols for image analysis, and event-related differences between encoding and retrieval.

More specifically, in McIntosh's paper, two different analytical methodologies are presented which are optimised for quantifying the operation of neural systems, namely structural equation modelling and partial least squares. These two methodologies are presented with specific empirical examples. Structural equation modelling is used to explore shifting prefrontal and limbic interactions from the right to the left hemisphere in a delayed match-to-sample memory task, using faces as the experimental stimuli. At short delays, a right hemisphere functional network emerged comprising hippocampus, inferior prefrontal, and anterior cingulate cortices. At longer delays, the same three areas were strongly linked, but this time in the left hemisphere. This change in neural representation over delay may have reflected a change in task strategy from perceptual to more elaborate encoding with increasing task delay. In another episodic memory

---

Requests for reprints should be sent to Jonathan K. Foster, Department of Psychology, University of Manchester, Oxford Road, Manchester M13 9PL, UK.

retrieval study, incorporating different levels of retrieval success, covariances of location within the right prefrontal cortex and the left hippocampus were estimated using partial least squares. The findings of this analysis indicate that activity in regions of the right prefrontal cortex can reflect either memory retrieval mode or retrieval success, depending on other brain regions to which right prefrontal regions are functionally linked. This finding is taken by McIntosh to imply that regional brain activity must be evaluated within the neural context in which it occurs: i.e. he argues that learning and memory are emergent properties of network interactions, such that a given brain region can play a different role across different mnemonic functions, and its role within a given context is mediated by its interactions with anatomically related regions. One significant implication of this paper is that we should move away from the use of the simple subtraction methodology and instead focus on the possible inter-relationships between diverse brain regions across different task conditions if we are to use neuroimaging techniques to their full potential in future for characterising the neural basis of cognition.

In the paper written by Van der Linden et al., the focus shifts to verbal working memory. In particular, the authors are interested in re-examining the cerebral areas involved in subserving the updating function of the postulated central executive, using a running span task in which participants are required to watch strings of consonants of unknown lengths and then to recall serially a specified number of recent items. In order to dissociate more precisely the memory updating process from the memory storage process, a four-item rather than a six-item memory load was used. In addition, a serial recall procedure was used instead of a recognition procedure, in order to suppress the use of visuospatial strategies. The most significant increases in cerebral blood flow in this study were noted in the left frontopolar cortex, spreading to the left middle frontal region. These findings imply that frontopolar activation underlies general updating functions in working memory. Importantly, this study applied the techniques of modern neuroimaging to an investigation of the working memory central executive system, a system that has previously been considered by some theorists to be non-modular. Research of this kind thus significantly extends the potential scope and value of neuroimaging investigations within the domain of working memory.

The paper by Markowitsch reports the neuroimaging correlates of functional amnesia: i.e. amnesia without any previously clear biological correlates. Markowitsch argues that the findings of functional neuroimaging studies have provided new insights into anatomico-functional interactions, particularly in the area of memory encoding and retrieval. The author argues that this is especially the case concerning the role of the prefrontal cortex in episodic memory, regarding the contribution of the two hemispheres in different types of information processing, and for our thinking about impaired information processing after neurological and psychogenic forms of memory impairment.

This paper stresses the insights that may be obtained from neuroimaging investigations into environmentally triggered deficits in information processing and discusses the possible subtle neuroanatomical correlates of functional amnesias. Markowitsch's paper especially emphasises that stressful situations and depressive states may modify the release of glucocorticoids and neurotransmitters, causing selective memory disturbances that may manifest as "mnestic block syndrome". Markowitsch's paper nicely complements the others presented in this special issue, by considering the interaction of functional and neurological aspects of human memory functioning. Indeed, it is suggested on the basis of Markowitsch's paper that rather than thinking about functional and neurological impairment of memory as a dichotomy, we should instead start to think about them as lying on different points of a continuum.

Nyberg's paper begins by arguing, non-contentiously, that functional neuroimaging studies are beginning to identify the neuroanatomical correlates of diverse cognitive functions. This wide-ranging paper then proceeds to present empirical findings that are relevant to several different theories of episodic memory, including component processes of episodic retrieval, encoding specificity, inhibition, item versus source memory, encoding–retrieval overlap, and the picture-superiority effect. By revealing specific activation patterns (for example, in regions of the prefrontal cortex that are putatively mediating different encoding- and retrieval-related processes), Nyberg argues that the results reported not only support some existing theoretical views of memory functioning, but also provide some unique information which may be important to consider in attempts to develop further our cognitive theories of episodic memory. This position can perhaps be contrasted with that proposed by other contributors to the special edition, who argue that neuroimaging research findings have to be interpreted in the context of other data, using a converging operations methodology.

Reed et al. investigated patients who had previously shown evidence of medial temporal lobe atrophy on MRI. However, when their PET data were analysed in the present study, they showed bilateral thalamic hypometabolism, and there was also evidence of bilateral retrosplenial hypometabolism. Cognitively, the patients performed like other patients with medial temporal lesions. Taken together these findings suggest that structural lesions to the medial temporal lobe can have distal metabolic effects, extending into the diencephalon. Reed et al. interpret their findings in terms of parallel anatomical projections between medial temporal lobe structures and the thalamus (some of which seem to pass via the retrosplenium). More generally, the authors advocate caution regarding the neuropsychological interpretation of neuroimaging data. They argue that the site of focal hypometabolism may represent (i) the critical site for a cognitive function or (ii) a specific node within a network, or (iii) it may be spurious. Therefore, it is argued, the site of regional hypometabolism should be interpreted only after examining the findings of different forms of image analysis, and in conjunction with the findings of detailed cognitive analyses, as conducted in this study. One corollary of these findings is that one cannot make a strong inference or diagnosis on the basis of one form of neuroimaging data used in isolation, but instead both structural and functional techniques should be used in parallel, so that both anatomical and physiological indices of the brain can be derived. This point has significant implications not only in clinical applications, but also seeking to interpret imaging data obtained from cognitive studies of controls (see also Foster et al., this issue).

In strongly advocating a convergent operations approach between different methodologies, the paper by Mayes and Montaldi argues that there needs to be more interaction between the lesion and functional neuroimaging literatures in order to explore apparent inconsistencies and conflicts: notably, the central issue surrounding the role of the medial temporal lobe in mediating long-term memory for novel information. The authors focus on a discussion of episode and fact encoding. It is argued that functional neuroimaging can potentially be highly informative in distinguishing between differential hypotheses that have been advanced from the findings of lesion studies. However, the authors suggest that, to date, these differential hypotheses have been underexplored because neuroimaging studies of encoding have been insufficiently hypothesis-driven and have not controlled adequately for incidental encoding-related processes so that clear interpretation of results can be made. Mayes and Montaldi argue that there is good evidence that specific kinds of associative encoding and/or consolidation are sufficient to activate the medial temporal lobes, and preliminary evidence suggests that some kinds of associative priming may reduce activation in this region. Medial temporal lobe activation consequent upon attentional orienting to certain kinds of novel information remains, according to the authors, a more open question. In contrast to other papers presented in the special edition, the paper written by Mayes and Montaldi is, importantly, critical of the theoretical interpretation of some current neuroimaging data, specifically the HERA framework, citing evidence that it is incorrect. Mayes and Montaldi further argue that prefrontal cortex encoding activations are probably due to effortful cognitive processes and that encoding sometimes also activates parietal regions as well as frontal and medial temporal cortex.

McDermott et al. use event-related fMRI to investigate the relationship between intentional encoding and subsequent retrieval of visually presented words. Their findings highlight both similarities and differences between these two sets of activations. In particular, when comparing encoding and retrieval, areas that were more active in encoding include the left parahippocampal gyrus, the posterior cingulate, the left inferior frontal cortex, the left superior frontal cortex, the medial frontal cortex, and the left superior temporal cortex. By contrast, regions that were more active in retrieval include the bilateral precuneus, the bilateral inferior parietal cortex, and the right superior frontal, anterior frontal, and insular cortices. The authors especially note the significance of the parietal cortex in episodic recognition of verbal materials, as indicated by their findings. Although accepting the significance of these findings, the authors concede that other similar comparisons, using different types of study and test materials, will be necessary to reveal the extent to which these findings generalise across test domains (for example, using verbal versus non-verbal test materials). Another relevant distinction is likely to be that between activation patterns shown to different forms of retrieval (e.g. different subtypes of recall and recognition). Nevertheless, as the authors point out, compared with previous blocked trial PET and MRI methodologies, event-related fMRI methodologies are likely to represent a considerable advance in delineating the neural substrates of different elements of episodic memory. One intriguing finding of this encoding/retrieval theory-driven study is that brain activation does not apparently differ when ''old'' versus ''new'' items are being evaluated at test. This finding clearly requires further exploration.

In their study, Conway et al. investigate the neurobiology of autobiographical memory using PET. They find that a large network of the left frontal cortical region, together with the left inferior temporal and occipital areas, is significantly active during retrieval of autobiographical memories, compared with paired associate recall. Furthermore, these activations are observed irrespective of the age of the remembered events. The authors propose that the left frontal lobe activation reflects the operation of control processes that modulate the construction of representations of autobiographical memories in posterior cortical networks. Of additional theoretical significance for theories of the neural representation of memory, the hippocampal system was significantly active in all task conditions, regardless of whether the participant was recalling recent or more remote autobiographical memories. These theoretically important findings would therefore seem to support the more recent proposal that the hippocampal memory system is involved in the retrieval of both recently and remotely acquired information (Nadel & Moscovitch, 1997), at least regarding memories for autobiographical events. Once more, as in several other neuroimaging investigations of memory, it is the prefrontal regions that are the most active across the different experimental conditions.

Fletcher and Dolan explore the neural changes associated with increasing familiarity of studied materials encoded as word pairs. In particular, they demonstrate that the neuronal response in the right ventrolateral prefrontal cortex is preferentially sensitive to an experimental condition in which both words are familiar (i.e. a condition in which all material has previously been presented prior to scanning). By contrast, a more dorsal right prefrontal region was found to be more active in a condition in which one familiar item is presented together with a novel associate. Fletcher and Dolan interpret their findings as indicating that sensitivity to stimulus familiarity is expressed in the right ventral prefrontal cortex, even within the context of an encoding task. The authors also argue that their findings present evidence for functional heterogeneity within the right prefrontal cortex, with a more ventral region responding to familiarity of complete word pairs and a more dorsal region responding to familiar single words occurring in the context of new associative relationships.

In the final paper included in the special issue, Foster et al. present the findings of a study that uses structural MRI to investigate the relationship between the volume of medial temporal lobe structures and memory performance, focusing on the relationship between hippocampal volume and delayed recall. Healthy young female participants were tested on their recall of a story vignette and then received volumetric MRI scans. Intriguingly, the volume of the left hippocampus was *negatively* associated with the level of delayed verbal recall performance. This relationship was confirmed in further testing and is consistent with a previous report of a similar relationship in healthy elderly individuals but not in patients with Alzheimer's disease, in whom the opposite relationship seemed to hold. The authors advance a speculative account of their findings in terms of impaired neural pruning of the hippocampus (whereby insufficient pruning of the hippocampus during childhood and adolescence may lead to reduced mnemonic efficiency). However, they acknowledge that other mechanisms, such as the ongoing influence of the hippocampal hormonal environment, may also play a role in their findings. Nevertheless, these findings (which run counter to a large body of received but somewhat underexplored wisdom) have important implications for the functional interpretation of differential hippocampal volumes in healthy young people.

SOME FINAL THOUGHTS

The collection of papers presented in this special issue covers a range of stimulating memory-related topics, from autobiographical memory, memory for novel information, and working memory (and their neural substrates) to important methodological issues. There are a number of important messages to take away from this special edition. One central theme is that we require a firm grasp on theory if we are to interpret the plethora of research findings that is now emerging from neuroimaging labs investigating memory. In addition, one critical goal that we should strive for is greater reliability and replicability: in addition to developing ever more ingenious test paradigms to derive novel research findings, we need to be able to cross-reference both behavioural and neuroimaging data across laboratories and centres, using transparent analytical protocols. This is a central goal if we are to avoid the trap of generating a wealth of data without the necessary organisational framework for their satisfactory interpretation: methodological consistencies across studies conducted in the same and different centres will inevitably lead us to a better understanding of the brain and cognitive mechanisms involved in subserving different elementary components of memory.

More specifically, although no one would deny that the subtraction methodology has proved extremely valuable and influential to date, as McIntosh points out in this issue, we may now need to focus more on interactive neural network models if we are to exploit neuroimaging technologies to their full potential in the future. This would seem especially relevant if we are to probe the functioning of regions such as the hippocampus—a central structure in lesion-based theorising about memory and amnesia—which may be active across a number of different cognitive challenge conditions. Since evidence was first put forward that the structures of the left prefrontal region are implicated in encoding information into long-term memory, while regions of the right prefrontal cortex appear to be more involved in retrieval, an overwhelming number of encoding and retrieval studies of memory have demonstrated prefrontal activations. In addition, previously undiscussed regions of the brain such as the precuneus have now been cited in several neuroimaging investigations as an important anatomical component of specific memory networks. However, together with hippocampal findings, we need to be able to reconcile these observations with those of pre-existing literatures (both human and non-human), using a convergent operations methodology, if we are to make substantial progress in the future, and the development and application of more interactive models of neural activation may well facilitate this process.

Taken together, the papers in this special edition indicate the range of theoretically informative neuroimaging studies currently being conducted into the neurological and cognitive architecture of memory, just a few years after serious cognitive challenge studies using functional imaging techniques began. This augurs well for the future of cognitive neuroimaging research into memory. Indeed, the parting message should probably be that, powerful as many contemporary neuroimaging technologies potentially are, with this power should come responsibility, and these techniques can only provide meaningful data if they are used to address appropriate psychological questions within a well designed and coherent experimental and theoretical framework. Indeed, it is in providing such a framework that experimental psychologists play an essential role.

To reiterate, neuroimaging techniques must be used carefully and within a clearly defined frame of reference if they are to generate cognitively meaningful data. We need to conduct hypothesis-driven and clearly planned and structured investigations, with careful task selection and debriefing of research participants, and we need to control carefully for processes such as attention, arousal, and emotional responses elicited by target materials, if we are to be confident that we are probing memory processes of central interest. However, this said, not only does neuroimaging provide an important source of novel information for memory researchers, but findings obtained using neuroimaging methodologies provide an important reciprocal constraint when one is considering the theoretical significance of data obtained from other types of investigation. It is, therefore, when interpreted within the context of complementary sets of experimental findings that neuroimaging data are likely to offer the greatest reward in future research.

REFERENCE

Nadel, L., & Moscovitch, M. (1997). Memory consolidation, amnesia, and the hippocampal complex. *Current Opinion in Neurobiology, 7*, 217–227.

Subject Index